PEACE THROUGH HEALTH

PEACE THROUGH HEALTH

How Health Professionals
Can Work for a Less Violent World

Edited by Neil Arya *and* Joanna Santa Barbara

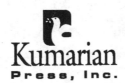

Kumarian
Press, Inc.

Peace through health: how health professionals can work for a less violent world

Published 2008 in the United States of America by Kumarian Press
22883 Quicksilver Drive, Sterling, VA 20166 USA

Copyedit by Connie Day
Proofread by Beth Richards
Design and production by Rosanne Schloss, NY
The text of this book is set in 11/13 Adobe Sabon

Printed in the USA on acid-free paper by Thomson-Shore, Inc.

∞ The paper used in this publication meets the minimum requirements of the American National Standard for Information Sciences—Permanence of Paper for Printed Library Materials, ANSI Z39.48-1984.

Library of Congress Cataloging-in-Publication Data

Peace through health : how health professionals can work for a less violent
    world / edited by Neil Arya and Joanna Santa Barbara.
        p.   cm.
    Includes bibliographical references and index.
    ISBN 978-1-56549-258-5 (pbk. : alk. paper)
1. Medical personnel—Professional ethics. 2. Violence—Prevention.
3. War—Health aspects. 4. Human rights—Health aspects. 5. Medical ethics.
6. Peace. I. Arya, Neil, 1962–   II. Santa Barbara, Joanna, 1943–
    [DNLM: 1. Health Personnel—ethics. 2. Delivery of Health Care—ethics.
3. International Cooperation. 4. Moral Obligations. 5. Professional Role.
6. Violence—prevention & control. W 21 P355 2008]
    R725.5.P42 2008
    174.2—dc22
                                                                    2007047305

Contents

PART IV: PREPARING TO ACT ON
PEACE THROUGH HEALTH

PART V: CASE STUDIES

CONCLUSION

Acknowledgments

We'd like to thank Jim Lance and Kumarian Press for their faith, confidence, and willingness to take risks in accepting the idea of an edited text on Peace through Health, a new thematic direction for them, or any press. Klaus Melf and Robbie Chase as our internal reviewers and our anonymous external reviewers provided many challenges and constructive criticism, stimulating our thinking and that of other authors. Heather Farrell and Eileen Nicolle volunteered untold hours, patience and grace in copy and style editing, but going much further in bringing their knowledge and skills and values to the project.

We appreciate the efforts of our Peace through Health colleagues, in particular Salim Yusuf who supported various endeavors for conferences and studentships, Rob Stevens who coordinated various *Peace through Health* projects and Vic Neufeld, who hosted us, guided us and shared from his extensive international experience.

Despite busy schedules as Peace through Health practitioners and academics our contributors have indulged us through many editing cycles. We also appreciate the inspirations of colleagues in the field, whose projects serve as beacons for us. Many academic colleagues supported us and challenged us as we developed the book. They will help the discipline grow and flourish in the future. Our students keep us alive intellectually, posing many challenges and offering the gift of their infectious, boundless enthusiasm.

Finally we'd like to acknowledge the love and support of our families—our parents who inculcated the values underlying our work and promoted our education, Jack Santa Barbara, who helped with the work in various phases, and our many friends for putting up with our endless discussions of Peace through Health over many years.

PART I

Basic Concepts in Peace through Health

1

Introduction

Joanna Santa Barbara and *Neil Arya*

The engagement of health professionals with war has a long history. We can assume, that throughout the 10,000-year history of human warfare (Fry 2006, 134–41), there have been healers trying to mend the injuries inflicted by those who did battle. But intertwined as these functions were, they came from two different systems in human society—warriors and healers—and from different castes, different social groups, and different spheres of decision making. There were those (whether warrior kings or civilian diplomats) who decided between war and peace, and there were those who knew how to heal. In this book, however, we propose that healers have a role in the prevention and mitigation of war and other violence. On what is such a proposition founded?

The answer lies partly in the success of the public health or community health model as a powerful factor in improving human health over the last several centuries. This model demands that even while the practitioner is healing injuries and illness, there must always be a drive to identify and act on prior causes, often seen as a chain or web of causes. Not only cure, but also prevention, becomes the imperative. As we will demonstrate, war is an important determinant of death, of injury, and of illness both physical and mental. How can the health professional act preventively on war and other violence?

This may seem a daunting prospect until the reader realizes that the path has already been lightly trodden. There is a short, innovative, and exciting history of defining war as a public health problem and attempting to act on it in various ways from the health perspective. This book will introduce you to these efforts and, we hope, encourage you to join them.

IMPACT OF WAR ON HEALTH

War and other violence have devastating effects on human health. There were well over 100 million deaths from war in the last century (Project

Ploughshares 1996; Elliot 1972). Each year over 1.6 million people world-wide lose their lives directly to violence, accounting for 14 percent of deaths among males and 7 percent of deaths among females aged 15–44 years worldwide—those in the prime of life (Krug et al. 2002). The World Health Organization and the World Bank predict that war will be the eighth leading cause of disability and death by 2020 (Murray and Lopez 1996). For every person who dies as a result of such violence, many more are injured and suffer from a range of physical and mental health problems.

Malnutrition and undernutrition occur with increased frequency during and after wars. Disruption of infrastructure allows the spread of waterborne cholera, dysentery, and typhus. HIV/AIDS may be spread as soldiers engage in unsafe sexual practices with multiple partners. New diseases such as Ebola "emerge" with greater frequency, and diseases such as measles, malaria, and tuberculosis are; difficult to reduce; as a direct result of war (Connolly and Heymann 2002, Diamond 1997, Holdstock 2002).

Women may suffer from sexual and physical abuse and may be at increased risk of sexually transmitted diseases including HIV/AIDS, increased reproductive complications, and mental health problems (Shanks and Schull 2000). Refugees and internally displaced persons (IDPs) suffer from increased mortality, disability, and psychological distress (Santa Barbara 1997).

Violence costs countries billions of US dollars each year in health care, law enforcement, and lost productivity. The Inter-American Development Bank in Latin America has estimated the direct and indirect cost of (direct) violence for Latin America at US$140–170 billion per year, up to 15 percent of GDP (GIIS 2001); some claim figures up to 25 percent of GDP in Colombia (Vieira 1998). These figures may be somewhat lower now.

In 1986 public health specialists and health promoters determined, and stated in what became known as the Ottawa Charter (WHO 1986), that the fundamental conditions and resources for health are (in this order) peace, shelter, education, food, income, a stable ecosystem, sustainable resources, social justice, and equity. Not only is peace the first prerequisite for a "secure foundation" for health, but war also undermines each of the other conditions fundamental to health. We believe then, that to improve the health of populations, it is our responsibility to reduce violence and promote peace, especially in settings of impending, actual, or recent violent conflict.

WHAT IS PEACE THROUGH HEALTH?

Throughout the world, clusters of people working in the health sector (physicians, nurses, psychologists, sociologists, anthropologists) are attempting to address, in their own ways, issues related to the impact of violence on human health, and, in particular, violence at its largest scale—war. In doing so, they have found that there are ways in which health workers can actually contribute to peace. These new approaches go by several names, including Peace through Health, Health as a Bridge to Peace, and Medical Peace Work. We use the first of these names in this text. **Peace through Health, then, refers to those ways that peace is advanced through work from the health sector.**

In a search for solutions, health professionals have found themselves in dialogue with peace scholars and arriving at new approaches together. This text attempts to synthesize over fifteen years of applied work and thought in this area and to provide a roadmap of how to do Peace through Health work.

FOR WHOM ARE WE WRITING THIS VOLUME?

We are writing this book for all health practitioners (and students of health practice) who adopt a public health approach to the impact of war and other violence on health. This includes those in regions not at war who are concerned with the potential for massive violence by the use of weapons of mass destruction, those who are working in war and postwar zones, those who are dealing with violence at a scale where it falls under the heading of human rights abuse, those who are providing humanitarian assistance in conflict situations, and those who are dealing with the health effects of oppression and exploitation. Three possible scenarios follow.

Health professionals in zones of violence

> *You work in the emergency department in a Central American city hospital. You are astonished by the number of gun injuries you see, many of them fatal. Some quick research reveals that gun injury mortality in your country is far higher than in neighboring countries and forty times higher than in the least violent countries in the world. Your country is only six years from the end of a vicious war that left huge quantities of firearms distributed throughout the population. As your research deepens, you find other factors that may contribute to the high rate of gun violence. These include a "macho" culture assigning positive value to male violence, high rates of poverty and inequality,*

unemployment, gang formation around the drug trade, and a sense of lack of political participation. Political polarization and concerns about a resumption of political violence also exist. You decide that you can no longer continue just to bandage victims, but want to look at how to prevent such violence.

Those providing humanitarian assistance

You are a health worker or humanitarian aid worker in a country that has just had an earthquake. This disaster has occurred during a civil war between the government and ethnic factions in the province. Ongoing differences in religion, social class, economics, and urbanization were fueling the violent conflict. You feel that you are too busy dealing with acute problems to think about abstract concepts such as peace.

Yet the issues intrude in your work anyway. Will you remain neutral? Will you cooperate with the government? Will you demonstrate solidarity with the population? Will you use armed guards to secure your aid so it can be delivered? Does the natural disaster offer any opportunities to deal with the violent conflict?

Those involved in rebuilding after violent conflict

Let us move a few years later. The civil war has abated, and direct violence has been reduced. You are looking for ways to support those who want to knit the social fabric together again and diminish the likelihood of recurrent eruption of violence. The health system needs to be rebuilt, and there is international aid to accomplish this—but, as usual, little for peacework. Nationalist factions are discussing the creation of parallel ethnically segregated health systems. You see a potential role for yourself here in strengthening the social fabric, and you must make your case to the international funding agency What do you have to offer?

Peace Studies Students and Peace Workers

Those who have specialized in the dynamics of violence, nonviolence, conflict, conflict transformation, and reconciliation may find themselves working in alliance with various sectors of society, such as the media, representatives of religious institutions, and (in the case of the work highlighted here) the health sector. (This topic is explored further in Part III of this book.) An example:

You are a student of peace studies working for the summer as part of a government-funded rural health team. In this area, 95 percent of inhabitants are indigenous people. They are a minority in most of the country and have been so since the arrival of Europeans in the seventeenth century. For the next three centuries, the indigenous people suffered violence, expropriation of their land,

and attempted extinction of their culture through a residential school system in which punishment discouraged use of the indigenous language and practice of its customs.

Measured by all indicators, the health of this population is much worse than that of the majority population. The indigenous people's housing, water system, sanitation, and school infrastructure are all substandard compared to the rest of the population. Unemployment is high. A nearby mining development employs very few of these people, although the land was expropriated from them with an agreement to offer employment opportunities.

Recently, an aboriginal group occupied a piece of land on which a business entrepreneur was building a new suburb. The protestors' ongoing land claims demonstration was conducted nonviolently, but it elicited a massive police response in which two indigenous people were shot dead.

Your health team genuinely wants to help these young people. You are aware, from the youth who come to the clinic, that there is hopelessness and despair among them—and an attraction to guns and violence. Accident, homicide, and suicide rates are very high among youth. What are your skills and limitations in helping to address the situation?

The aim of this volume is to help promote the improvement of health and the restoration of peace in large-, medium-, and small-scale conflict situations. We hope that it leads to further training of future health professionals in peace and conflict transformation principles. We hope that it helps those working internationally and domestically to clarify their own goals and values; to recognize their knowledge, skills, assets, and deficits; and to apply the principles of Peace through Health to their work and even to other aspects of their lives. We have tried to provide you with the tools to enlist your own unique knowledge, skills, and values in the quest for peace.

Before we proceed, however, we should make sure that we have a common understanding of several terms.

WHAT IS PEACE?

We define it thus: **Peace is an attribute of a relationship between two or more entities in which, at least, no harm is being done to any party, and conflicts are resolved nonviolently; at most, it is a harmonious relationship of mutual benefit and cooperation.** The "entities" in the relationship can be aspects of your self, two or more people, or two or more groups, nations, states, or regions. We sometimes extend this idea to consider peace between humans and Nature and peace between the present generations of humans living on Earth and those who will live here in the future.

The opposite of peace is not conflict, which can be constructive and creative as well as violent and destructive.[1] Rather, the opposite of peace is **violence,** which we now must consider.

WHAT IS VIOLENCE?

Here we call upon the thinking of peace researcher Johan Galtung.[2] He defined violence as **avoidable insults to basic needs** (1996, 1997), **diminishing life potential.** Continuing with Galtung, we think of basic needs as fourfold: **security, well-being, identity,** and **freedom.** It is easy to see that killing or injuring someone will insult their need for security and obliterate or diminish their potential for a happy life. What about someone who is persistently undermined and denigrated by others? He or she is also losing potential for a happy life—words can do violence too. What about a situation in which the way a society is structured means that whole groups of people have lower potential for a happy life, perhaps because they are too poor to fulfill their well-being needs or because they adhere to a particular religion or belong to an ethnic group that is excluded from certain opportunities? Is this violence too? Galtung included such factors in his definition. He spoke about **direct violence,** wherein there is a conscious action directed by one entity against another, with intent to harm—hitting someone, dropping a bomb on a village. Then he described **structural violence,** in which the structures of society prevent certain people from fulfilling their potential for a happy life. This could occur in a family in which girls and women are oppressed, or it could refer to economic globalization, which causes some to grow ever richer while others are hungry. Structural violence can quite often be measured in life expectancy differences. Galtung added a third category, **cultural violence,** by which he meant those attitudes, values, and beliefs that justify direct and structural violence. Perhaps the most prevalent form of cultural violence is the belief that the lives of one's own group (religion, ethnicity, nation) are more worthy and valuable than the lives of others.

Those who work in the framework of Peace through Health may focus on any or all of these types of violence, especially the large-scale, direct violence of war.

WHAT IS WAR?

We use a definition derived from one of the founding thinkers in Peace through Health, Graeme MacQueen. **War is mutual, mass, persistent, lethal**

direct violence engaged in by two or more groups. It can be useful to think of war not as a sporadic event, but as a phase of a **war system,** in which the politics, economies, and cultures of countries are engaged in ongoing preparation for war, which periodically erupts in spasms of killing. We can also envisage a **peace system,** in which the politics, economies, and cultures of countries are engaged in the maintenance of harmonious, cooperative relationships by means of conflict transformation systems, minimal or absent threat levels, respect for law, and multiple relationships of mutual benefit.

Because violence, and especially war, often ensue from conflict, we must return to consider this complex idea.

WHAT IS CONFLICT?

Conflict occurs when two or more entities pursue apparently incompatible goals. Here again, these entities may be aspects of oneself, small groups, or regions of the world with populations of billions of people. Goals may be pursued with such intensity that people are willing to inflict violence on others to try to get what they want. A great deal of knowledge has accumulated about how to deal with conflict constructively and non-violently. Much of it resides in each culture; some of it is consciously taught as **conflict resolution** or **conflict transformation**—for example, in peer mediation[3] in some schools or in courses at the college level.

Those who work in the challenging environments of war zones need, at the very least, to understand the dynamics of the situations in which they work. Sometimes their demonstrable knowledge of peace processes is put to use, as when one of the McMaster University team members working in Afghanistan was appointed to that country's Independent National Commission on Strengthening Peace and worked to bring excluded parties into the peace process in Afghanistan.

WHAT IS HEALTH?

The Constitution of the World Health Organization (WHO 1992) defines health as "**not merely the absence of disease or infirmity**" but, more holistically, as a "**state of complete physical, mental and social well-being**" (WHO 1946).

What determines health, in an individual or a population? Good genes, good nurturance, and good lifestyle provide a foundation. We can then consider **exposures** to aspects of the human environment that may adversely affect health: insufficient housing and clothing, injuries, toxins, microorganisms, and experiences that cause mental stress. It is clear that different populations, and different portions of the same population, incur different degrees of exposure to these factors that diminish health. Some people's lives are more protected than others'.

What influences these different degrees of exposure? We think about the following six phenomena as especially important and as interwoven in complex ways: **Poverty, war and other violence, environmental degradation, disintegration of community, poor governance, and poor human rights observance.**[4] All of these factors are known to be correlated with lower levels of population health. In this book, we focus on war, but war, most unhappily, brings the other five lethal factors in its wake. Protective influences in the environment include the availability of education and health care.

PEACE AND HEALTH

Peace and health are both widely agreed-upon human goods; both are often proposed as human rights. Both are supported by disciplines founded on value structures (unlike "hard sciences" such as physics). The structure of health science thinking in terms of the sequence **diagnosis, prognosis, therapy** is also very useful in application to war, violence, and other conflict. In transposing this structure, the health worker's emphasis on therapy—the imperative to search for solutions to the problem—may be helpful in encouraging political analysts to think creatively beyond diagnosis, or beyond a single (military) solution for every problem.

Another conceptual transposition from health studies to peace studies is elaboration of the idea of prevention. In the health arena, **primary prevention** applies to action on the chain of causes preceding the onset of illness or injury. In the peace arena, it means acting on the multiple causal factors leading to the eruption of violence. **Secondary prevention** in health involves actions to shorten the course of illness or to lessen its ill effects on the body. In peace processes, it means to shorten the course of a war or to mitigate its effects on populations. **Tertiary prevention** applies to actions to rehabilitate the person after illness or injury, or the population and the society after the damage of war. In each case—that is, in the primary, secondary, and tertiary prevention of war and other violence—there are roles appropriate to health professionals, as we shall show.

In each of the scenarios described above, you could choose to treat only the problem under your nose—gun injuries, humanitarian needs, health system reconstruction, or hopeless, angry, indigenous youth. Or you could turn your gaze "upstream" to the sources of the health deficits in the hope of acting preventively. What part has violence, in any of its forms, played in the problems before you? As soon as you expand your vision in this way, you are likely to discover gaps in your knowledge. You will want to be able to analyze what you are seeing and to devise constructive ways of lessening the suffering incurred. This book aims to fill those gaps. But first, we must identify them.

Where you begin will depend on whether you are approaching the problem as a health worker or a peace worker, so you may choose your point of entry accordingly. You will want to analyze the **health deficits** in this situation, actual or potential. It will be helpful to do a **violence analysis**, taking into account direct, structural, and cultural violence, as defined above. This analysis will be informed by knowledge of the **impact of violence on health.**

You may wonder, at this point, about the role of the health worker in addressing peace. The concept of **multisector peacework** may help you see how it fits with the responsibility of all sectors of society to work toward peace.

Each of our scenarios illustrates a different kind of conflict underlying the violence. You will understand your context for action better if you do a **conflict analysis,** including identifying the **stage** of conflict. In complex, large-scale violence, this analysis will frequently benefit from the training of peace specialists or political scientists and from learning from more than one expert. Part of this analysis will be understanding important elements of the history and culture of the arena where you are working. An ideal team for generating the understanding of context would include health workers, peace experts, political scientists, anthropologists, and human rights advocates, with as many as possible of these from the local population (quite possibly not with formal training).

At this point, you are ready to consider whether, as a health worker, you may be able to work "upstream" to improve some of the peace deficits causing ill health; or whether, as a peace worker, you can work with a health team in a useful way. You will need, from at least this point, to work closely in a team with people from the area of focus and to know something about forming good **partnerships** and good **teams.** You will benefit from hard-won knowledge gained in this area and summarized in several analytic **tools** to apply when approaching a problem.

Now comes the most creative part of peace-health work: considering what processes might be helpful in expanding both health and peace. It will help to have some knowledge of previous Peace through Health work and the **mechanisms** by which it operates. Strategies applied in other situations may or may not be relevant to yours. For example, the "Ceasefires for Immunization" strategy described in "Humanitarian Ceasefires" in Chapter 17 has been used in El Salvador, the Philippines, Afghanistan, and many other places, but it probably is not relevant to any of our scenarios. We need to make explicit the **values** that underlie our work and to remind ourselves of **ethical principles.** Respect for universal **human rights** will be part of our value set. Among declarations of human rights, and in particular among those intended to apply in war, we may find principles that act as valuable levers to move governments to take actions that we believe will promote peace and health.

We hope that when you finish this book, you will have the knowledge, inspiring examples, and evaluative tools to design and implement these ideas for your own peace and health projects. Part I continues with a chapter on the history of Peace through Health and introduces basic concepts in the area. Part II looks at the impacts of war and the weapons of war now and in the future. Part III examines principles and values in Peace through Health. In Part IV we describe ways of approaching problems. Part V presents case studies at each level—primary, secondary, and tertiary prevention. These are examples from which you might learn how to design your own interventions before, during, and after the violent phases of conflict. Part VI deals with evaluation of the peace component of Peace through Health work. Part VII shows how we expand the scope of what is commonly considered violence prevention and health work. Finally, in Part VIII, we conclude with a few other special topics. We hope that the methods and examples provided are both inspiring and practical, demonstrating how you might work whether you are a student, a health professional, or a peace practitioner.

REFERENCES

Connolly, M. A., and D. Heymann. 2002. Deadly comrades: war and infectious diseases. *The Lancet*, 360:23–4.

Diamond, J. 1997. *Guns, germs and steel: The fates of human societies.* New York: W. W. Norton.

Elliot, G. 1972. *Twentieth century book of the dead: Charles Scribner.* New York: Ballantine Books.

Fry, Douglas. 2006. *The human potential for peace: An anthropological challenge to assumptions about war and violence.* New York and Oxford: Oxford University Press.

Galtung, Johan. 1996. *Peace by peaceful means.* London: Sage Publications.

Galtung, Johan, Carl G. Jacobsen, and Kai Brand-Jacobs. 2002. *Searching for peace: The road to transcend.* Ann Arbor: University of Michigan Press.

Graduate Institute of International Studies (GIIS). 2001. Small arms survey 2002: Counting the human cost. Geneva: Oxford University Press, 4.

Holdstock, D. 2002. Morbidity and mortality among soldiers and civilians. In I. Taipale et al., eds. *War or health? A reader.* London and New York: Zed Books.

Krug, E. G., L. L. Dahlberg, J. A. Mercy, A. B. Zwi, and R. Lozano. 2002. World report on violence and health, Abstract. Geneva: WHO.

Murray, C. and Lopez, A., eds. 1996. *The global burden of disease: A comprehensive assessment of mortality and disability from diseases, injuries, and risk factors in 1990 and projected to 2020.* Cambridge, MA: Harvard School of Public Health.

Project Ploughshares. 1996. Armed conflict reports 1996–2000. Waterloo see www .ploughshares.ca website.

Santa Barbara, J. 1997. The psychological effects of war on children. In B. S. Levy and V. W. Sidel, eds. *War and public health.* 168–85. Oxford: Oxford University Press.

Shanks, L., and M. J. Schull. 2000. Rape in war: The humanitarian response. *Canadian Medical Association Journal,* 163, 9:1152.

World Health Organization. 1946. Constitution of the World Health Organization. Geneva: WHO.

———. 1986. The Ottawa Charter for Health Promotion. Available online at www.who .int/healthpromotion/conferences/previous/ottawa/en

———. 1992. *Basic documents.* 39th ed. Geneva: WHO.

Vieira, O. 1998. Workshop on International Small Arms/Firearms Injury Surveillance and Research. Toronto: Ryerson Polytechnic University, 18 June.

NOTES

1. An example of a creative conflict outcome is the resolution of a border conflict between Peru and Ecuador. These two countries went to war over their border in the Condor mountains in 1941, 1981, and 1995. Shortly after the last war, peace researcher Johan Galtung remarked to a diplomat of one of the countries that their conflict could be transformed by establishing a binational park in the area. This has been done, greatly to the benefit of the Amazonian indigenous people in the mountains, whose families were previously divided by the violent conflict (Galtung et al. 2002).

2. Johan Galtung was born in Oslo in 1930. He is widely regarded as a founding father of peace research. He generated the Transcend method of conflict transformation and has applied it in 45 major conflicts. His concept of "structural violence" has been fruitfully applied by many thinkers. He has held professorships in numerous universities, has 12 honorary degrees, and has published over 1000 articles and 100 books on peace-related topics.

3. **Peer mediation** is a system of conflict resolution in an organization where some members are trained as mediators. They perform that function, sometimes working in small teams, when conflicts arise among members of the organization. This approach to conflict is often found in schools.

4. This list is a little different from the factors prominent in the current studies of the World Health Organization's Commission on the Social Determinants of Health. Most of the factors in these studies would be subcategories of our typology. For example, poor housing, urban slum-dwelling, and unemployment would fall under our broad category of poverty. On the other hand, the Commission on the Social Determinants of Health does not include war, poor governance, or environmental degradation in its arena of study.

2

History of Peace through Health

Simon Rushton

The ending of the Cold War brought with it seismic changes in the international security environment and also profoundly affected international approaches to issues of war and peace. As the urgency of the threat posed by the nuclear standoff between the superpowers receded, a new wave of challenges came to the fore. Latent grievances that had been suppressed by the heavy hand of inter-bloc rivalry erupted in a series of fierce internal armed conflicts, particularly in sub-Saharan Africa and the Balkans. At the same time, prominent Western states—now acting in a new strategic environment, and with less chance of limited military engagements escalating out of control—began to show more willingness to intervene militarily in other countries, either out of humanitarian concern or in pursuit of perceived security interests. As a result, there was a wave of new thinking on the potential of the international community to engage in conflict prevention and peacebuilding activities; these ideas were most prominently expressed by the UN Secretary-General in *An Agenda for Peace* (Boutros-Ghali 1992). Such new thinking has been increasingly reflected by medical and public health scholars and practitioners who have sought to address the question of what they can contribute to promoting peace.

The claim that health professionals have a part to play in preventing war and bringing about peace is not in itself a new one. Health work and peacework have not always gone hand in hand—indeed, health professionals have been complicit in some of the worst humanitarian atrocities the world has seen, the most high-profile example being the revelations, made at the Nuremberg trial of Karl Brandt and other German doctors, that medical trials were conducted on concentration camp inmates (for example, Schmidt 2004). But even so, there is a relatively long history of attempts to bring the efforts of health workers and peace workers together. Perhaps the highest degree of international recognition has been

15

achieved by the International Committee of the Red Cross, which, in addition to its humanitarian work, has played a major campaigning role, not least in regard to the development of international humanitarian law. Many other organizations have also worked in this area. The Association Médicale Internationale Contre la Guerre was founded in 1905. A number of organizations with a variety of different aims and approaches followed: the Medical Peace Campaign in the 1930s, the Medical Association for the Prevention of War in the 1950s, and International Physicians for the Prevention of Nuclear War in the 1980s (Jenssen 2002; Lewer 1992; Maddocks 1996). Each of these organizations and many others like them sought to encourage a broader view of the role of health professionals in relation to violent conflict, and to move away from a narrow focus on "military medicine" toward an engagement with war as a major determinant of the health of individuals and populations.

The Peace through Health framework on which this volume focuses originated at McMaster University in the early to mid-1990s. The Centre for Peace Studies and the Centre for International Health came together around issues that arose during the Gulf War of 1991 and the subsequent wars in the Balkans. As well as leading to a number of practical initiatives (discussed below and in subsequent chapters), this cooperation has inspired a reassessment of the broader intellectual and theoretical underpinnings of the health sector's peacebuilding potential. The organizations discussed above—from the Association Médicale Internationale Contre la Guerre to IPPNW—generally emphasized what is referred to here as primary prevention (Levy and Sidel 1997), engaging in advocacy and diplomacy to raise awareness of the health impacts of armed conflict and/or the use of particular types of weapons. In his 1992 survey of the historical involvement of physicians in the peace movement, Nick Lewer raised the possibility of moving beyond this advocacy role toward a more direct involvement in mediation, whereby health workers could exploit the traditional neutrality of medical personnel in war "to help facilitate the removal of psychological barriers and so help bring belligerents together for meaningful talks" (Lewer 1992, 96–97).

Work on Peace through Health at McMaster has taken up this challenge, building on these previous efforts by health workers to bring about peace and seeking to explore more fully the potential to engage in secondary prevention (peacemaking) and tertiary prevention ("post 'hot' war peace-building") (Arya 2004, 246). In addition to examining these different forms of prevention, the Peace through Health framework has been intellectually located within a school of thought that holds that promoting peace is a job not for governments and international organizations alone, but for a whole range of actors at a variety of levels. In particular, the Peace through Health concept has been linked to the idea of "Multitrack Diplomacy" (Diamond and McDonald 1993). The argument has been made that the health sector has a particular contribution to make to creating and maintaining peace (Peters 1996, 7) and that health deserves to be treated as a "track" in its own right, with appropriate recognition given to its distinctive approaches and strengths (MacQueen, McCutcheon, and Santa Barbara 1997, 180). McMaster has not been alone in these endeavours, and related activities by a variety of others (not least Paula Gutlove, who has been responsible for a considerable amount of work on "Health Bridges for Peace") have complemented and contributed to the development of Peace through Health. The result has been a concerted attempt over a decade or more to develop the intellectual and theoretical basis of the framework. A body of academic work has been published. Two conferences held at McMaster in 2001 and 2005 brought together individuals working in this area. All this activity has added to the growing sense that Peace through Health can be considered an emerging discipline in its own right (MacQueen et al. 2001).

The guiding concern has been to create a dialogue within the medical and public health communities over the extent to which, and the variety of ways in which, health workers can contribute to bringing about and sustaining peace. These ideas have not, however, been entirely free from controversy within those communities. In particular, attention has focused on the difficulty of providing evidence of the effectiveness of such activities, especially given the supposedly slim track record of Peace through Health initiatives (Vass 2001). Yet it is by necessity that the development of the framework has been a two-part process, with theorizing and practical action taking place simultaneously and to mutual benefit. The two Peace through Health conferences were held partly in an effort to bring these two elements together. Indeed, the 2005 conference was titled "Learning from Action." Even so, much work remains to be done in this area, particularly in terms of documenting the impacts of Peace through Health interventions.

There have, however, been enough examples of actions successfully linking health initiatives to peace outcomes to give reasonable cause for optimism. These initiatives have been both large and small in scale and have been undertaken by a variety of actors ranging from international organizations and national governments to small groups of concerned individuals.

One of the earliest of the large-scale initiatives (and one that predated the Peace through Health framework) was the Pan American Health Organization's "Health as a Bridge for Peace" program in the 1980s. A key element of this program was the negotiation of temporary ceasefires to allow for polio vaccination of children in war-affected areas, and it met with success (in health terms at least) in El Salvador and Peru (de Quatros and Epstein 2002). The wars of the 1990s in the Balkans witnessed a concerted attempt by the World Health Organization (in partnership with the UK's Department for International Development) to extend this earlier PAHO strategy and to integrate conflict resolution across the range of its activities in Bosnia and Herzegovina. This initiative—the "WHO/DFID Peace through Health Programme in Bosnia-Herzegovina"—included a wide range of elements, focusing in particular on postwar intercommunity reconciliation. Although it remains difficult to determine how much these types of activities contribute to a broader peacebuilding process, the internal evaluation of the Bosnia-Herzegovina program found it to have been effective in addressing a number of obstacles to a stable peace (WHO Europe 1998, 33–39). There is also anecdotal evidence to suggest that these types of initiatives have opened up the possibility of dialogue between warring parties in other cases. For example, the Sierra Leonean minister of health reportedly told the WHO Director General in 2001 that the immunization ceasefire program in that country had indeed been a "bridge to peace" and had opened the way for negotiations in other areas (Griekspoor and Loretti 2001).

Along with these large-scale attempts to engage the health sector in peacemaking (secondary prevention) and peacebuilding (tertiary prevention), health professionals were also closely involved, through the 1990s, with successful campaigns to prevent conflict and/or to delegitimize particular types of weapons (both of which are examples of primary prevention). The International Campaign to Ban Landmines provides a striking illustration of the potential influence of medical peace organizations, in this case working in conjunction with a variety of other civil society groups. Crucial to the progress made toward the signing of the Ottawa Treaty[1] was the successful reframing of the landmine issue as a humanitarian crisis rather than a question of military effectiveness (Price 1998). The presentation of the health impacts of antipersonnel landmines was a central part of this strategy: a classic example of deploying health as a "superordinate goal," and a demonstration that this can be effective even within the realm of defense policy—an area usually guarded jealously by states.

In addition, there is now a significant repertoire of practice accumulated through many smaller-scale Peace through Health initiatives. Early examples that arose directly from the work at McMaster include the "Health of Children in War Zones" project, which sought not only to address the impact of war on children's health (both physical and mental) but also to include actions specifically designed to contribute to postwar peacebuilding and reconciliation. Projects were carried out in Gaza, Croatia, and Sri Lanka. In the Croatian case in particular, there was a significant reduction in inter-ethnic hatred among those children who were part of the project (Santa Barbara 1999). A large number of other examples of Peace through Health initiatives both large and small are detailed in subsequent chapters.

It may still be too early to assess the potential of Peace through Health approaches, and more evidence is needed to show the effectiveness of such initiatives. We hope that this text represents a step forward in this respect. There remains a pressing need for further research—not to mention further action—in this field. Yet, as this volume shows, it is not a discipline without a history. Indeed, considerable progress has been made in understanding the ways in which actors in the health sector can contribute to peace, and there have been a variety of attempts to put such ideas into practice. As a result of this earlier work, there are clear grounds for optimism that health professionals can indeed make a distinctive and worthwhile contribution to peace.

REFERENCES

Arya, Neil. 2004. Peace through health I: Development and use of a working model. *Medicine, Conflict and Survival* 20 (3): 243–57.

Boutros-Ghali, Boutros. 1992. *An agenda for peace: Preventive diplomacy, peacemaking and peacekeeping.* New York: United Nations.

De Quatros, Ciro A., and Daniel Epstein. 2002. Health as a bridge for peace: PAHO's experience. *The Lancet* 360 (1): 25–26.

Diamond, Louise, and John McDonald. 1993. *Multi-track diplomacy: A systems approach to peace.* Washington, DC: The Institute for Multi-Track Diplomacy.

Griekspoor, Andre, and Alessandro Loretti. 2001. Health and peace: An opportunity to join forces. *The Lancet* 358:1183.

Jenssen, Christian. 2002. Medicine against war: An historical review of the anti-war activities of physicians. In *War or health? A reader,* ed. Ilkka Taipale et al., 7–29. London and New York: Zed Books.

Levy, Barry S., and Victor W. Sidel. 1997. Preventing war and its health consequences: Role of public health professionals. In *War and public health,* ed. Barry S. Levy and Victor W. Sidel, 388–93. Oxford: Oxford Univ. Press.

Lewer, Nick. 1992. *Physicians and the peace movement*. London: Frank Cass.

MacQueen, G., R. McCutcheon, and J. Santa Barbara. 1997. The use of health initiatives and peace initiatives. *Peace and Change* 22 (2): 175–97.

MacQueen, G., and J. Santa Barbara. 2000. Peace building through health initiatives. *BMJ* 321:293–6.

MacQueen, Graeme, J. Santa Barbara, V. Neufeld, S. Yusuf, and R. Horton. 2001. Health and peace: Time for a new discipline. *The Lancet* 357:1460–61.

Maddocks, I. 1996. Evolution of the physicians' peace movement: A historical perspective. *Health and Human Rights* 2 (1): 88–109.

Peters, Mary Anne, ed. 1996. *A health to peace handbook*. Hamilton, Ontario: McMaster University War and Health Program. Available online.

Price, R. 1998. Reversing the gun sights: Transnational civil society targets land mines. *International Organization* 52 (3): 613–44.

Rodriguez-Garcia, James Macinko, F. Xavier Solórzano, and Maria Schlesser. 2001. *How can health serve as a bridge for peace?* Washington, DC: George Washington University School of Public Health and Health Sciences. Available online.

Santa Barbara, Joanna. 1999. Health reach: Helping children affected by war. *Peace Magazine* 15 (5): 26.

Schmidt, Uli. 2004. *Justice at Nuremberg: Leo Alexander and the Nazi doctors' trial*. Basingstoke: Palgrave Macmillan.

Vass, Alex. 2001. Peace through health: This new movement needs evidence, not just ideology. *BMJ* 323:1020.

WHO Europe. 1998. WHO/DFID Peace through Health Programme: A case study prepared by the WHO field team in Bosnia and Herzegovina. Copenhagen: WHO Europe.

NOTE

1. Formally known as the Convention on the Prohibition of the Use, Stockpiling, Production and Transfer of Anti-Personnel Mines and on their Destruction. The treaty, which outlaws antipersonnel landmines, became binding in international law in March 1999.

3

Setting the Role of the Health Sector in Context: Multi-track Peacework

Graeme MacQueen

News media persist in discussing the achievement of peace as though it were the responsibility of a small subgroup in society—leaders of states, of nations, of insurgent groups or factions. So-and-so meets in a secluded location with what's-his-name, and they sign a paper. Peace ensues. As for the bulk of the affected populations, they may mill about in the streets, they may wave placards or raise their fists in the air, but this is all backdrop for the real action.

This understanding of how peace is achieved and maintained is inaccurate and insulting. To accept it is to show our ignorance of the historical role of ordinary human beings in the achievement of peace and to resign ourselves to our own irrelevance.

Multi-track peacework (MTP) is a recent development, but it takes its place in a long tradition that challenges the narrow view of peacework that dominates the news media. It is important that we understand MTP if we wish to appreciate and contribute to the health track to peace.

MULTI-TRACK PEACEWORK

MTP seeks to set free as much of society's intelligence and creativity as possible for the tasks of achieving and maintaining peace. It does so by drawing on the different functions of a society (such as healing, building, teaching, and cultivating), and on the sectors or communities who specialize in these functions, to make use of multiple, specific forms of knowledge, skill, and analysis, as well as resources, social legitimacy, and networks. MTP need not be antigovernmental, nor need it be wholly independent from government and government leaders, but it must not be restricted to or dependent on government: it must include approaches to peace significantly different from the governmental.

MTP derives from the concept and practice of multi-track diplomacy developed by two members of the Washington, DC–based Institute for Multi-Track Diplomacy (IMTD). Louise Diamond and John McDonald had been stimulated by Joseph Montville's 1981 discussion of the distinction between "official governmental actions to resolve conflicts (track one) and unofficial efforts by nongovernmental professionals to resolve conflicts within and between states (track two)" (IMTD 2006). Diamond and McDonald developed a model that expanded the total number of tracks to nine, among them such social functions as business, education, and religion (Diamond and McDonald 1993). The power of the model is that it encourages disciplined reflection on the specific contributions that different sectors of society can make to the achievement and maintenance of peace.

Since the pioneering work of IMTD, several organizations involved in Peace through Health (PtH) have adopted a multi-track analysis, making additions and changes as appropriate. Most obviously, they have repaired a major deficiency in the IMTD model by adding health as a separate track. Moreover, some PtH organizations found themselves uncomfortable with the word *diplomacy,* which traditionally refers to the "soft" methods used by states to influence other states for their own ends. The deeper and more humane concept of *peacework* encompasses all the work that society does to bring about and maintain positive peace. Use of this comprehensive term has therefore become common.

HOW THE TRACKS WORK

To see how the tracks work, let us take as an example the social function of *building.* The community associated with this function (architects, engineers, artisans, and workers in the building trades) knows that its tasks respond to basic human needs, especially the need for shelter. As it approaches peacework, this community will begin by applying its central metaphors to the new tasks, which in this case respond to the basic human need for security. The term *peacebuilding* will be attractive to this community. All illusions about peace springing into being naturally as soon as two heads of state sign an agreement are swept away by the metaphor of *building.* It reflects an awareness of the many forms of intelligence, skill, and labor that will be required to *build* peace; of the fact that a plan will be needed; of the necessity of a building process with stages, at each of which different skill-sets will be needed; of the need to build resilient structures able withstand the forces that will challenge them; of the escape routes and emergency measures that must be planned from the outset; and so on.

In addition to the new metaphors, this community will offer many practical skills and resources. After all, modern war typically targets the built environment of a population: its homes, businesses, government buildings, and transportation and energy systems. To undertake peace-through-building in a practical way, a group would need, for example, to be able to undertake postwar physical reconstruction in a manner sensitive to social context and to the goals of peacework. The group would have to see physical reconstruction as a part of social reconstruction. It would need some knowledge of conflict analysis and conflict transformation, and it would need to be able to adapt the basic principles of these learning areas to the specific demands of its professions. For example, it would need to know whether, and at what point, to have former adversaries work together in teams to rebuild each other's communities. It would need to know whether one particular group needs to be empowered in the reconstruction process, and how this might be managed. Finally, the group would need to be able to use its identity as a group of builders to access resources—calling on associations, unions, and global contacts for assistance.

THE HEALTH TRACK

Advantages

Each track to peace covers distinctive terrain. The list of mechanisms by which a track reaches its goal will give it a unique profile, even though several of the items in the list will be shared among different tracks. There is, however, another way to grasp the uniqueness of a track, and that is to ask what values, areas of concentration, and social characteristics typify the sector of society in question.

Here are six elements—two values, one area of concentration, and three social characteristics—that typify the health sector and make its track to peace uniquely effective.

Values. Health workers, as individuals, may be no more altruistic than workers in any number of other sectors, but they work in organizations that formally place the highest value on, and have attempted to institutionalize, *altruism.* To the extent that health workers live up to this formal commitment, compassion and caring will be supported, funded, appreciated, and given legitimacy in this sector in a way that will be rare in many sectors. This is an enormous advantage for peacework.

Health work, as dominated and shaped by developments in Western civilization over the last century and a half, is formally committed to *scientific procedure*. To the extent that this commitment is honored, hypotheses not supported by evidence and by an appropriate chain of reasoning will not be accepted. The valuing of science, given that war making creates an environment where myth, propaganda, and lies flourish, is very important.

Area of Concentration. Anyone working with definitions of peace and of health rapidly discovers so many common themes that distinguishing these two human goods becomes problematic. Health and peace can be pictured as greatly overlapping circles within the wider circle of human well-being. The area of *peace-health overlap* can be characterized as "restoration and maintenance of harmonious human functioning." It is because of this substantial overlap between the concepts of peace and health that the sharing of understanding, metaphor, analysis, and skills between the sectors of society devoted to these goods is natural.

Social Characteristics. Because health is one of society's most highly valued goals, it will typically be granted both social legitimacy and various kinds of *support, including funding*. Such support can be very helpful when it can be extended to the pursuit of peace.

Health workers typically achieve an *access to war zones* denied to most social sectors. They are present, in some form, even in the midst of intense, violent conflict, and this access makes them invaluable aids to peacemaking.

Through international journals, conferences, common standards, and technology, the international health community is *a strongly integrated community*. A thing learned here can quickly be communicated there; an initiative developed there can be tried here. The international health community is a powerful learning community. It has the potential to adapt quickly to new conditions and put new ideas into practice rapidly.

Disadvantages

All tracks to peace face challenges, and it would be irresponsible to ignore them. Three challenges to PtH stand out.

Health workers who engage in peacework may be perceived as going beyond their area of expertise. They may also be seen as "politicized"— as having their true healing function corrupted by involvement in political commitments and alliances. These perceptions may reduce their perceived legitimacy and consequently their effectiveness for both health and peace.

Health workers are typically not trained in the skills necessary for peacework. They may attempt peacework and fail, thereby betraying the confidence that others have placed in them and, again, losing trust and legitimacy.

If PtH is simply added to an already overburdened health team in a zone of conflict and stress, especially in the absence of institutional support and the sympathetic understanding of other agencies in the field, that team is again likely to fail, with similar consequences.

These challenges confront many of the tracks to peace, not merely the health track. They are, in fact, common to nearly all interdisciplinary innovation. Time, patience, adequate training and standards, the building of institutional support, the gradual growth of understanding and respect from other organizations, and the demonstrated effectiveness of the method will combine to reduce these difficulties.

Dynamism

MTP offers a stimulus to creative thinking, not a template. PtH should be seen less as a static set of procedures than as an evolving and dynamic system, wherein two social goods, health and peace, join to power an upward spiral that can replace the downward spiral of war and disease.

REFERENCES

Diamond, Louise, and John McDonald. 1993. *Multi-track diplomacy: A systems approach to peace*. Washington, DC: Institute for Multi-track Diplomacy.

Institute for Multi-track Diplomacy. November 2006. Available online at the www.intd .org website.

4

Mechanisms of Peace through Health

Graeme MacQueen and *Joanna Santa Barbara*

In developing theory on Peace through Health, it seemed important to understand the ways in which health sector actors sought to influence peace in their arena of action. The McMaster group attempted a finer-grained examination of the fundamental mechanisms by which changes might be induced. By examining accumulated case studies, we developed the following typology (MacQueen et al. 1997):

1. Redefinition of the situation
2. Superordinate goals
3. Mediation and conflict transformation
4. Dissent and noncooperation
5. Discovery and dissemination of knowledge
6. Rebuilding the fabric of society
7. Solidarity and support
8. Social healing
9. Evocation and extension of altruism
10. Limiting the destructiveness of war

REDEFINITION OF THE SITUATION

War is a complex phenomenon. Its meaning is not obvious beyond the fact that war is an arena of contention and struggle. Peace through Health (PtH), as a form of multi-track peacework, seeks to develop the intelligence and resources of societies in ways that allow them to deal humanely with war and conflict. Its practitioners must therefore be willing to challenge certain understandings of war and to propose others.

There are many meanings assigned to war (Rapoport 1968, 13). They include

- the rational continuation of policy by other means
- a zero-sum game with a clear winner

- a manly contest
- the fulfillment of national or religious destiny
- an instance of the cosmic conflict between good and evil
- a non-zero-sum game, which often ends in lose-lose
- a nonrational mode of behavior now endangering human civilization
- a crime
- a disaster
- public health problem

There is no need to hold that any one of the above definitions expresses the full meaning of war and that all others are false depictions. But if PtH is to contribute to peacework at this point in history, it must be prepared, like other participants in the movement for peace, to challenge the first five meanings. This will require assertiveness, since these five understandings are rooted in a long tradition of epic, myth, and national self-understanding, and since they are often promoted powerfully by governments and national military institutions.

Here is a common example. Two belligerents have a series of battles. A newspaper favoring belligerent A reports the battles as though they were engagements in a lengthy game. The players (combatants), decked out in their uniforms, take to the field and try to score goals—to kill each other. There are rules to the game; there are cheerleaders and spectators. The newspaper sees its job as a combination of score keeping ("party A killed 12 of party B's players while party B killed only 6 of party A's") and cheerleading ("party A behaved with courage and professionalism against the ruthless murderers of party B").

Accounts much like the above are common in news accounts from Sri Lanka to Canada. Descriptions of battles and their outcomes may differ little from reports on cricket or football. The game proceeds; military people are called on to analyze the state of play; editorials romanticize government forces and eulogize the "fallen" among them, while excoriating official enemies as "nihilists" whose death in large numbers is supposed to be a cause for celebration.

Now suppose a health organization inserts itself into this discourse. Suppose it carries out a study focusing on the misery experienced by the "players" on both sides and their families; the massive injury and devastation inflicted on ordinary civilians in the war zones and the undermining of their livelihood and sanity; the wounded and the lost homes; the impoverishment and despair. Suppose the study demonstrates that the children of the society in the war zone are losing all opportunity for education and are dying of preventable diseases. Declining to cheer for either side, the health study makes it clear that to the extent this activity may be called a game, the score is negative for both sides.

The organization makes its report public, challenging not only specific facts given in newspapers but the entire way the newspapers have constructed the war. The organization says, in effect, "Maybe this war is not like cricket or hockey; maybe it is more like a hurricane. Maybe we need to shift our approach to it and consider it as a massive public health problem."

The World Health Organization's magazine *bridges,* which aims to show, through health research, the ongoing cost of the Israeli–Palestinian conflict to both parties, is a remarkable example of the attempt to redefine a violent conflict. (See "The Role of Medical Journals" in Chapter 17.)

When viewing war as a disaster in which most if not all participants are injured, and where the losses outweigh the gains, we draw back from taking sides, draw back from blaming, draw back from seeing glory and success as likely outcomes. We see war as, at best, a semirational activity associated with many risks, much harm, and multiple unintended consequences. As we measure the human costs of war and make our results public, we contribute to the accumulation of knowledge about war and peace so that our society—and global society at large—becomes a "learning society," which matures through growing knowledge and intelligence and, therefore, does not have to keep repeating the Battle of the Somme.[1]

At some point, health research then moves to the next step and carries out such analyses before a war begins, as Medact did prior to the 2003 Anglo-American invasion of Iraq (Medact 2002). By making the results of its study known before the invasion, Medact gave society crucial data on which to base an informed, intelligent decision about whether to choose the option of going to war. This process is necessary not only to the building of learning societies but also to the building of genuine, informed democracies.

Seeing war as a disaster is, of course, just one way of seeing. If it is our only way of seeing, we will be blind to certain important facts. For war, unlike natural disasters, does involve human decision making and human will and, at least to some extent, rational aims and purposes. PtH is able to accommodate this. Civil society organizations (CSOs) involved in PtH may, for example, join other CSOs, as well as international organizations, in holding the architects and initiators of war accountable to international law. The distinction between aggressors and defenders is sometimes a valid one, and those participating in PtH are not barred from recognizing this. In such a case, they might choose to contribute their skills in the measurement of human costs to the support of criminal proceedings.

Yet war-as-disaster is, overall, probably the most distinctive and appropriate approach to war for PtH practitioners. It was pioneered in recent decades by the various national organizations within International Physicians for the Prevention of Nuclear War (quite appropriately, since nuclear war is the form of war that most closely fits the model of war as an unmitigated disaster causing catastrophic public health problems). The model and the analysis can be adapted, with qualifications as necessary, to other forms of war.

SUPERORDINATE GOALS

In experiments carried out in the 1950s, researchers discovered that through the introduction of superordinate goals into a situation, cooperation could be encouraged, and tensions reduced, between antagonistic groups. Superordinate goals were understood as goals that appealed to, or were compelling to, members of both the antagonistic groups but could be attained only if the groups cooperated. For example, two groups of boys, antagonistic toward each other, might be confronted with a situation where a truck useful to both groups was stuck in a rut in the road and could be set free only by the combined efforts of both groups. Getting the truck out was, in this case, the superordinate goal (Sherif et al. 1961).

In addition to these experimental observations, historical studies have yielded examples of such superordinate goals arising naturally and having similar effects. For instance, it was discovered that opposing military forces in the trenches of World War I had sometimes worked out unspoken agreements about when each party should shell the other. In this way, each party was able to make preparations and avoid taking heavy casualties. The superordinate goal in this case was survival, the soldiers having recognized that this goal could be achieved only through cooperation (Axelrod 1984).

Not surprisingly, peace workers have come to regard superordinate goals as a vital resource for their work. A classic example of the use of a health-related superordinate goal for peacemaking is the humanitarian ceasefire. (See "Humanitarian Ceasefires" in Chapter 17.) Parties A and B both want their own children to be healthy. This is a compelling goal, but they come to see that their children cannot be immunized against infectious diseases under conditions of war and that it is, therefore, in their interests to agree with their opponent on "days of tranquility" during which children of both populations will be immunized. There is no requirement that the separate populations care about the children of their opponents (Peters 1996).

Here it is necessary to make a point about superordinate goals. There is nothing about superordinate goals *per se* that ensures that they will promote large-scale or sustainable peace. All they do is promote cooperation, and reduce tension, for a certain time and at a certain level.

Suppose Party A covets the resources of Party B. Party A realizes it does not have the military strength to take these resources. It therefore builds a military alliance with Parties C and D, with the aim of invading B, stripping it of its wealth and resources, and sharing the spoils—to the extent necessary—with its allies. Here a superordinate goal (getting hold of B's wealth) draws A, C, and D together, but although it promotes cooperation at a certain level and for a certain period, it certainly does not promote large-scale or sustainable peace. Far from being unusual, cases of this kind are to be found everywhere. We must remember that all large-scale warfare depends on large-scale cooperation; cooperation and war are not opposites.

Why, then, should superordinate goals be promoted as a PtH mechanism? Health-related superordinate goals have greater potential than most for peacemaking. Typically, health-related superordinate goals are seen as more noble than military goals. And they can be used to promote not only small-scale and temporary cooperation but also humane values, feelings, and actions.

For example, if a humanitarian ceasefire is to be useful to peacemaking, it will be guided by those who understand its long-term potential and who understand, and are prepared to make explicit to the parties, the rules crucial to its peacemaking success (Hay 1990; Peters 1996). As a mediator trusted by all parties takes them through a process of negotiation and agreement leading to the ceasefire, the mediator will attempt to extend and deepen the peace process. Although superordinate goals do not require altruism, it is certainly true that altruism may be nurtured during the period of cooperation stimulated by the pursuit of the ceasefire, and this will make sustained peace far more likely.

Humanitarian ceasefires are a means of reaching the superordinate goal of health for one's children, but in the process of achieving this goal, all sorts of complex social interactions may be initiated and several PtH mechanisms employed. Other processes linked to health-related super-ordinate goals, many of which have been actively encouraged in conflict zones, include common health planning among former or current belligerents and the sharing of vital health resources, training, and skills.

MEDIATION AND CONFLICT TRANSFORMATION

Suppose the PtH practitioner has identified humane superordinate goals that have the potential to induce cooperation, and even a sustainable peace, among belligerents. Then what? Is it sufficient to point out the superordinate goals to the contestants? No, this will seldom do the job. Discovering such goals and bringing the belligerents together into a peaceful relationship are two different things, and the path connecting them is long and fraught with peril.

We frequently hear of the humanitarian ceasefire initiated in El Salvador in the 1980s through UNICEF's James Grant and with trusted local mediating institutions such as the Roman Catholic Church. We hear less often about the initiatives that ran into difficulties. I (GM) was an observer in one such case in Sri Lanka in the mid-1990s. The idea of launching a humanitarian ceasefire in that country at that time was greeted with several objections. One of these had to do with the perceived unreliability of the Liberation Tigers of Tamil Eelam (LTTE), the government's opponent. Not only government spokespersons, but also several intergovernmental organizations (IGOs) and CSOs with experience in Sri Lanka, said the LTTE had shown itself over time to be unreliable as a partner in such initiatives. The LTTE, they said, could be expected to agree to the ceasefire but to then use it, in violation of the formal rules guiding such initiatives, to better position its forces and to gain advantages. Whether this judgment was accurate or not, it was sufficiently pervasive to impede the process.

In a case such as this, a trust-building exercise involving both parties may be useful, and to this end, people who are trusted by both parties and who have expertise in mediation and conflict transformation may be crucial.

Mediation

Mediation is a voluntary process guided by an impartial party outside the conflict formation—often called a "third party," although this mistakenly implies that there will always be just two parties in the conflict.

Especially when war is involved, good mediation requires a grasp of the psychology of severe conflict—what happens to the minds of leaders of armed groups, for example, after they have been involved in fighting for a long time, and what happens to groups themselves and their sense of identity and security after involvement in armed conflict.

Mediators may assist parties in initiating cooperation and in working through problems; they may, when permitted, report the needs, perceptions, and proposals of parties to other parties; they may sometimes be in a position to provide important information unavailable to any of the parties.

It is crucial that a mediator be trusted by all parties and be seen as unbiased. If the mediator feels he or she can no longer be unbiased but must move to a position of advocacy for one party, the only responsible thing to do is to step down from the position of mediator. There are many different roles a person may adopt in peacework, but it is important to know what role is appropriate at a given moment and to be honest about which role one is adopting.

Because health practitioners are frequently "in the field" in the midst of serious conflicts, there are several reasons why they should receive mediation training. First, they will be required to carry out their health work within groups and organizations that are experiencing great stress, when conflicts inside the group will be common and, often, more destructive than in everyday life. Second, they will typically be working in an environment overwhelmed with governmental and nongovernmental aid organizations of all kinds, and it is important that these groups work effectively together. And finally, the PtH practitioner may have opportunities, both large and small, to promote peace between belligerents. The ability to perceive such opportunities is as important as the skill to make use of them. If PtH practitioners do not have the required mediation skills, by all means let them bring in someone who does, whether that person is from the health field or not. They will have contributed a great deal simply by seeing the opportunity and seizing it.

Good mediation requires a sense of when it is helpful to bring opponents together and when they are not yet ready to come together. It requires a sense of when an outside actor can offer something of use and when it is time to rely on local resources, traditions, and practitioners. It is a skill all mature human beings need and all groups and organizations require in order to be humane and efficient. Mediation skills should therefore be widely shared, and there are dangers in the current tendency in North America to professionalize mediation and have the field dominated by lawyers. Mediation skills are required by governments, by IGOs, and by CSOs.

But PtH practitioners may find themselves in the midst of a conflict that is complex, has deep roots, and seems intractable. Or, as mentioned earlier, they may find themselves drawn to take sides in a conflict, as they conclude that justice favors one of the parties. There is no need to feel guilty when this happens, but it is important to know how to respond. It is helpful to understand that each of the numerous roles of peace workers may contribute to a just peace within an overall framework of conflict transformation.

Conflict Transformation

Conflict transformation (CT) is a term that many practitioners now prefer to *conflict resolution*. Although different practitioners have slightly different understandings of the term, CT generally implies at least the following beliefs (Galtung 2000; Lederach and Maiese 2003).

1. Conflict is a natural part of human interaction. It is not necessarily bad; in fact, it can often be part of the growth and improvement of both individual and social life.
2. We do not, therefore, necessarily want to "resolve" all conflicts, and we are especially wary of methods of resolving conflicts that are quick and superficial and of methods that involve suppressing the conflict parties' true needs and feelings or denying and obscuring the causes of the conflict.
3. We do, however, recognize that conflicts can sometimes be very destructive, especially when they involve violence or when they become "frozen."
4. We therefore seek to transform conflicts, and to let conflicts transform us, in ways that are positive—that are humane and lead to mature, compassionate, and just relations. The process of transformation may or may not lead to resolution of a conflict.

What does this mean concretely for the PtH practitioner? Suppose a physician in a war zone regularly treats patients who are victims of torture by government forces. The physician wants to see the war end, but she has to admit to herself that resistance, and even vigorous struggle, against the government are legitimate and necessary. She comes to see that although she may not want to resolve the conflict (at least not prematurely), she can help the resisters wage the conflict more humanely as well as more effectively. She may point out to resistance forces that assassinating government leaders both puts the resisters on the same moral level as the government and is apt to strengthen the most negative and self-perpetuating aspects of the conflict (mutual demonization, brutalization of all conflict participants, distortion of the self). Suppose she finds that she is able to help resistance forces see that there are other modes of struggle, which are nonviolent, dialogical, and efficacious in the long term. Perhaps she finds herself able to facilitate the responsible documentation and publication of human rights abuses, and suppose this results in governments, CSOs, and IGOs putting pressure on the government to change its behavior. In this case she has not sacrificed her feelings of indignation at the torture of her patients, but she has been able to help the resisters to increase their social intelligence and preserve their humanity while pursuing justice. This is a case of the transformation of conflict.

DISSENT AND NONCOOPERATION

There is a tendency in some literature to characterize PtH as wholly devoted to increasing cooperation among individuals and groups. This is simplistic. In the history of the struggle for peace, noncooperation has been as important as cooperation. Just as cooperation does not necessarily lead to peace, noncooperation does not necessarily promote long-term conflict, much less violence.

The "Health: A Bridge for Peace" initiative of the Pan American Health Organization (PAHO), which began in Central America in 1984, is rightly recognized as a pioneering effort in PtH, and it involved the promotion of cooperation in pursuit of superordinate goals (Rodriguez-Garcia et al. 2001). But during the same period, Physicians for Social Responsibility (PSR) in the United States was tackling a different aspect of the struggle for peace through dissent and noncooperation. It was advocating that physicians refuse to take part in civil defense exercises that were part of their government's preparation for nuclear war (MacQueen et al. 1997). It said that such exercises were a sham—that after major nuclear war there would be little if any health care remaining in the societies of the belligerents. The public, PSR said, must be told this. PSR said that the only position with either scientific or moral credibility was advocacy of the prevention of nuclear war. This position will strike most of us as reasonable and moderate, but we must remember that adopting it involved dissent and noncooperation.

To be willing to dissent is no more than to be willing to think, and speak, for oneself. It is the lifeblood of civil society and of the CSOs that have risen to prominence in the last half of the twentieth century. Nowhere has dissent been more important than in the movement for peace, where age-old traditions of war, as well as a massively funded, interlocking global military system (now consuming more than US$1 trillion per year), have had to be challenged.

It does not follow that dissenters are opponents of all tradition or that they are unruly rebels acting in ad hoc ways. The peaceful traditions of which they are the inheritors are just as old as the warlike traditions. They should make use of these traditions. When PSR spoke out against nuclear war in the 1980s, it did so by announcing that it was drawing on "the most hallowed traditions of medicine" (Lown and Pastore 1985).

But how do dissent and noncooperation fit with the other PtH mechanisms? (Especially, how can noncooperation be made to fit with cooperation?) And where, analytically, do they fit within peacework?

All of PtH, insofar as it carves out a new role for health workers and insists on the legitimacy of this role, is an exercise in dissent. Redefinition of the situation, the basis of all PtH work, where this involves challenging mainstream thinking, involves dissent and may involve serious levels of noncooperation. Although it may sound contradictory, even the promotion of superordinate goals, altruism, and cooperation frequently involve dissent and noncooperation. There is no contradiction: to promote cooperation between A and B, one may need to engage in noncooperation with respect to C. We have no doubt that the PAHO pioneers wishing to promote cooperation among health departments in Central America had, at some point, to engage in serious dissent with respect to certain institutions and parties.

None of this implies that dissent and noncooperation, especially in dramatic and public forms, should be resorted to lightly. Credibility is a coin that can be spent until it is gone. If physicians or medical organizations are perceived as acting outside their areas of expertise, or if they are seen as inappropriately "politicizing" health care, they may sacrifice long-term influence for short-term gains.

It is tempting to try to resolve this tension by assigning different roles to different sorts of groups. IGOs such as WHO and the ICRC, for example, which depend for their efficacy on maintaining good relations with governments, might be assigned the roles of building bridges and fostering cooperation, whereas small, feisty, and perhaps short-lived CSOs might be expected to take on the more confrontational duties involved in "speaking truth to power." To some extent this is probably appropriate, but we must be careful not to take this differentiation of roles too far. No organization can entirely give up the right to dissent if it is to maintain its integrity. Moreover, it must be remembered that losing legitimacy in one sphere may mean gaining it in another.

The World Health Organization has at times dissented from powerful states in remarkable ways. An example is its decision to take nuclear weapons to the World Court for a ruling on their legality (Peters 1996). WHO had to assert itself as having the competence and legitimacy to undertake this action. It needed to redefine the situation; it needed to disagree with certain governments that challenged its right to carry out this action and tried to de-legitimize it; it needed to persevere under pressure. Whatever legitimacy WHO may have lost during the process among certain governments, it gained in the eyes of civil society. It dared to honor the hopes and fears of world society at large, rather than the interests of powerful governments and elites. It needed to break free of a certain defined role to do this, but it did not need to break free from the traditions of health care. On the contrary, it built on the traditions of health care in the same way that PSR had done earlier, insisting on the importance of preventive measures for the protection of public health.

Many peace studies theorists argue that the various mechanisms listed in the PtH toolkit are relevant at different stages in the evolution of a just peace. Some have argued that dissent and protest are needed at a stage of a conflict where general awareness of the conflict or of its causes is low and where there is severe power imbalance among the parties to the conflict. Protest and dissent raise awareness of the issues and of the need to address them. They also strengthen the weak or exploited parties in the conflict, creating a more balanced relationship, after which the process of mediation has a much greater chance of success. It is not a question of dissent versus mediation, therefore, but of each having a role to play at different stages and in different types of conflicts (Curle 1971).

When health workers or organizations feel they must refuse the invitation to collaborate in wars or preparation for wars, or in the development of inhumane or brutal technology or policy, they may invoke not only international law but their own health traditions as formally expressed in such documents as the Declaration of Geneva, the International Code of Medical Ethics, the Declaration of Tokyo, Regulations in Time of Armed Conflict, and Statement of Nurse's Role in Safeguarding Human Rights. Moreover, they will make it their business to propose and advocate new health codes where they see the need for them.

DISCOVERY AND DISSEMINATION OF KNOWLEDGE

Knowledge can be used to show what war does to people. In October 2006, *The Lancet* published an article on mortality figures during the three-year war of the US and UK against Iraq (Burnham et al. 2006). This peer-reviewed study used the best available epidemiological methods and produced an estimate of 655,000 excess deaths in this period. Most were by direct violence, and most of those were by gunshot. About 85,000 deaths were from air strikes, and only the invading forces were capable of air strikes.

These figures were of great significance to politicians either defending or criticizing the war, and to citizens taking a moral position on the war. It is common knowledge that truth is distorted in war. Governments need to find pretexts for attacking other states, in order to maintain the morale of soldiers and public support of a situation in which citizens' lives are being lost and public treasure is being spent in huge amounts. Telling the truth about the health effects of war can be a powerful intervention discrediting its supposed benefits. So powerful is it, in fact, that heavy resistance to such efforts can be expected. In the case of the Iraq mortality study, the president of the United States chose to question the methodology of the study, with no stated basis for doing so. Clearly, disseminating this knowledge had struck a nerve.

Knowledge counters lies and propaganda. It also counters official "forgetting." Where marginalized communities are attacked, there are sometimes official attempts to obscure or deny what has happened. The keeping of records or evidence may be important in eventually reaching a state of reconciliation after atrocities have been perpetrated. The work of forensic pathologists is not usually regarded as PtH work, but it has its place in the recording of truth about atrocities. The Documentation Center of Cambodia has attempted to perform such a function, intending eventually to contribute this knowledge to a reconciliation process based on acknowledgment of what really happened in that genocide.[2] Discovering crucial facts about an ongoing violent conflict may be difficult, especially if one of the belligerents has control over access to information, which is more and more likely in modern war. The special access of international health actors, such as Médecins sans Frontières (as in Chechnya and many other places) or of local health professionals' groups (such as Medipaz, the Nicaraguan affiliate of IPPNW) may provide unique knowledge, not otherwise obtainable, about the health impact of war.

Knowledge may lead to action. Beginning with the International Red Cross/Red Crescent (ICRC) in the 1980s, knowledge of the impact of landmines was disseminated by an increasing number of nongovernmental organizations. Much of this was epidemiological knowledge (see Chapter 15), but knowledge of another kind was conveyed in images of child amputees. It is not possible to weigh accurately the importance of various elements in the campaign to ban landmines, but both statistical data and "emotional knowledge" of the impact of landmines on victims played a part in its success. The Mine Ban Treaty was achieved in Ottawa in 1996.

Knowledge is globalized, as is the moral response to it. Anyone, anywhere with access to modern news services, and particularly to the Internet, can know what is happening in other parts of the world. People react with compassion to the suffering of others. Those with a sense of empowerment may feel impelled to act on that knowledge, even if the site of the suffering is half a planet away. There is, for example, a global response to the suffering of people in Darfur, Sudan, with much pressure on governments by citizens who insist on trying to mitigate a genocide.

We can become habituated to knowledge of horrifying impacts on human health if we are forced to live with such knowledge for long periods. This has been the case with our desensitization, over six decades, to the appalling potential of nuclear weapons to cause massive human death and destruction. The presence of these devices fades from the consciousness of most people, most of the time, just as the threat posted by an active volcano slips out of the minds of those who live on its slopes and have nowhere else to go. The thankless task of keeping this knowledge alive falls to a few who cannot forget it and need to keep reminding the rest of us. The health sector plays a prominent part in accomplishing this task.

REBUILDING THE FABRIC OF SOCIETY

War, when the direct violence has ended, leaves a society with depleted "social capital." Groups' attitudes toward other groups have hardened; trust is at a low ebb. The society may have physically rearranged itself into more ethnicized ghettoes. Most people are much worse off financially than before. The society is at risk for the recurrence of violence.

A great deal needs to be done in resolving the original grievances that gave rise to the violence, in reconstruction of all that was damaged, and in reconciliation of the groups between whom violence occurred. The health system needs to be built or rebuilt. This can be done in divisive ways or in ways that connect people and strengthen the social fabric. The latter approach involves bringing groups together to plan the health system, forming multiethnic teams for this task and for subsequent health delivery, making care equally accessible to all, and respecting the cultural needs of all groups in the design of health care and its facilities. These considerations can make such decisions as the siting of clinics a matter of great delicacy. The Peace-Health Filter deals with this dimension in some detail (See also "Healing Across the Divides: American Medical Peacebuilding" in Chapter 13).

After violence ended in Bosnia-Herzegovina in 1995, the health system needed reconstruction. WHO and the British Department for International Development applied such principles in developing the health system. On the basis of qualitative evidence, they claimed that this reduced ethnic antipathy (WHO/DFID 1999). Such a reconstructed health system signals to people that the government cares about their well-being and strengthens civic identity. It encourages displaced people to return home. Postwar governments that invest early in health care may be less likely to revert to political violence (Collier et al. 2006, 87).

SOLIDARITY AND SUPPORT

In some situations of conflict, a health team may take great care not to align itself with any "side," but, rather, to carefully clarify that it serves the needs of all. If it is working on superordinate health goals, it may attempt to do this by bringing the several "sides" together for this purpose, again taking great care to be seen as nonaligned. However, there are other situations in which the power imbalance between the "sides" is so great that the voice of one side is scarcely heard while it suffers large-scale injustices and human rights abuses. These injustices may include deficits in health care. In such a situation, a health team may deliberately act in solidarity with the oppressed group, attending to its health deficits and making its plight known to the oppressor and to the world at large.

Physicians for Human Rights–Israel[3] is such a group, acting on behalf of Palestinian rights to health care. It provides some of the missing care itself but, in particular, agitates authorities when there is severe denial of health care by the state of Israel. It defends the rights of any person to health care; most of its attention goes to the serious difficulties of Palestinians. Many societies with aboriginal populations are not at peace with those populations. Structural and cultural violence persists—and, in some cases, severe direct violence. There is in these cases a marked power imbalance in the conflict, sometimes so severe that the issues remain hidden. Health professionals may act in solidarity with such groups, extending health care, mediating with authorities, and exposing injustices. In acting in this mode, they throw a spotlight on the conflict and its impact on people, increasing social awareness. These are necessary steps toward just resolution of the conflict, and they are part of the spectrum of peacework. Some solidarity groups also offer education in nonviolent ways to address the conflict.

SOCIAL HEALING

The treatment of injuries and illnesses in war must obviously be carried out both at an individual and a public health level. The same might be said for biologically based mental illness, including that resulting from head injury. The increase in psychological illness resulting from the stress of war presents a more controversial problem. Anxiety, depression, and posttraumatic stress disorder (PTSD) are examples of such problems that commonly afflict adults and children. Arguments are made against individualized treatment for such problems (which may be severe and disabling) on the basis of inadequate resources in the face of the huge numbers of people affected, the stigma attached in many societies to having a psychiatric diagnosis, and the greater importance attached to, and greater availability of, social support in some societies (see "A Model for Improving Mental Health in Palestine—An Alternative View on Peace and Health?" in Chapter 17).

For such reasons, some programs to address mental health of war-affected children, in particular, have been designed for group delivery. In Croatia (Woodside et al. 1999) and Afghanistan these programs are delivered as part of the school curriculum. In Sri Lanka, the healing is delivered through play and creative arts (see "Butterfly Peace Garden—Healing War-Affected Children in Sri Lanka" in Chapter 18). In all cases, the program is intended to be delivered to groups of children that include several ethnicities previously hostile to each other. The content of the program deals with problems beyond those suffered by children individually, and it extends to helping children cope with diversity, especially ethnic differences. Children learn nonviolent conflict resolution, concepts of human rights, reconciliation, and a vision of a peaceful society. These are elements of social healing, the components of a culture of peace.

In Afghanistan, when these elements were delivered to adults and included conflict analysis to help people understand the chaos they experienced, they asked for this educational material to be taken to higher levels of decision-makers. The peace process aspects of the material were then brought to many political players, some currently in the cabinet at the time of writing.

Evaluation revealed that the Croatian program achieved modest success in reducing children's ethnic antipathy (see "Peace Education as Primary Prevention" in Chapter 16). Work with adults in the former Yugoslavia is described in "Psychosocial Healing" in Chapter 18.

EVOCATION AND EXTENSION OF ALTRUISM

Health care, in its purest sense, is an expression of altruism—caring for others, sometimes at expense to oneself. The ethical obligations of health workers demand impartiality in providing health care to all who need it, irrespective of the many categories that divide humans. In a war zone, the salient category is the side of the conflict the patient is on. An ethical physician may not discriminate on this basis. Such altruism extends over a broad circle, including all who need and have access to services.

This impartiality flies in the face of the tendency to polarize factions during war into "them" and "us." This is accompanied by the universal human tendency to regard one's own side as fundamentally good and well-intentioned and the other side as bad, with evil intentions. This polarization easily descends into dehumanization, in which the "other" is expelled beyond the boundaries of moral consideration and stripped of human dignity. This makes it easier to kill and injure the "other" and to torture and commit atrocities. The health professional's impartial care for all who are suffering undercuts this malignant tendency. Further, the health professional confronts human suffering, whose dimensions are the same across divisions of politics, soldier or civilian status, and every other basis of categorization; the patient is rehumanized. Health care affirms the value that all humans are equally worthy.

These principles are expressed in medical organizations that operate in war zones, such as Médecins sans Frontières; in organizations that care for those injured in war and prisoners of war, such as the Red Cross/ Red Crescent; and in organizations involved in postwar reconstruction of health systems, such as WHO. They are institutionalized in treaties recognizing the essential humanity of all involved in war, no matter what "side" they are on, such as the Geneva Conventions and their additional protocols, initiated by the Red Cross.

Such principles may be threatened by ruling authorities, as in Nepal in 2005, when health professionals were ordered not to treat members of the armed insurgency challenging the government. Dissent from such commands on the basis of medical ethics and human rights enables the health professional to depoliticize the situation and to reaffirm extended altruism.

The Medical Action Group was a group of Filipino health professionals acting in solidarity with internally displaced communities during a communist insurgency in the 1990s. The people they served had fled to remote places in the mountains and lacked health services. Doctors, dentists, and children's workers hiked into the mountains on a regular basis to serve them. The communities were harassed by the state armed forces from time to time. The Medical Action Group had a consultation on whether, if confronted with the need, they would treat a member of the armed forces. They concluded that they must do so, despite their orientation of solidarity with the displaced people. At the same time, in their interactions with the military as they traversed the country, they hoped to arouse their altruism by humanizing the supposed enemy.

LIMITING THE DESTRUCTIVENESS OF WAR

There is a long history of attempting to restrict war by banning abhorrent weapons. The second Lateran Council of 1139 outlawed the crossbow for use against Christians (the narrowly limited altruism will be evident to readers) (Wikipedia 2006). When proposals to ban particular weapons or tactics are based on health effects or promoted by health professionals, it is reasonable to consider them as PtH initiatives. Measures against nuclear weapons, landmines, cluster bombs, napalm, phosphorus, and/or poison gas on the basis of their horrific health effects belong in this category. So do measures against food and crop destruction, deliberate starvation, physical and mental torture, destruction of health facilities, and destruction of water treatment facilities.

The International Committee of the Red Cross, in particular, has a long history of institutionalizing some of these proscriptions in the Geneva Conventions. Others—nuclear weapons, landmines, and chemical and biological agents of war—have been the subject of separate treaties. More such treaties are needed—for example, agreements covering water-treatment facilities, which were deliberately targeted by the United States in Iraq (MacQueen et al. 2004). The Red Cross has conducted research and developed criteria for a medically based definition of "superfluous injury or unnecessary suffering." Use of these criteria can lead to banning the development of some weapons—for example, blinding lasers.

There is a risk in efforts to limit the destructiveness of war. Some interpret legal restrictions on war as implying that war is a civilized, professional institution directed against only military targets, though occasionally and accidentally damaging civilians and their infrastructure—a matter of "collateral damage" to be regretted. That this is very far indeed from the truth is known to anyone who follows actual wars even superficially. Yet, at their best, such restrictions can be seen as one possible means of drawing attention to the atrocities of war and eradicating some of them.

CONCLUSION

Health workers can be creative in making use of whatever mechanisms are available to them to lessen human suffering from war. We have listed those approaches we have become aware of, from our own work and that of others, in the hope of increasing the repertoire of those who share the conviction that this is avoidable suffering, to be treated just as other massive public health problems are—through prevention.

REFERENCES

Axelrod, Robert. 1984. *The evolution of cooperation.* New York: Basic Books.

Burnham, G., S. Doocy, R. Lafta, and L. Roberts. 2006. Mortality after the 2003 invasion of Iraq: A cross-sectional cluster sample survey. *The Lancet* 368:1421–28.

Collier, P., V. L. Elliott, H. Hegre, A. Hoeffler, M. Reynal-Querol, and N. Sambanis. 2006. *Breaking the conflict trap: Civil war and development policy.* Copublication of the World Bank and Oxford University Press: 87.

Curle, Adam. 1971. *Making peace.* London: Tavistock Publications.

Documentation Center of Cambodia. www.dccam.org

Galtung, Johan. 2000. *Conflict transformation by peaceful means.* United Nations Disaster Management Training Program.

Hay, Robin. 1990. *Humanitarian ceasefires: An examination of their potential contribution to the resolution of conflict.* Ottawa: Canadian Institute for International Peace and Security. Working Paper 28.

Lederach, John Paul, and Michelle Maiese. 2003. *Conflict transformation.* Available online at the www.beyondintractability.org website.

Lown, Bernard, and John Pastore. 1985. A medical prescription for survival. *The Lancet* 2 (8467): 1285–87.

MacQueen, G., R. McCutcheon, and J. Santa Barbara. 1997. The use of health initiatives as peace initiatives. *Peace and Change* 22 (2): 175–97.

MacQueen G., T. Nagy, J. Santa Barbara, C. Raichle. 2004. "Iraq water treatment vulnerabilities": A challenge to public health ethics. *Medicine, Conflict and Survival* 20 (2): 109–19.

Medact. November 2002. *Collateral damage: The health and environmental costs of war on Iraq.* London. Available online at the www.ippnw.org website.

Peters, Mary Anne, ed. 1996. *A health-to-peace handbook: Ideas and experiences of how health initiatives can work for peace.* Hamilton, Ontario, Canada: McMaster University. Available online at www.jha.ac/Ref/r005.htm

Rapoport, Anatol, ed. 1968. *Carl Von Clausewitz: On war.* London: Penguin Books.

Rodriguez-Garcia, Rosalia, James Macinko, F. Xavier Solorzano, and Marita Schlesser. 2001. *How can health serve as a bridge for peace?* Washington, DC: The George Washington Center for International Health.

Schroeder, H. J. 1937. *Disciplinary decrees of the General Council: Text, translation and commentary.* St. Louis: B. Herder. Available online at the Internet Medieval Resource Book. Available online at www.fordham.edu/halsall/basis/lateran2.html

Sherif, Muzafer, O. J. Harvey, B. J. White, W. R. Hood, and C. W. Sherif. 1961. *Intergroup conflict and cooperation: The Robbers Cave experiment.* Norman, OK: University Book Exchange.

WHO/DFID Peace through health programme. Copenhagen: WHO, 1999.

Wikipedia 2006. Second Council of the Lateran.

Woodside, D., J. Santa Barbara, and D. G. Benner. 1999. Psychological trauma and social healing in Croatia. *Medicine, Conflict and Survival* 15:355–67.

NOTES

1. The Battle of the Somme, July to November 1916, was one of the largest battles of World War I, pitting British and French forces against Germans. Intended to be a decisive breakthrough, instead it became a byword for indiscriminate slaughter, resulting in 1,265,000 deaths on all sides.

2. Documentation Center of Cambodia, www.dccam.org

3. Physicians for Human Rights–Israel, www.phr.org.il

PART II

War and Its Impact on Human Health

5

The Health Effects of War

Victor W. Sidel and *Barry S. Levy*

War has an enormous and tragic impact—both directly and indirectly—on health. War causes death and disability; destroys families, communities, and the environment; diverts resources; destroys infrastructure that supports human health; violates human rights; and begets further violence (Levy and Sidel 2008).

An estimated 200 million people died directly or indirectly as a result of wars during the twentieth century (Rummel 1994). Through the early part of the century, up to the start of World War II, the preponderance of deaths during war occurred among uniformed combatants, usually members of national armed forces. Although many noncombatants suffered social, economic, environmental, and health consequences of war and may have been the victims of what is now termed the collateral damage of military operations, noncombatants were generally not directly targeted and were largely spared death and disability directly resulting from war.

World War II brought a dramatic weakening of constraints on targeting of, and "collateral damage" to, civilians and noncombatants. In recent wars, the definition and identification of "civilians" and "noncombatants" have become increasingly difficult. The percentage of all deaths directly caused by war that are deaths of people who are unarmed, are not in uniform, and are generally considered noncombatants or civilians is increasing. Since 1937, when Nazi forces bombed the city of Guernica in the Basque region of Spain, military operations have increasingly killed and maimed civilians through purposeful targeting and "carpet bombing"[1] and through the collateral damage of heavy attacks on military targets. It is estimated that during World War I between 10 and 20 percent of all direct war-related deaths were civilian deaths; during World War II, the percentage of war-related deaths that were civilian deaths rose considerably. During wars near the end of the twentieth century and the beginning of the twenty-first century, the percent of direct and indirect war-related deaths among civilians increased further.

Many of the civilians who died were innocent bystanders, caught in the crossfire of opposing armies or killed by the chaos, starvation, and disease that accompany war; others were civilians who were specifically targeted during wars. Today, armed conflicts largely consist of civil wars (conflicts within countries, to which other countries sometimes contribute military troops) that continue to rage in many parts of the world. During the post–Cold War period of 1990–2001, there were fifty-seven major armed conflicts in forty-five locations—all but three of which were civil wars (World Health Organization 2002). The Stockholm International Peace Research Institute (SIPRI) publishes an annual yearbook that documents military conflict around the world. The 2006 edition provides the location of seventeen major armed conflicts during 2005 (Stockholm International Peace Research Institute 2006); see Table 5.1.

Data on deaths related to war are largely unknowable because of the problem of defining the relationship of death to war, generally poor recordkeeping in many countries, and the failure of recordkeeping in times of war (Zwi, Ugalde, and Richards 1999). More than 3.8 million people have died during the civil war in Congo, a catastrophic impact that might not have been recognized were it not for epidemiologic investigations (Roberts et al. 2001). Over thirty years of civil war in Ethiopia have led to the deaths of a million people (Kloos 1992).

Many people survive wars, only to be physically scarred for life. Millions of survivors are chronically disabled from injuries sustained during wars or the immediate aftermath of wars. "Improvised explosive devices,"

Table 5.1 Location of the Seventeen Major Armed Conflicts in 2005

Africa	Americas	Asia
Burundi	Colombia	Afghanistan
Sudan	Peru	India (Kashmir)
Uganda	United States*	Myanmar
		Nepal
Europe	**Middle East**	Philippines†
Russia	Iraq	Sri Lanka
(Chechnya)	Israel	
	Turkey	

Notes: *This refers to conflict between al-Qaeda and the United States and its coalition partners.
†There were two conflicts in the Philippines.

such as those used in Iraq, and antipersonnel landmines are a particular threat. For example, in Cambodia, one in 236 people is an amputee as a result of a landmine (Stover et al. 1994). More than one-third of the soldiers who survived the civil war in Ethiopia were injured or disabled, and at least 40,000 individuals lost one or more limbs during the war (Kloos 1992).

Another major impact of war is the creation of many refugees and internally displaced persons, whose basic human needs may not be met. A substantial number of the more than 12 million refugees and approximately 20 million internally displaced persons in the world today have been uprooted from their homes as a result of war or the threat of war (Hampton 1998; Reed, Haaga, and Keely 1998; Toole 2000). An important example is the situation in Darfur, a western province of Sudan, Africa's largest country, where violent conflict began in 2003. More than 2 million people have fled their homes, and about 200,000 refugees have crossed the border into Chad (Refugees International 2007).

Wars often have an especially devastating impact on women (Ashford and Huet-Vaughn 2008), children (Santa Barbara 2008), and other vulnerable populations. Wars also destroy the health-supporting infrastructure on which people, particularly vulnerable people, depend, thus increasing the health disparities in a society (Levy and Sidel 2006).

Since September 11, 2001, there has been increasing concern in the United States and other countries about violence inflicted by individuals and groups to create fear and advance a political agenda. These individuals or groups are commonly called terrorists, although some who believe such actions justifiable under certain circumstances refer to those who commit them in more positive terms, such as freedom fighters. Others believe that actions of nation-states designed to target civilians and create fear should be termed state terrorism (Levy and Sidel 2007).

A classified assessment by US intelligence agencies found evidence that the threat of individual and group terrorism has grown since the attacks of September 11, 2001 (Mazzetti 2006). This threat has grown despite what has been termed the "war on terror," and particularly since the US invasion and occupation of Iraq. We believe there should be greater public discussion of the nature and causes of individual and group terrorism and of state terrorism. There should also be a balanced approach to strengthening systems and protecting people in response to the threat of terrorism—an approach that strengthens a broad range of public health capacities and preserves civil liberties (Levy and Sidel 2007).

WEAPONS OF INDISCRIMINATE MASS DESTRUCTION

The term *weapons of mass destruction* (WMD) is generally used to refer to nuclear, chemical, and biological weapons. However, many analysts believe that the inclusion of chemical and biological weapons within the term has been used by the United States and other nuclear-weapons states to draw attention away from the especially devastating effects of nuclear weapons and to justify their use against nations (Weapons of Mass Destruction Commission 2006). Radiologic weapons ("dirty bombs"), antipersonnel landmines, and massive bombing using conventional explosives and incendiaries can also be indiscriminately and extensively destructive.

Nuclear Weapons

The nuclear weapons used by the United States to bomb Hiroshima and Nagasaki in 1945 were based on nuclear fission and had an explosive force equivalent to about 15,000 tons (15 kilotons) of TNT. During the 1950s the United States and the Soviet Union developed thermonuclear weapons, commonly called hydrogen bombs, that were based on nuclear fusion; these bombs had an explosive force equivalent to as much as 20 million tons (20 megatons) of TNT, 1000-fold greater than the force of the nuclear weapons used in 1945 (Rhodes 1995). Physicians in Boston published a series of articles in the *New England Journal of Medicine* on the medical consequences of the use of these new weapons on cities and concluded that there would be little health workers could do to meet the needs of the victims if these weapons were used (Ervin et al. 1962; Nathan et al. 1962; Sidel, Geiger, and Lown 1962). This work led to the formation of Physicians for Social Responsibility (PSR) in the United States in 1961 and, 20 years later, to the formation of International Physicians for the Prevention of Nuclear War (IPPNW) (Forrow and Sidel 1998).

There are approximately 27,000 nuclear warheads in at least eight nations—the United States, Russia, the United Kingdom, France, China, Israel, India, and Pakistan—and it is possible that some have been stockpiled in North Korea. Iran is using a nuclear power reactor to prepare fissile material that might be usable in the production of a nuclear weapon; the United States and other nuclear-weapons states are exploring ways to halt this development (Hirsch 2006; Physicians for Social Responsibility 2006). The weapons summarized in Table 5.2 have an aggregate explosive force of over 200,000 Hiroshima-sized bombs, a

Table 5.2 Approximate Size of Nuclear Arsenals

	Strategic	Total
United States	5,235	10,000
Russia	3,500	16,000
France	288	350
China	20	200
United Kingdom	200	200
Israel	N/A	100
India	N/A	70–110
Pakistan	N/A	50–110
North Korea	N/A	<10

Source: Sutton and Gould 2008, p. 169.

force equivalent to that of 11 billion tons of TNT, almost 2 tons for every human on the planet.

The historic high in explosive capacity of nuclear-weapons stockpiles worldwide was reached in 1960, with an explosive capacity equivalent to 20 billion tons (20,000 megatons) of TNT, the force of 1.4 million Hiroshima-sized bombs. In the United States, the number of nuclear weapons had reached approximately 32,000 by 1967, with nuclear warheads of thirty different types. By 2003, US nuclear weapons had been reduced to about 10,400, equivalent to about 2000 megatons of TNT. Other warheads had been dismantled or were being held in reserve. Approximately 2000 to 3000 nuclear warheads, mounted on missiles in the United States, Russia, and possibly other countries, are still on hair-trigger alert, ready to be launched on a few moments' notice.

The detonation of nuclear bombs over Hiroshima and Nagasaki in August 1945 at the end of World War II led to the immediate deaths of approximately 200,000 people (primarily civilians), the lasting injury and later death of many others, massive devastation of buildings and facilities, and widespread radioactive contamination of the environment in these two cities (Sutton and Gould 2008). The use of nuclear weapons by the United States that was threatened in the 2002 U.S. Nuclear Posture Review included their possible use under a wider range of circumstances. In addition to the threat of "state terrorism"—the use of nuclear weapons by nation-states—there appears to be a possible threat of the use of nuclear weapons by individuals and groups.

Production of nuclear weapons has led to major environmental contamination. For example, the area around Chelyabinsk in Russia has been heavily contaminated with radioactive materials from the nuclear-weapons production facility in that area. The level of ambient radiation in and near the Techa River in the area has been documented to be as high as twenty-eight times the normal background radiation level. As another example, leakage of radioactive materials from storage of wastes from nuclear-weapons production at Hanford, along the Columbia River in Washington State, has led to extensive radioactive contamination (Levy and Sidel 2005).

Open-air testing of nuclear weapons by the United States, the Soviet Union, and other countries has led to environmental contamination, with increased rates of leukemia and other cancers among populations who were downwind from these tests. The effects on children of exposure to iodine-131, a radioactive isotope of iodine produced by the tests, have been documented by the National Cancer Institute (2006).

The dismantling and disposal of nuclear weapons has also led to environmental contamination. The primary site for the disassembly of US nuclear weapons is the Pantex Plant, located seventeen miles northeast of Amarillo in the Texas panhandle. The United States has dismantled about 60,000 nuclear warheads since the 1940s; during the 1990s, over 11,000 warheads were dismantled. Plutonium from these weapons represents a long-term hazard. Plutonium, an element first produced by the Manhattan Project in 1942, has a half-life[2] of 24,000 years. More than 12,000 plutonium pits (hollow shells of plutonium, encased in steel or other metal, that are essential components of some nuclear weapons) are stored in containers at Pantex.

Production of as many as 80 new pits annually is planned at the Los Alamos National Laboratory, and the Bush administration advocates building a modern pit facility capable of producing 250 to 900 pits annually by 2018. The administration's 2002 Nuclear Posture Review proclaims a continuing role for nuclear weapons into the future. It lists five nation-states as potential targets of US nuclear weapons: Iraq, Iran, North Korea, Libya, and Syria. In addition, Russia and China remain potential nuclear-weapons targets. The Nuclear Posture Review reshapes the US nuclear-weapons arsenal from one intended mainly for deterrence to one that may be used for fighting a nuclear war, and the distinction between nuclear and non-nuclear missions and weapons has become blurred (Gordon 2002; Nuclear Posture Review Report 2002; Sidel et al. 2003). Attempts to halt nuclear-weapons production and to abolish nuclear weapons, although mandated by the International Court of Justice in 1996, have been largely ineffective (Forrow, Mutalik, and Christ 1995; Forrow and Sidel 1998).

Radiologic Weapons

"Dirty bombs," which are conventional explosive devices mixed with radioactive material, and attacks on nuclear power plants with explosive weapons could scatter highly radioactive materials widely (Sutton and Gould 2006). Radiation released by these explosives could have serious immediate effects on people exposed to it and long-lasting impacts on populations and on the environment if long-lived radioisotopes were released.

Chemical Weapons

Although nations that signed the 1899 Hague Declaration promised not to use chemical weapons, during World War I these weapons—including tear gas, chlorine gas, phosgene, and mustard gas—were employed. During World War I, 125,000 tons of chemical weapons were used, resulting in 1.3 million casualties. One-fourth of all casualties in the American Expeditionary Force in France were caused by such weapons (Harris and Paxman 1982; Sidel and Goldwyn 1966).

In 1925, twenty-eight nations negotiated the Geneva Protocol for the "prohibition of the use in war of asphyxiating poisonous or other gases and of all analogous liquids, materials or devices and of bacteriological methods of warfare." But the Protocol prohibited only the use of these weapons, not their development, production, testing, or stockpiling. Furthermore, many of the nations ratifying the Protocol reserved the right to use such weapons in retaliation, and the Protocol became, in effect, a "no first use" treaty with no verification or enforcement provisions. The United States was one of the initial signatories, but the US Senate did not ratify the treaty until 1975.

Despite the Protocol, use of chemical weapons continued. Italy used mustard gas during its invasion of Abyssinia (Ethiopia), and Japan used mustard and tear gases in its invasion of China. Germany developed acetylcholinesterase inhibitors to be used as nerve agents. The United States and Britain stockpiled chemical weapons during World War II; transportation and storage accidents caused deaths, but there was no direct military use. Following World War II, chemical weapons were used by Egypt in Yemen; mustard and nerve gases were used in the Iran–Iraq War; and Iraq used chemical weapons against Kurdish villages in its own territory. Chemical-weapons stockpiles and production facilities in Iraq were ordered destroyed by the United Nations following the 1991 Persian Gulf War. The United States and Russia are known to maintain chemical-weapons stockpiles, and several other countries have either stockpiles or facilities for rapid chemical-weapons production (Lockwood 2000).

During the Vietnam War, the United States military used herbicides on mangrove forests and other vegetation, which not only defoliated and killed trees and other plants but also caused birth defects and malignancies (Allukian and Atwood 2008). In addition, the development and production of conventional weapons involve the use of many chemicals that are toxic and can contaminate the environment. Furthermore, there is now a plausible threat of nonstate agents using chemical weapons. A Japanese cult, Aum Shinrikyo, used sarin in the subway system of two Japanese cities in the mid-1990s, accounting for the death of nineteen people and injuries to thousands (Lifton 1999).

Troops can be protected against these weapons for limited periods by the use of gas masks and impenetrable garments. Such protective gear, however, reduces the efficiency of troops by as much as 50 percent and damages morale, so the use or threat of chemical weapons may continue to be considered effective against troops. Civilian populations, on the other hand, cannot be adequately protected. Israel, for example, provides every civilian in the country with a gas mask and a self-injectable syringe filled with atropine, a temporary antidote to nerve gas. But this limited protection is inadequate against weapons such as mustard gas that attack the skin or against longer-term exposure to nerve gas. Furthermore, poorly trained civilians are likely to injure themselves with equipment such as self-injectable syringes.

Production of chemical weapons has been associated with serious accidents to workers and with high levels of pollution in the production sites and nearby communities. The potential for exposure exists not only for military and civilian populations who may be exposed during the use of chemical weapons in wartime, but also for workers involved in the development, production, transport, and storage of these weapons and for people living near facilities where these weapons are developed, produced, transported, and stored. Disposal of these weapons, including their disassembly and incineration, can be hazardous. Even destruction of the weapons is dangerous, since toxic ash is produced by their incineration (Levy and Sidel 2005).

The Chemical Weapons Convention (CWC), which took effect in 1997, prohibits all development, production, acquisition, stockpiling, transfer, and use of chemical weapons. It requires each state party to destroy its chemical weapons, its chemical-weapons production facilities, and any chemical weapons it may have abandoned on the territory of another state party. The verification provisions of the CWC affect not only the military sector, but also the civilian chemical industry worldwide through certain restrictions and obligations regarding the production, processing, and consumption of chemicals that are considered relevant to the objectives of the convention. These provisions are to be verified through a combination of reporting requirements, routine on-site inspection of declared sites, and short-notice challenge inspections. The Organization for the Prohibition of Chemical Weapons (OPCW) in The Hague, established by the CWC, ensures implementation of the provisions of the CWC. The disposal of chemical weapons required by the CWC has raised controversy about the safety of two different methods of disposal: incineration and chemical neutralization. The controversy about safety and protection of the environment has delayed completion of the disposal beyond the date required by the CWC (Levy and Sidel 2005).

Biological Weapons

Biological weapons depend on the ability of microorganisms to infect and multiply in the attacked organism. These weapons are very hard to defend against and are not as controllable or predictable in their use as are chemical weapons (Sidel and Goldwyn 1966).

Use of biological warfare dates at least to the sixth century BC when Persia, Greece, and Rome used diseased corpses to try to contaminate sources of drinking water. In 1346, Mongols besieging the Crimean seaport of Kaffa placed cadavers on hurling machines and threw them into Kaffa. In 1710, Russian troops used cadavers of plague victims to start an epidemic among enemy Swedes. During the French and Indian War in the mid-1700s, British commander Sir Jeffrey Amherst sent smallpox-infected blankets to Native Americans. During the US Civil War, dead animals were left in wells and ponds to deny fresh water to retreating troops (Metcalfe 2002).

During World War I, Germany is alleged to have used the equine disease glanders[3] against the cavalries of Eastern European countries. During World War II, according to testimony at the Nuremberg trials, prisoners in German concentration camps were infected during tests of biological weapons. Great Britain and the United States, fearing the Germans would use biological weapons in World War II, developed their own. Gruinard Island, off the coast of Scotland, was contaminated during a test use of anthrax spores by the United Kingdom and the United States; the island remained uninhabitable for decades. The United States developed anthrax spores, botulinum toxin, and other agents as biological weapons but did not use them (Guillemin 2005).

In the 1930s, Japanese troops dropped from planes rice and wheat mixed with plague-carrying fleas, resulting in plague in areas of China that had been previously free of it. During World War II, Japanese laboratories conducted extensive experiments on prisoners of war using a wide variety of organisms selected for possible use as biological weapons, including the agents that cause anthrax, plague, gas gangrene, encephalitis, typhus, typhoid, hemorrhagic fever, cholera, smallpox, and tularemia (Wright and Kelcham 1990). Unlike the Soviet Union, which in 1949 prosecuted twelve people involved in this work, the United States never prosecuted any of the participants. Instead, US researchers met with Japanese biological-warfare experts in Tokyo and urged that the experts be "spared embarrassment" so the United States could benefit from their knowledge (Powell 1981).

Development of biological weapons continued after World War II. None of the numerous allegations of biological-weapons use has been confirmed or even fully investigated, but it is known that extensive biological weapons testing has been done. In the 1950s and 1960s, for example, the University of Utah conducted secret, large-scale field tests of biological weapons, including the agents that cause tularemia, Rocky Mountain spotted fever, plague, and Q fever, at the U.S. Army Dugway Proving Ground in western Utah. In 1950, US Navy ships released as simulants (materials believed to be nonpathogenic that mimic the spread of biological agents) large quantities of bacteria in the San Francisco Bay Area to test the efficiency of their dispersal. Some analysts attributed subsequent infections and deaths to one of these organisms, *Serratia marcescens* (Cole 1988). During the 1950s and 1960s, the United States conducted 239 top-secret, open-air disseminations of simulants, involving such areas as the New York City subways and Washington National Airport (Cole 1988). The US military developed a large infrastructure of laboratories, test facilities, and production plants related to biological weapons. By the end of the 1960s, the United States had stockpiles of at least ten different biological and toxin weapons (Geissler 1986). In 1979, the accidental release of anthrax spores near Sverdlovsk in the Soviet Union resulted in at least seventy-seven cases of inhalation anthrax and at least sixty-six deaths (Guillemin 2001).

In 1969 the Nixon administration—with the concurrence of the Defense Department, which declared that biological weapons lacked "military usefulness"—unconditionally renounced US development, production, stockpiling, and use of biological weapons and announced that the United States would unilaterally dismantle its biological-weapons program. In 1972 the Soviet Union, which had urged a more comprehensive treaty including restrictions on chemical weapons, ended its opposition to a separate biological-weapons treaty. The United States, the Soviet Union, and other nations negotiated the Convention on the Prohibition of the Development, Prevention and Stockpiling of Bacteriological (Biological) and Toxin Weapons and on Their Destruction (BWC). The BWC prohibits— except for "prophylactic, protective and other peaceful purposes"—the development or acquisition of biological agents or toxins, as well as weapons carrying them and means of their production, stockpiling, transfer, or delivery. The US Senate ratified the BWC in 1975, the same year it ratified the Geneva Protocol of 1925 (Falk 1990; Wright and Ketcham 1990). As of February 2008, 158 nations had ratified the BWC, and an additional 16 nations had signed but not yet ratified it.

Invoking the specter of possible new biological weapons and unproven allegations of aggressive biological-weapons programs in other countries, the Reagan administration initiated intensive efforts to conduct "defensive research" permitted under the BWC. The budget for the US Army Biological Defense Research Program (BDRP), which sponsors programs in a wide variety of academic, commercial, and government laboratories, increased dramatically during the 1980s. Much of this research work is medical in nature, including the development of immunizations and of treatments against organisms that might be used as biological weapons (King and Strauss 1990; Miller, Engelberg, and Broad 2001; Novick and Shulman 1990; Piller and Yamamoto 1988).

Although research and development of new biological weapons is outlawed by the BWC, it is possible that it will still occur (Alibek 1999). Novel dangers lie in new genetic technologies, which make possible the development of genetically altered organisms not known in nature. Stable, tailor-made organisms used as biological weapons could travel long distances and still be infectious, rapidly infiltrate a population, cause debilitating effects very quickly, and be resistant to antibiotic treatment (Piller and Yamamoto 1988, 1990).

Antipersonnel Landmines

There are now approximately 80 million antipersonnel landmines still deployed worldwide in at least 78 countries. These landmines have been termed "weapons of mass destruction, one person at a time." They have often been placed in rural areas, posing a threat to residents of these areas and often disrupting farming and other activities. Civilians are the most likely to fall victim to landmines, which continue to injure and kill 15,000 to 20,000 people annually. Since the entry into force of the Mine Ban Treaty in 1997, production of landmines has been markedly reduced, and many implanted landmines have been removed. Millions of mines are still buried, however, and additional resources will be required to continue unearthing and destroying them, tasks that pose inherent risks to demining personnel (Stover et al. 1994; Sirkin, Cobey, and Stover 2008).

CONVENTIONAL WEAPONS

Conventional weapons consist of explosives and incendiaries of various sizes, ranging from "small arms and light weapons" to heavy artillery and bombs. Conventional weapons have accounted for the overwhelming majority of deaths and of adverse environmental consequences due to war. During World War II, for example, extensive carpet bombing of cities in Europe and Japan accounted not only for many deaths and injuries but also for widespread devastation of urban environments. Use of conventional weapons indiscriminately can, in effect, turn them into weapons of mass destruction (Cukier and Sidel 2006).

Explosives

Explosives used in war range from the carpet bombing of cities during World II to improvised explosive devices (IEDs) used by insurgents in Iraq. One example is the US Guided Bomb Unit-28, a 5000-pound laser-guided "bunker buster," developed to penetrate hardened Iraqi command centers located deep underground. Explosive weapons include "cluster munitions," miniature explosives packed into a bomb, rocket, or artillery shell and designed to scatter over a wide area (No place for cluster bombs, 2006). US forces used cluster munitions in Iraq, Russia used them in Chechnya, and Israel used them in Lebanon. Militias, other groups, and individuals in Iraq and Afghanistan have used improvised explosive devices.

Incendiaries

Incendiary weapons used in the carpet bombing of cities during World War II (as in Dresden, Germany, and Tokyo, Japan) also constituted indiscriminate mass destruction. Incendiaries, like explosives, are relatively easy to obtain and use and are therefore often employed as weapons by individuals and groups.

Napalm, a form of jellied gasoline, was used extensively in Vietnam by US forces and has been used in other wars (Reich and Sidel 1967). It has been alleged that white phosphorus was used as a weapon, which is different from its use to light up a battlefield or a target, but this use is still being debated.

Small Arms and Light Weapons

Small arms and light weapons (SALW), which include pistols, rifles, machine guns, and other hand-held or easily transportable weapons, are the weapons most often used in wars (Cukier and Sidel 2006). Some restrictions have been imposed, such as the outlawing of the use of "dum-dum bullets," which cause extensive injuries when they strike a person, but few effective measures have been taken to outlaw the use of SALW in war.

DIVERSION OF RESOURCES

Governmental and societal preoccupation with war and preparation for war—often known as militarism—lead to massive diversion of resources needed to promote human health and welfare. The United States has spent, and continues to spend, billions of dollars on its nuclear arsenal (Schwartz 1998). Militarism is a problem in many countries but is especially serious in developing countries. Many developing countries have substantially higher military expenditures than health-related expenditures. For example, in 1990 Ethiopia spent $16 per capita for military expenditures and only $1 per capita for health, and Sudan spent $25 per capita for military expenditures and only $1 per capita for health (Foege 2000). A report in August 2005 estimated that the $204.4 billion initially appropriated for the Iraq War could have purchased *any* of the following desperately needed services in the United States: approximately 3.5 million elementary school teachers, 24,000 new elementary schools, 27 million Head Start places for children, 40 million scholarships for university students, 1.8 million affordable housing units, 3.2 million port container inspectors, or health-care services for the 46 million people in the United States who are uninsured. Internationally, these monies could have been used to do *all* of the following for almost three years: cut world hunger in half, launch a global comprehensive program to respond to HIV/AIDS, fully immunize all children in the developing world, and provide clean water and functioning sewage systems to respond to current unmet needs throughout the world (Bennis and Leaver 2005). By 2007, only two years later, more than twice as much money had been appropriated for the war in Iraq, and some economists estimate that the ultimate cost of the war will be more than $2 trillion—more than ten times as much money.

IMPACT ON THE ENVIRONMENT

War and other military activities also cause serious health consequences through their impact on the physical, economic, social, and biological environments in which people live. The environmental damage affects not only people in nations directly engaged in war, but people in all nations. Much of the morbidity and mortality during war, especially among civilians, results from devastation of societal infrastructure, including destruction of food and water supply systems, health-care facilities and public health services, sewage disposal systems, power plants and electrical grids, and transportation and communication systems. Destruction of infrastructure has led to food shortages and resultant malnutrition, contamination of food and drinking water and resultant food-borne and waterborne illness, and health-care and public health deficiencies and resultant disease.

Damage to the physical environment—water, land, air, and space—and use of nonrenewable resources may also result from preparation for war. Lakes, rivers, streams, aquifers, land masses, and the atmosphere may be polluted through the testing and use of weapons. Space may be contaminated through placement and use of weapons beyond Earth's atmosphere. Nonrenewable resources may be employed in weapons production, testing, and use (Levy and Sidel 2005).

The social environment may be affected by increasing militarism, by encouragement of violence as a means of settling disputes, and by infringement on civil rights and civil liberties. In addition, preparation for war, like war itself, can promote violence as a means for settling disputes. Militarism and military spending also have important impacts on national foreign and domestic policies, divert resources from health services and other human services, and encourage domestic and community violence.

PREVENTION

There are a number of roles that health workers can play in reducing the impact of collective violence and war on human health (Carnegie Commission 1997; Sidel and Levy 2008). Many are detailed in this book and in Chapter 26 ("Preventing War and Its Health Consequences: Roles of Public Health Professionals") in the second edition of *War and Public Health* (Levy and Sidel 2008). These roles include efforts in surveillance and documentation of the health effects of war and of the factors that may cause war; participation in education and awareness-raising programs to prevent or end war; advocacy of widespread use of these programs; and. direct engagement in effective actions to prevent and end war (Sidel and Levy 2008).

CONCLUSION

War is the most serious threat to public health. Health workers can do much to prevent war and its health consequences. As the World Health Assembly declared in 1981, "The role of health workers in promoting and preserving peace is the most significant factor for achieving health for all" (World Health Assembly 1985). Preventing war and its consequences should be in the curricula of schools of public health, on the agendas of public health organizations, and in the practice of public health professionals. Activities by health workers to prevent war and its health consequences are, in our view, essential parts of our professional obligations.

REFERENCES

Alibek, Ken. 1999. *Biohazard.* New York: Random House.

Allukian, Myron, Jr., and Paul Atwood. 2008. The Vietnam War. In Levy and Sidel 2008, 313–36.

Ashford, Mary-Wynne. 2008. The impact of war on women. In Levy and Sidel 2008, 179–206.

Bennis, P., and E. Leaver. 2005. IPS Iraq Task Force. The Iraq quagmire: The mounting costs of war and the case for bringing home the troops. Washington, DC: Institute for Policy Studies and Foreign Policy in Focus, August 31.

Carnegie Commission on Preventing Deadly Conflict. 1997. *Preventing deadly conflict: Final report.* New York: Carnegie Corporation.

Cole, Leonard. 1988. *Clouds of secrecy: The army's germ warfare tests over populated areas.* Totowa, NJ: Rowman and Littlefield.

Cukier, Wendy, and Victor W. Sidel. 2006. *The global gun epidemic: From Saturday night specials to AK47s.* Portsmouth, NH: Praeger Security International, 2006.

Ervin, Frank R., J. B. Glazier, S. Aronow, et al. 1962. The medical consequences of thermonuclear war. 1. Human and ecologic effects in Massachusetts of an assumed nuclear attack on the United States. *New England Journal of Medicine* 266:1127–36.

Falk, Richard. 1990. Inhibiting reliance on biological weaponry: The role and relevance of international law. In *Preventing a biological arms race,* ed. Susan Wright, 241–66. Cambridge, MA: MIT Press.

Foege, William. 2000. Arms and public health: A Global Perspective. In Levy and Sidel 2008, 3–11.

Forrow, Lachlan, Guraraj Mutalik, and Michael Christ, eds. 1995. *Abolition 2000: Handbook for a world without nuclear weapons*. Cambridge, MA: International Physicians for the Prevention of Nuclear War.

Forrow, Lachlan, and Victor W. Sidel. 1998. Medicine and nuclear war: From Hiroshima to mutual assured destruction to Abolition 2000. *JAMA* 280:456–61.

Geissler, Erhard. 1986. A new generation of vaccines against biological and toxin weapons. In *Biological and toxin weapons today*, ed. Erhard Geissler, 36–65. Oxford: Oxford University Press.

Gordon, M. R. 2002. U.S. nuclear plan sees new targets and new weapons. *New York Times*, March 10.

Guillemin, Jeanne. 2001. *Anthrax: The investigation of a deadly outbreak*. San Francisco: University of California Press.

———. 2005. *Biological weapons: From the invention of state-sponsored programs to contemporary bioterrorism*. New York: Columbia University Press.

Hampton, J., ed. 1998. *Internally displaced people: A global survey*. London: Earthscan, Norwegian Refugee Council and Global IDP Survey.

Harris, Robert, and Jeremy Paxman. 1982. *A higher form of killing: The secret story of chemical and biological warfare*. New York: Hill and Wang.

Hirsch, Seymour M. 2006. The Iran plans: Would President Bush go to war to stop Tehran from getting the bomb? *New Yorker*, April 8.

King, Jonathan, and Harlee Strauss. 1990. The hazards of defensive biological warfare research. In *Preventing a biological arms race*, ed. Susan Wright, 120–32. Cambridge, MA: MIT Press.

Kloos, H. 1992. Health impacts of war in Ethiopia. *Disasters* 16:347–54.

Last, John M. 2007. *A dictionary of public health*. New York. Oxford University Press.

Levy, Barry S., and Victor W. Sidel. 2005. War and other military activities. In *Environmental health: From local to global*, ed. Howard Frumkin, 269–97. San Francisco: Jossey-Bass.

———. 2006. *Social injustice and public health*. New York: Oxford University Press.

———. 2007. *Terrorism and public health: A balanced approach to strengthening systems and protecting people*. Updated paperback edition. New York: Oxford University Press.

———. 2008. *War and public health (second edition)*. New York: Oxford University Press.

Lifton, Robert Jay. 1999. *Destroying the world to save it*. New York: Henry Holt.

Lockwood, Alan H. 2000. The public health effects of the use of chemical weapons. In Levy and Sidel 2000a, 84–97.

Mazzetti, Mark. 2006. Spy agencies say Iraq war worsens terror threat. *New York Times*, September 24.

Metcalfe, N. 2002. A short history of biological warfare. *Medicine, Conflict and Survival* 18:271–82.

Miller, Judith, Stephen Engelberg, and William Broad. 2001. *Germs: Biological weapons and America's secret war*. New York: Simon & Schuster.

Nathan, David G., H. Jack Geiger, Victor W. Sidel, and Bernard Lown. 1962. The medical consequences of thermonuclear war: Introduction. *New England Journal of Medicine* 266:1126–7.

National Cancer Institute. 2006. Understanding the legacy of nuclear testing. *NCI Cancer Bulletin* 3 (2): 3.

No place for cluster bombs. 2006. Editorial. *New York Times,* August 26.

Novick, Richard, and Seth Shulman. 1990. New forms of biological warfare. In *Preventing a biological arms race,* ed. Susan Wright, 103–19. Cambridge, MA: MIT Press.

Nuclear Posture Review Report, submitted to Congress on December 31, 2001. Global Security.org, January 8, 2002. Available online at the www.globalsecurity.org website.

Physicians for Social Responsibility. 2006. *Medical consequences of an attack on Iran.* Washington, DC: Physicians for Social Responsibility. Available online at the www .psr.org website.

Piller, Charles, and Keith R. Yamamoto. 1988. *Gene wars: Military control over the new genetic technologies.* New York: Beech Tree Books.

———. 1990. The U.S. Biological Defense Research Program in the 1980s: A critique. In *Preventing a biological arms race,* ed. Susan Wright, 133–68. Cambridge, MA: MIT Press.

Powell, John W. 1981. A hidden chapter in history. *Bulletin of the Atomic Scientists* 37, no. 8:45–49.

Reed, H., J. Haaga, and C. Keely, eds. 1998. *The demography of forced migration: Summary of a workshop.* Washington, DC: National Academy Press.

Refugees International. 2007. The Crisis in Darfur. Available at the www.refugees international.org website.

Reich, Peter, and Victor W. Sidel. 1967. Napalm. *New England Journal of Medicine* 277:86–88.

Rhodes, Richard. 1995. *Dark sun: The making of the hydrogen bomb.* New York: Simon and Schuster.

Roberts, Lee, Charles Hale, Fathi Belyakdoumi et al. 2001. *Mortality in eastern democratic Republic of Congo: Results from eleven mortality surveys.* New York: International Rescue Committee.

Rummel, R. J. 1994. *Death by government: Genocide and mass murder since 1900.* New Brunswick, NJ, and London: Transaction Publications.

Santa Barbara, Joanna. 2008. The impact of war on children. In Levy and Sidel 2008, 179–92.

Schwartz, S. I. 1998. *Atomic audit: The costs and consequences of US nuclear weapons since 1940.* Washington, DC: Brookings Institution Press, 1998.

Sidel, Victor W., H. Jack Geiger, and Bernard Lown. 1962. The medical consequences of thermonuclear war. II. The physician's role in the post-attack period. *New England Journal of Medicine* 266:1137–45.

Sidel, Victor W. and Robert M. Goldwyn. 1966. Chemical and biologic weapons—a primer. *New England Journal of Medicine* 274:21–27.

Sidel, Victor W., H. Jack Geiger, Herbert L. Abrams, R. W. Nelson, and John Loretz. 2003. *The threat of low yield earth penetrating nuclear weapons to civilian populations: Nuclear "Bunker Busters" and their medical consequences.* Cambridge, MA: International Physicians for the Prevention of Nuclear War. Available online at the www.ippnw.org website.

Sidel, Victor W., and Barry S. Levy. 2008. Collective violence: Health impact and prevention. In Institute of Medicine (IOM). *Violence prevention in low- and middle-income countries: Finding a place on the global agenda.* Washington, DC: National Academies Press, pp. 171–99.

Sirkin, Susannah, James C. Cobey, and Eric Stover. Landmines. In Levy and Sidel 2008, 102–16.

Stockholm International Peace Research Institute. 2006. *SIPRI yearbook 2006: Armaments, disarmament and international security.* New York: Oxford University Press.

Stover, Eric, A. S. Keller, J. Cobey, and S. Sopheap. 1994. Letter from Phnom Penh: The medical and social consequences of land mines in Cambodia. *JAMA* 72:331–6.

Sutton, Patrice M., and Robert M. Gould. 2006. Nuclear, radiological and related weapons. In Levy and Sidel 2008, 220–42.

Sutton, Patrice M., and Robert M. Gould. 2008. In Levy and Sidel 2008, 152–76.

Toole, Michael J. 2008. Displaced persons and war. In Levy and Sidel 2008, 207–26.

Weapons of Mass Destruction Commission. 2006. Final report. *Weapons of terror: Freeing the world of nuclear, biological, and chemical arms.* Stockholm, Sweden, June 1.

World Health Assembly. 1985. WHA34.38. In *Handbook of resolutions and decisions of the World Health Assembly and the Executive Board, Vol. II.* 1973–1984, 397–8. Geneva: WHO.

World Health Organization. 2002. *World report on violence and health.* Geneva: WHO.

Wright, Susan, and Stuart Ketcham. 1990. The problem of interpreting the U.S. Biological Defense Research Program. In *Preventing a biological arms race,* ed. Susan Wright, 243–66. Cambridge, MA: MIT Press.

Zwi, Anthony, Antonio Ugalde, and Patricia Richards. 1999. The effects of war and political violence on health services. In *Encyclopedia of violence, peace and conflict,* ed. L. Kurtz, 679–90. San Diego, CA: Academic Press.

NOTES

1. According to a Wikipedia article on carpet bombing, the term refers to the use of large numbers of unguided gravity bombs, often with a high proportion of incendiary bombs, to attempt the complete destruction of a target region either to destroy personnel and materiel or as a means to demoralize the enemy.

2. "Half-life is the time in which the concentration of a substance, such as the radioactive content of an element or the body burden of a toxic chemical, is reduced by half" (Last 2007).

3. Glanders is a disease of horses, donkeys, and mules caused by *Buricholderia* (formerly *Pseudomonas*) *mallei.* It occasionally infects humans, in whom it can cause a fatal bronchopneumonia (Last 2007).

6

Future Wars

Joanna Santa Barbara

This chapter will discuss the issues likely to provoke future wars and the fomenting and "permissive factors" that increase their probability. It will examine possible changes in the means of waging wars, the impact of future wars on health, and some factors that constrain wars and offer alternatives. This rather dark prognosis is sketched in the hope that, looking ahead, we will develop more enlightened policies to change this trajectory.

THE CONFLICT ISSUES

We can project into the future a continuation of those factors that cause current wars. The United States, it can be predicted, will continue its drive for geopolitical domination, particularly in regions producing fossil fuels and other strategic resources. The United States may find itself in increasing competition with China and India for oil. There is likely to be other regional competition over remaining reserves of fossil fuels—for example, between Japan and China and between India and China. There will continue to be violent conflict over land, water, and valuable exportable commodities in many countries.

Water is likely to be an issue that generates serious conflict in the future (Klare 2001). The basins of the Jordan, the Ganges-Brahmaputra, the Mekong and the Nile, among many others, are sites of competition over use of water and hence are possible sites of violent conflict (UN Office for the Coordination of Humanitarian Affairs 2006). Darfur, Sudan, is the site of a recent genocide partly caused by competition between agriculturalists and pastoralists over the use of water (Sachs 2006).

Water scarcity and soil degradation combine to threaten food production in some areas, as does the collapse of ecosystems such as fisheries. Such factors stress populations and increase the probability of violent conflict.

It is likely that we have reached global peak production of oil (Campbell and Laherrere 1989; Campbell 2002/2003), and the gap between demand and supply will increasingly widen. The advancing oil scarcity has enormous implications for sudden shocks to the financial, social, and political structures of all modern societies. There is reason to believe that these shocks will provoke violent conflicts in the future over access to and control of fossil fuels (Klare 2004) and over the currency in which they are traded (Clark 2005), as well as between factions within oil-producing countries. Because of likely financial, social, and political strains to all societies, those states already stressed by social divisions will also be at greater risk of violent conflict, whether or not they are major oil producers or consumers.

We are seeing some of this conflict already, with wars in Afghanistan and Iraq being fought at least partly (and perhaps mainly) to ensure control of oil and gas supplies. There is also tension within Venezuela, Uzbekistan, Mindanao in the Philippines, Saudi Arabia, and Nigeria—all fossil fuel-producing areas.

These problems will be exacerbated by the projected impacts of climate change. Global ecosystems are already showing negative impacts of global warming due to increased levels of carbon dioxide produced by human use of fossil fuels. Rising sea levels, increased desertification, extreme weather patterns, and unbalanced ecosystems will have direct impacts on human health, some effects being mediated by epidemic illness. In many areas, populations already exceed their areas' "carrying capacity"—that is, the ability of a region to sustainably support a certain population. The advent of peak oil and climate change will make this "overshoot" more evident as dependence on imports becomes more problematic. All of these effects are also likely to increase large-scale movements of populations to escape from areas that can no longer support them, and to provoke violent conflicts in stressed populations.

FOMENTING AND PERMISSIVE FACTORS

Fomenting factors are those factors that, although they are not core causes of war, add fuel to the flames. An example is the deliberate polarization of people in conflict by stimulating ethnic or religious hatred. *Permissive factors* are those factors that, although they are not core causes of war, facilitate the waging of violent conflict. An example is the geography of an area that enables guerrilla forces to disperse and hide easily.

Human population, a fairly stable several million for most of human history (Cohen 1995; Smil 2001), has swung upward extremely dramatically in the last several hundred years, especially since access to cheap energy from fossil fuels greatly increased food production. In some densely populated areas, competition for limited land and water has resulted in war. As a cause of war, this factor can be expected to increase in importance as the human population continues to grow—and needed resources, damaged by human activity, continue to shrink. Most frightening, the expected mid-century population plateau at 9 to 10 billion depends on rising standards of living, which may not occur. Population growth may therefore shoot beyond 10 billion if the demographic transition to lower fertility associated with higher living standards does not occur.

War has always involved dehumanization of the "enemy" in order to overcome normal human inhibitions against killing other people. Skin color, ethnicity, and religion are common dimensions of devaluing. A current version likely to increase in importance is the Western–fundamentalist Islam divide. Dehumanization proceeds on both sides of this divide, and the outcomes in violent conflict are likely to grow more dangerous.

In theory, the increasing democratization of many countries in the world should bring decisions about whether to go to war increasingly under the control of the people who will pay the multiple costs of war, and therefore they will not wage war. In reality, however, such decisions are made with little accountability to the people. Loopholes in governance systems are found to enable elites to make these decisions. Modern armies are relatively smaller than before because of advances in weaponry; recruitment is from the poorer classes of societies. Thus the children of the elite are unlikely to be found among the combatants. Those who decide to go to war are likely to benefit rather than pay the costs of war. These factors make war more likely, not less.

MEANS OF WAGING WAR

Resorting to war as a means of dealing with conflicts is influenced by, among other things, the *opportunity* to do so. The availability of arms is a major multiplier of opportunity. The arms trade, dominated by the nuclear-armed powers, is an important source of revenue for suppliers. Modern arms of high lethality, both small (can kill with the efforts of one or two persons) and large (can kill with the efforts of a team) are widely distributed throughout the world, with a concentration in countries that are the site of present or recent warfare.

The so-called revolution in military affairs has increased the lethal accuracy of modern weaponry via satellite and other information technology, an aspect of the militarization of space. The United States, in particular, is moving toward the weaponization of space, attempting to enhance its military domination of all parts of the planet (US Government 2006).

The reduced availability of oil will increasingly affect the means of waging war as we now know it. The modern army is intensely oil-dependent (Klare 2007). Global military use of oil accounts for a significant proportion of consumption, and armies are likely to receive high priority in rationing supplies. Nonetheless, air and tank warfare will be compromised, and armies will become less mobile (Crowley et al. 2007). Guerrilla warfare will be least affected. It is seriously worrying to consider the possibility that decreasing capacity for other means of high technology warfare could result in states resorting to nuclear, chemical, and biological weapons. Attacks on an enemy's vital infrastructure might be used—for example, destruction of crops, water supplies, water purification capacity, or even electronic communication capacity.

Alongside the diversion of economic resources from human welfare to military use, we will see a parallel diversion of dwindling fossil fuels to military purposes. Uses that should take priority over military use include building infrastructure for alternative energy production, use in the manufacture of plastics and pharmaceuticals, and use for health care.

Compliance of home populations with all these measures may be secured by further constriction of civil liberties, especially that of free speech, as we have seen in the "war on terror."

IMPACT ON HUMAN HEALTH

It is possible to draw a very dark scenario from the above projections: more of the same kinds of impacts of war on human health; new, catastrophic impacts from the use of weapons of mass destruction; and health-compromised populations as a consequence of the ever worse diversion of resources away from human welfare. Added to this will be the multiple adverse health impacts of climate change, oil and water scarcity, population movement, new pandemic illnesses, and political instability.

THE FUTURE OF CONSTRAINING FACTORS
AND ALTERNATIVES TO WAR

In the last decade, the number of wars has been diminishing (Human Security Centre, 2005). Among other causes, this is attributed to the quiet diplomacy and the peacekeeping functions of the United Nations, and to the even quieter efforts of nongovernmental organizations working to prevent war in myriad ways, from arms control to peace education.

International law has been steadily developing, alongside the international institutions that implement it—the United Nations, the International Court of Justice, and the International Criminal Court. Knowledge of how to prevent war has steadily expanded; examples include the strategies of creative conflict transformation and of nonviolent struggle. The culture of peace has perhaps become more pervasive, judging by the number of peace organizations, peace education programs, conflict resolution centers, and reconciliation processes. This means that there are more people to promulgate the above ideas and to insist on them, even under future stresses.

Oil scarcity is likely to mean a devolution of decision making from national to local levels. This may mean diminished likelihood of resorting to political violence.

Recent experience of improving violent conflict situations during reconstruction after the tsunami in Aceh, Indonesia, gives rise to hope that we can use knowledge of peace dynamics constructively in situations of natural disaster (Renner and Chafe 2007)

How these negative and positive trends will evolve is impossible for us to predict.

CONCLUSION

The convergence of multiple trends in human-caused stress on Earth's resources, together with denial and slow response by most governments, leaves civil society[1] in the position of not only blowing the warning bugle but also attempting to generate action. The enormity of the phenomena and of their present and future impact on human health and well-being suggests that these issues are within the mandates of organizations dealing with the environment, public health, social justice, development, human rights, and peace. Devising a mechanism for concerted work from all such organizations might create some possibility of mitigating these impacts.

REFERENCES

Campbell, C. J. 2002/2003. Forecasting global oil supply 2000–2050. *Hubbert Center Newsletter.* M. King Hubbert Center for Petroleum Supply Studies.

Campbell, C. J., and J. H. Laherrere. 1989. The end of cheap oil. *Scientific American,* March: 78–83.

Clark, W. R. 2005. *Petrodollar warfare: Oil, Iraq and the future of the dollar.* Gabriola Island, BC, Canada: New Society Publishers.

Cohen, Joel. 1995. *How many people can the earth support?* New York: Norton.

Crowley, T. D., D. C. Corrie, D. B. Diamond, S. D. Funk, W. A. Hansen, A. D. Stenhoff, and D. C. Swift. 2007. *Transforming the way DOD looks at energy: An approach to establishing an energy strategy. Report FT602T1.* LMI Government Consulting.

Human Security Centre. 2005. *Human security report: War and peace in the 21st century.* Oxford University Press. Available online at the www.humansecurityreport.info website.

Klare, M. T. 2001. *Resource wars: The new landscape of global conflict.* New York: Henry Holt.

———. 2004. *Blood and oil: The dangers and consequences of America's growing dependency on imported petroleum.* New York: Henry Holt.

———. 2007. *The Pentagon v. peak oil: How wars of the future may be fought just to run the machines that fight them.* Available online at the www.alternet.org website.

Renner, M., and Z. Chafe. 2007. *Beyond disaster: Creating opportunities for peace.* Washington, DC: Worldwatch Institute.

Sachs, J. 2006. Water climates. Global Policy Forum, October. Available online at the www.globalpolicy.org website.

Smil, V. 2001. *Feeding the world: A challenge for the twenty-first century.* Cambridge, MA: MIT Press.

UN Office for the Coordination of Humanitarian Affairs. 2006. Water is running out: How inevitable are international conflicts? In *Running dry: The humanitarian impact of the global water crisis.* October. Available online at the www.irinnews.org website.

US Government. 2006. US national space policy, August. Available online at the www .ostp.gov website.

NOTE

1. *Civil society:* the aggregate of nongovernmental organizations that manifest the interests and will of citizens; individuals and organizations in a society that are independent of the government (*Webster's New Millennium Dictionary of English,* Los Angeles: Lexico, 2003–2006).

PART III

Values and Ethics in Peace through Health

7

What Values Underlie Our Actions?

Graeme MacQueen

INTRODUCTION

Ethics, or rules of moral conduct, guide our relationships and are typically taught during the socialization that prepares young humans for group life. Those whose role in life involves intervening in the lives of others in terms of their bodily integrity, their most intimate secrets (in the case of health workers), or their security and well-being (in the case of peace workers) have extra reasons for disciplining their behavior by ethical principles, because their potential to do harm is greater. Such principles are derived from values—what we hold to be worthy and good. Thus it is important for Peace through Health workers to reflect on values.

VALUES AWARENESS

Values awareness, as the expression is used here, simply means conscious awareness of our values, of the values of the people with whom we interact, and of the relationship between these values and behavior. There are three main reasons it is important for PtH practitioners to develop an awareness of values and the role of values.

Motivating Values of the Self

Although it is always useful to gain awareness of one's motivating values, awareness is especially important for people who may be entering into war zones or other places of desperation and severe conflict. Motivating values include values directed toward others, such as compassion, empathy, respect, honesty, and a sense of fairness. Few of us go to work motivated only by these values, but if, on reflection, we find that our goals are mainly dictated by self-interest (be it a quest for glory, adventure, career advancement, or a need to punish ourselves), we can do everyone a favor by staying home.

Normal human beings have mixed motivations, and we do not need to be perfect to help others, but if we are aware of what values are dominant in us at a given moment and a given stage of our lives, we can act more honestly and confidently. It is irresponsible to focus unnecessarily on one's own confusion in places of great suffering.

Values Awareness and Conflict Transformation

In conflict work, such as is common in PtH, an awareness of the values that motivate ourselves and others is crucial. We have a tendency to assume that those who disagree strongly with us have no values or have values completely different from our own. Dialogue, listening, and careful exploration of motivations and passions will usually make it clear that our opponent also has values and that there is at least some overlap (and often great overlap) between their motivating values and our own. Recognizing this can help us, and our opponent, to perceive commonality and to focus on the problem of how similar values have led to opposing positions in a conflict.

> **Example:** *During the conflict between Canadian forces and Taliban forces in Kandahar, a prominent Canadian journalist cited the blowing up of girls' schools by the Taliban as proof that the Taliban were "nihilists" and must be utterly defeated, with no compromise, dialogue, or negotiation.*
>
> *Labeling our opponent a nihilist cuts off genuine curiosity about the opponent and undermines empathy, reducing the possibility of a solution to the conflict acceptable to all parties. This labeling supports the refusal to admit that those opposing us violently may be doing so on the basis of their own moral values—values different from ours, but values all the same. In this case the journalist's indignation at the practice of blowing up schools for girls expressed her own values. The indignation was an appropriate starting point for a discussion, but it was not an appropriate end point.*

Denying that our opponent has moral values is one of the surest methods of dehumanization, and affirming that our opponent has only evil values takes things the next step to demonization. The dehumanized *may* be killed; the demonized *must* be killed.

There are numerous methods of gaining awareness of the values of self and others during conflict work. These may be subtle and indirect, and they may or may not involve typical values clarification exercises.

Building PtH as a Discipline

The moral values that underlie PtH work are not significantly different from those that underlie other forms of humanitarian work, but the concrete ethical guidelines formulated from these underlying values should be distinctive. The guidelines should show an awareness of fundamental concepts of both health work and peacework. If PtH is to mature as a discipline, it will need such statements.

VALUE DILEMMAS

Value dilemmas are common in PtH work, and they lead to confusion and conflict—between official opponents, between co-workers, and even within the self. Let's consider five of the most common dilemmas.

Dilemma 1: Compassionate desire to help vies with respectful nonintervention.

Compassion and respect are two of the great motivating values that underlie ethical rules, yet there will be times when they seem to impel us in different directions.

> *Example: A humanitarian crisis is developing in a country, and there are international calls for immediate assistance. The humanitarian imperative urges us to reach out—quickly, effectively, and without ideological or political interference—to those in need. But many parties, organizations, groups and subgroups in the country in question are opposed to intervention. The country has in the past been a plaything of colonial powers and is now struggling to attain the ability to deal with internal crises through its own institutions and its own cultural methods. The government declines assistance, even while the international community readies itself to intervene.*

Compassion urges us to intervene, while respect appears to say, "Not so fast." What will our position be?

Dilemma 2: A desire for peace urges us to be nonpartisan in a conflict, while a sense of justice urges us to take sides.

> *Example: Two parties—a government and an insurgent group—are in direct and violent conflict. We wish to encourage conflict transformation, and we set out to find ways to help the groups problem-solve together. But*

we become aware that the government is funding death squads and that the toll in human misery from these groups is many times higher than that from the insurgents. Moreover, the death squads are also engaging in torture, which is largely hidden from internationals because the government controls the press. Suddenly, we find our nonpartisan stance disappearing. We find ourselves on the side of the insurgents. We stop speaking of mediation and nonpartisanship and begin speaking of "solidarity."

Respect, compassion, empathy, and a sense of fairness have given rise to particular concepts of peace and justice that now appear to be at war in us.

Dilemma 3: A desire for uniform and widespread peace and justice urges us to establish and promote universal principles and laws, while at the same time we wish to pay attention to the uniqueness of cultures, religions, and societies.

> *Example: Leaders of a country reject the Universal Declaration of Human Rights as a Western document expressing an unacceptable mixture of Christian and secular political ideas. These leaders say that they have moral values and that a system of rights can be constructed on the basis of these values, but they are not prepared to recognize the authority of the UDHR.*

What position do we take?

Dilemma 4: Compassion can move us to reject violence, but it (along with other values) can also move us to support armed intervention where populations are threatened with death and oppression.

The dilemma is old and has not gone away. The examples are numerous. What will be our position?

Dilemma 5: Our sense of justice may lead us to insist on equity, but this may conflict with our desire to respect traditional (and often inequitable) traditions and social structures in particular cultural groups.

> *Example: A government says it will allow UN agencies and NGOs into its country only if they respect the country's traditional culture. This will mean that women who are part of the UN and NGO teams will be severely*

restricted in their behavior. The UN and NGO communities say this is unacceptable and refuse to enter under these conditions. But the country's population is suffering from extreme deprivation.

What is our position?

AN APPROACH TO THE DILEMMAS

I will not attempt here to formulate universally applicable solutions to these dilemmas. But I wish to draw attention to three attributes that we will need as we face these dilemmas: awareness, respect, and creativity.

The case for *awareness* has already been made. Without it we may expend great passion and goodwill without necessarily helping those who are suffering. We may become part of the problem rather than part of the solution. It is essential that we make a point of discovering and reflecting on values—our own and those of others—and that we go into these dilemmas with our love and indignation guided by intelligence and, where appropriate, self-criticism. We may not always find it easy to become aware of the values of others. We may find at times that we have been cast abruptly into a violent and confused situation where we must interact with people whose cultures are new to us. It may take special effort and considerable patience to understand the values of the actors in such situations, but if we ignore this step, we may lose sight of the welfare of those we wish to help.

Respect plays an important role in many of the value dilemmas above. There are historical reasons for this. Western societies, to which many of the readers of this volume will belong, have been dominant forces in the world for several centuries. This dominance has frequently been associated with cultural arrogance, a sense of "chosenness" and entitlement, and high levels of militarism and force. It is not surprising that many peoples in the world currently have ambivalent feelings about Western intervention, even when it takes place via NGOs apparently motivated by the highest moral values. It is becoming widely understood that such NGOs can become vehicles of ongoing control and enforced dependency, whereby the West maintains its dominance. Under these circumstances, a responsible discipline of PtH will take care to be multinational and multicultural from the outset, so that no PtH initiative will be determined, either in its concepts or in its execution, solely by Western perceptions. Respect for others, combined with the habit of self-awareness and self-criticism, are essential.

Creativity is a key to facing all of the above dilemmas. When combined with dialogue, it often enables us to respect all the values that appear to be in conflict and to come up with solutions that suit the needs of all parties.

> *Example: We enter into a dialogue with the host country in Dilemma 1 about forms of assistance that might satisfy that country's autonomy needs. Let us assume that Islam is a dominant religion in this country. We agree that Muslim countries will take the lead in humanitarian assistance efforts, that Muslim aid agencies will be the lead agencies, and that Islamic concepts of debt and financing will be respected as the aid effort is put together.*

> *Example: In facing Dilemma 2, we bear in mind, from our study of conflict transformation, that there is room for different roles and types of work in the transformation of a conflict and that roles may be different at different stages of the conflict. (See the discussion of PtH mechanisms in chapter 4.) We therefore formulate a plan that allows solidarity and mediation to play valid and complementary roles.*

> *Example: We accept that the country in Dilemma 3 has a valid point, but we do not give up our quest for universal principles. On the basis of an appreciation of history and culture, we enter into dialogues that allow us to improve the UDHR. We include in our dialogues activists of this country who do support universality of human rights principles.*

> *Example: With respect to Dilemma 4, we make a distinction between a global, cooperative peace system, in which police work plays an important part, and a global war system in which competing armed forces fight each other. Recognizing that the similarity between national armed forces and international police forces is superficial, and that their aims, nature, and underlying values are radically different, we follow—and, where necessary, formulate—guidelines for the implementation of international police work.*

> *Example: We respect the values of the traditional culture in Dilemma 5 and enter into a dialogue on that basis. We exercise patience, knowing that forceful insistence on having our way may actually make things worse for women in the country in question. But we also make it clear to leaders in the traditional country that we too have values, that we are not merely opportunists and secular moneymakers, and that there are moral boundaries we will not cross. We demonstrate through our actions our willingness to sacrifice material gain and our desire to act on the basis of values. We attempt to evoke their respect for our values, not for our power, and on that basis we enter into ongoing, gentle dialogues.*

8

Human Rights

Lowell Ewert and *Dabney Evans*

THE LINK BETWEEN HUMAN RIGHTS AND PEACE

The observance of human rights is a fundamental condition for peace. The priority of this principle is best illustrated by the Universal Declaration of Human Rights (UDHR), which was adopted by the United Nations on December 10, 1948. Having recently emerged from the consequences of two horrific world wars in less than thirty years, the world community was sick of war and wanted the cycle of violence to stop. Therefore, the drafters of the Universal Declaration were tasked with trying to articulate a new kind of relationship between a government and the governed. In writing the Universal Declaration, they believed that they had finally found the key to peace.

"Whereas it is essential, if man is not to be compelled to have recourse, as a last resort, to rebellion against tyranny and oppression, that human rights should be protected by the rule of law" (United Nations 1948). "Respect human rights," the drafters can be paraphrased to have stated in the Preamble, and war will no longer be necessary. And with this simple statement, the UDHR became known as the antidote for war. What is most interesting, at least as it pertains to the topic of this book, is the role that health was seen to play as an essential element of peace.

The Declaration itself was just that—a Declaration. It claimed no direct legal impact and indeed was sold to the delegates at the United Nations on the basis of its nonbinding character. Don't worry, Eleanor Roosevelt, chair of the United Nations Commission on Human Rights said shortly before delegates voted on the UDHR, the Declaration "is not a treaty; it is not an international agreement. It is not and does not purport to be a statement of law or of legal obligation" (Kirgis 1977, 782). With this statement, she was trying to reassure delegates that a vote in favor of the Declaration would not let the human rights genie out of the bottle. In hindsight, however, we now know that she could not have been more wrong.

Not only have various articles of the UDHR since become accepted as part of customary international law, but even more important, the UDHR has inspired hundreds of millions of people to claim rights in a way that their governments never imagined at the time. "It is precisely the Declaration's language—at once eloquent, expansive and simple—that allowed it to express universal truths in words human beings all over the world could understand and wanted to hear. No formal legal instrument could have achieved that result and had quite the same inspirational impact on the human rights movement" (Buergenthal 1998, 91).

THE LINK BETWEEN HEALTH AND HUMAN RIGHTS

The right to health figures prominently in the UDHR's goal of attempting to set rules that make war unlikely and in the myriad of other legal documents that breathed life into its vague provisions and applied them in a more concrete way.

This inspiring perspective on health was stated most clearly by Article 25 of the UDHR, where it was written that "everyone has the right to a standard of living adequate for the health and well-being of himself and his family, including food, clothing, housing, and medical care and necessary social services, and the right to security in the event of unemployment, sickness, [or] disability" (United Nations 1948). While these words are so vague as to be unenforceable, their hortatory character led to greater definition in those documents that followed. Thus the UDHR is like the bedrock upon which large buildings are constructed—never seen, but utterly essential to the successful construction of the edifice.

What are some representative examples of the health principles that have been built on the solid foundation provided by the UDHR? While there is not space here to provide a comprehensive listing, several examples will illustrate how the UDHR's influence has changed our understanding of health. Prior to 1948, it was unthinkable to claim a right to health. Today, it is a mainstream idea, and in addition, health is now far more broadly interpreted than most people even one generation ago would ever have imagined.

First, and most important, is the International Covenant on Economic, Social and Cultural Rights (ICESCR), which, in contrast to the UDHR, is a legally binding treaty and does give rise to specific rights (United Nations 1966). Article 12 of the Covenant provides that "the States Party to the present Covenant recognize the right of everyone to the enjoyment of the highest attainable standard of physical and mental health. The steps to be taken by the States Parties to the present Covenant to achieve the full realization of this right shall include those necessary for: the provision for the reduction of the still-birth rate and of infant mortality and for the healthy development of the child; the improvement of all aspects of environmental and industrial hygiene; the prevention, treatment, and control of epidemic, endemic, occupational and other diseases; the creation of conditions which would assure to all medical service and medical attention in the event of sickness" (United Nations 1966).

Second, the World Health Organization provides a more expansive definition of health: "a state of complete physical, mental and social well-being and not merely the absence of disease or infirmity" (World Health Organization 2006a). Similar to the human rights paradigm itself, this definition recognizes the interdependence of health and social variables and reflects the complex interplay of health with other aspects of society.

Third, the Ottawa Charter for Health Promotion includes "peace, shelter, education, food, income, a stable ecosystem, sustainable resources, social justice and equity" in its definition of the fundamental conditions for health (World Health Organization 1986). This holistic health concept explicitly relates health to peace, which is the first determinant cited.

Fourth, the WHO Commission on the Social Determinants of Health seeks to address the social factors leading to ill health and health inequities (World Health Organization 2006a). The link between poverty and ill health is also reflected clearly in the prominence given to health within the Millennium Development Goals (MDGs) (United Nations 2006).

These four examples show how a vague and unenforceable idealistic standard first contained in the UDHR has slowly but steadily changed how we view the relationship among health, human rights, and peace. Although in the short-term we may lament that there is still a long way to go in promoting effective health practices and care, in the longer view we can see how very far we have come in six short decades.

THE LINK BETWEEN HEALTH AND THE LAW OF WAR

In contrast to the purpose of human rights law, which is to prevent war, the function of the law of war is to establish rules that regulate the conduct of the armed conflict so as to make the restoration of peace possible. The law of war, often referred to as humanitarian law, assumes that war (defined to be direct violence) is just a temporary condition. No nation or group has ever existed in a state of perpetual armed conflict. No nation or group can sustain war indefinitely. Historically, even after the most brutal of armed conflicts, peace (defined here as the absence of war) has eventually followed.

To recognize the temporary condition of war, the law of war evolved over time to "apply to the very situations in which laws have disappeared: wars, conflicts, major crises" (Bouchet-Saulnier 2002, 8). The humanitarian principles function to limit the destruction, killing, and humiliation that accompany war, so that society can more easily be rebuilt. Total war is banned. It has been replaced by an approach that in theory allows warriors to cause only the destruction that is necessary to accomplish the objective of war. Gratuitous or unnecessary violence is not permitted. Simply because one has the power and the means to cause suffering, death, and destruction does not give one the right to do so. "Laws [of war] do not spare us from conflicts, but they enable each actor to turn to clear definitions of what is just or unjust, normal or abnormal, behavior that is legitimate or unacceptable" (Bouchet-Saulnier 2002, 8).

The four Geneva Conventions and two Optional Protocols that were written to establish clear guidelines on how war is to be waged have emphasized the role of health in creating conditions that make the restoration of peace more likely. A few representative articles illustrate the role that the world community has determined health should play, even in times of war.

- Article 13 of Protocol II to the Geneva Conventions, which binds those states that have signed and ratified the Protocol, provides the widest scope of protection for victims of conflict when it specifies that (1) "[a]ll the wounded, sick and shipwrecked, whether or not they have taken part in the armed conflict, shall be respected and protected," and (2) "[i]n all circumstances they shall be treated humanely and shall receive, to the fullest extent practicable and with the least possible delay, the medical care and attention required by their condition" (Article 7, page 95 of Protocol).
- Article 3, which is common to all four Geneva Conventions and which most scholars would accept as customary law, thereby binding every state, mandates that "the wounded and sick shall be collected and cared for" (Geneva Convention 1949). No exceptions are given to this blanket statement.
- Article 55 of the Fourth Geneva Convention places on an occupying power "the duty of ensuring the food and medical supplies of the

population." The only limitation is that this duty must be carried out "to the fullest extent of the means possible" (Geneva Convention 1949).

These representative provisions illustrate the wide scale and scope of health protections that are contained in humanitarian law. There is no segment of the population that is not protected by humanitarian law. Active combatants who are no longer able to engage in hostilities; prisoners; civic, political, or religious leaders—all can claim rights under humanitarian law as can anyone else. This broad reach reflects the blanket priority that the world community ascribes to the provision of health care.

Clearly, it is not possible to separate health issues from the law of war or to ignore the link between providing basic health services and the goal of restoring peace. There is no space in this short chapter to outline the standard of care that is required for those who are under the military control of others, the ethical standards that medical personnel are required to follow, or the role of humanitarian organizations that provide health services. But health plays an important role in creating the context for a restoration of peace. Therefore, it is important for the health worker to understand the complex relationship that links health, human rights, the law of war, and peace. With such understanding will come insight into how the medical worker can best maximize each discipline to most effectively advocate improvement of health care for the marginalized.

WORKING FOR CHANGE

As other chapters of this book have sadly proved, the task that confronts the health and human rights advocate is not yet finished. Too many people in too many parts of the world continue to suffer from the consequences of unavailable or substandard practices of health care that continue to violate international law. What is the solution to this breach of human rights? How can one use a human rights or humanitarian law approach to advocate for changes in these circumstances?

Before one begins to answer this question, it is important to remember the profound change that international human rights law has caused in how humankind is viewed. Prior to the adoption of the UDHR, citizens were essentially viewed as the property of their nation of citizenship and as subject to almost absolute control by their government. In contrast, every subsequent human rights treaty or declaration affirms four fundamental principles that empower all advocates who are trying to create a better world. These four principals are the right of citizens to participate in the life of their community and nation; the right to hold those in power over them accountable; the right to work for change; and a reaffirmation of the dignity and value that all persons possess.

Within this framework of empowered advocates for justice, there are at least four different ways in which international law can be used to improve health rights. First, one can look to legal documents, determine what obligations these documents place on governments, and challenge those governments to live up to their obligations. When critiquing a nation's human rights performance, Chapman (1996) proposes a "violations approach" that outlines three types of violations of economic, social, and cultural rights such as the right to health: (1) violations as a result of actions and/or policies of the State, (2) violations related to discrimination, and (3) violations based on the State's failure to fulfill its minimum core obligations under the International Covenant on Economic, Social and Cultural Rights. Violations may include both acts of commission and acts of omission.

Chapman also argues that states have a primary obligation of conduct, as opposed to obligations of result. The Maastricht Guidelines provide examples of obligations of conduct and obligations of result in regard to the right to health. An obligation of conduct related to health could include the adoption and implementation of a national plan to reduce maternal mortality whereas an obligation of result could include the achievement of a milestone in the reduction of maternal mortality (Maastricht Guidelines 1998). In simple terms, obligations of conduct are related to State behaviors and processes, whereas obligations of result are demonstrated by outcomes.

One can also utilize a "violations approach" during times of war when humanitarian law applies. Maltreatment of detainees, whether they are civilians or combatants, during times of armed conflict is always prohibited. The new threats that we face today from terrorism do not justify cruel treatment, torture, humiliation, or outrages upon personal dignity. There are no excuses for the excesses of Abu Ghraib or Guantánamo.

Second, human rights and humanitarian law principles provide the legal and moral justification for individuals to refuse to follow illegal orders. There is no basis for persons to claim, as some did following the end of World War II, that they had no choice but to be complicit in war crimes.

Third, one can challenge international agencies to be more aware of their obligations under international law. For example, as a part of the 1997 United Nations Program for Reform, Secretary-General Kofi Annan called on UN agencies to mainstream human rights horizontally into their programs and activities. Although many of the UN agencies attempted to do this, a standardized conception of human rights–based approaches to programming did not exist. A 2003 interagency workshop resulted in the development of the "Common Understanding," which has now been adopted across many UN agencies. The Common Understanding makes three main points:

- All programs should further the realization of human rights set forth in the Universal Declaration of Human Rights and other international human rights instruments.
- Standards and principles put forth in the UDHR and other international human rights instruments should guide programming activities.
- Development cooperation assists in the development of both "duty-bearers" and "rights-holders."

All of these initiatives could involve a health component (United Nations Development Program 2006).

Fourth, the Geneva Conventions also assume a role for relief agencies that are attempting to provide humanitarian assistance during times of armed conflict. There are specific expectations about how this assistance may be provided, and a humanitarian role for nongovernmental organizations is anticipated. Nongovernmental organizations should be aware of their rights and duties as humanitarian actors and of how they can act on this authority to best assist civilians.

It is important to keep in mind that rights, laws, and customs change over time. Rights are not static and are not defined solely by what parliaments and international diplomats commit to writing. Rights become what people expect them to be as customs and societal expectations change. Often after customary interpretation and societal expectations have evolved, so too does legislation. In this way, new and evolving social expectations and customs can be seen as precursors to new legislation. Therefore, health advocates should not overlook the power of writing and public awareness campaigns that promote new interpretations of what the public should expect of health services.

CONCLUSION

The object of this chapter has been to demonstrate that there is a synergistic relationship between health and human rights, in times of war and peace. Health matters in issues of conflict. It plays an important role in preventing war and, if war has broken out, in restoring peace. When health workers are doing their medical jobs well, they are promoting peace. When human rights workers are doing their work well, they too are promoting peace, while simultaneously making it possible for health workers to be more effective. The health worker and the human rights worker are therefore colleagues in the common cause of peace.

REFERENCES

Bouchet-Saulnier, Francoise. 2002. *The practical guide to humanitarian law.* Boulder, CO: Rowman and Littlefield.

Buergenthal, Thomas. 1998. Centerpiece of the human rights revolution. In *Reflections on the Universal Declaration of Human Rights: A fiftieth anniversary anthology,* ed. B. Van der Heijden and B. Tahzib-Lie. The Hague: Martinus Nijhoff.

Chapman, A. 1996. A "violations approach" for monitoring the International Covenant on Economic, Social and Cultural Rights." *Human Rights Quarterly* 18.1:23–66.

Geneva Convention. 1949. *Geneva Convention relative to the protection of civilian persons in time of war of August 12, 1949.* 1986, 154, 174. Geneva: International Committee of the Red Cross.

Kirgis, Jr., Frederic L. 1977. *International organizations in their legal setting: Documents, comments and questions.* Portland, OR: Book News.

The Maastricht Guidelines on violations of economic, social and cultural rights. 1988. *Human Rights Quarterly* 20:691–705.

Protocol II. 1977. *Protocol additional to the Geneva conventions of 12 August 1949, and relating to the protection of victims of non-international armed conflicts.* Geneva: International Committee of the Red Cross.

United Nations. 1948. *Universal Declaration of Human Rights.* Available online at the www.un.org website.

———. 1966. *International Covenant on Economic, Social and Cultural Rights.* Adopted and opened for signature, ratification and accession by General Assembly resolution 2200A (XXI) of 16 December 1966.

———. 2006b. *United Nations Millennium Development Goals.* Available online at the www.un.org website.

United Nations Development Program. 2006. Indicators and standards for monitoring economic, social and cultural rights. Available online at the hdr.undp.org website.

World Health Organization. 1986. *Constitution, in basic documents,* 36th ed. Geneva: WHO.

———. 2006a. *Commission on social determinants of health.* Available online at the www.who.int/ website.

———. 2006b. *Ottawa charter for health promotion.* Available online at the www.euro .who.int website.

9

Medical Ethics

Neil Arya

ETHICS TO OPPOSE VIOLENCE AND PROMOTE PEACE

The term *medical ethics* refers to the study of moral values as they apply to medicine. Just as ethics represent a culture's distillation of guidelines for behavior, medical ethics represent such guidelines for health-care professionals. We cannot think of peace without justice and values. In promoting Peace through Health, we must look at the ethical bases of the health professions.

Since World War II, significant developments in the interpretation of medical ethics have forced physicians to confront their professional responsibilities. These guiding principles reflected in codes of behavior give moral weight to support and guide medical practitioners and enable them to be seen as legitimate, in their own eyes and to others, when they oppose the status quo and act against the power structures of their countries. This may enable them to overcome a culture that promotes direct and structural violence in the societies where they live.

Perhaps the most influential formulation of medical ethics is that of Childress and Beauchamp, in their seminal 1979 work *Principles of Bioethics*. Here they distilled four guiding principles: respect for autonomy, beneficence, nonmaleficence, and justice. Though usually conceived as applying to transactions between individuals, these principles can usefully be understood as governing relationships between aggregations of individuals—groups of various sizes. This becomes especially relevant when these ideas are applied to Peace through Health.

ETHICAL DILEMMAS FOR
PROFESSIONALS IN SITUATIONS OF VIOLENCE

As citizens and as professionals, doctors, nurses, medics, psychologists, and social workers who work with corrections officers, the police, or the military face tensions because of their many obligations—to themselves, their professions, and society. Physicians for Human Rights defines such conflicts as dual loyalty—as a "clinical role conflict between professional duties to a patient and obligations, express or implied, real or perceived, to the interests of a third party such as an employer, insurer or the state" (Physicians for Human Rights and University of Cape Town 2006). For example, to comply with the interests of authorities, health professionals can conceal human rights violations; can falsify findings, autopsy reports, or death certificates; and can be accomplices, accessories, or perpetrators in forced amputations, executions, or torture. Participation in such activities may be enforced or may contribute to material rewards, career advancement, or enhancement of reputation.

On the other hand, health workers can risk the displeasure of authorities by speaking out and exposing "disappearances," torture, or politically motivated murder and honestly documenting injuries. To live up to their moral obligations might be dangerous. If they do the right thing, they may face threats and persecution or may themselves be tortured. Sudfeld (1990) reports on cases of sixteen psychologists in Argentina, Chile, El Salvador, Kenya, Paraguay, Poland, Czechoslovakia, and Uruguay between 1977 and 1984 whose persecution was documented by the French Psychological Society. The Nepali doctors described in Chapter 16 faced imprisonment and beating solely for acting in accordance with professional ethics.

To choose to do what is right when faced with such a dilemma is even more difficult when these professionals support the goals of their nation-state against what they see as dangerous enemies. Health professionals have been complicit in torture in various settings, including Nazi Germany, Latin American dictatorships, the Soviet bloc, apartheid South Africa, and the United States in its war on terror. It is only after the fall of such regimes or when removed from their environment that they realize how horrific their actions have been. What codes of conduct can guide and assist professionals in making such decisions?

FROM HIPPOCRATES TO NUREMBERG AND GENEVA

The Hippocratic Oath (400 BC) states, "I will follow the system or regimen which according to my ability and judgment I consider for the benefit of my patients and abstain from whatever is deleterious and mischievous." Further principles of altruism, beneficence, and the primacy of patient welfare, as well as nonmaleficence or "do no harm" (primum non nocere) are found in the oath. However, such responsibilities were rarely considered in situations of armed conflict prior to World War II. But in 1946 in Nuremberg, Germany, twenty-three doctors, SS officials, and administrative bureaucrats were tried before the American military court for "crimes against humanity" for their participation in human experiments in concentration camps and research institutions, as well as in the murder or "euthanasia" of physically, mentally, and emotionally ill human beings.

Many defendants cited the exceptional situation of war, higher goals of science and truth, and acceptance of an ideology as mitigating factors that permitted them to dehumanize victims. In Buchenwald concentration camp, for instance, human experiments were conducted to develop a vaccination against typhus fever, an important military and civilian achievement since typhus epidemics were claiming German soldiers on the eastern front (Mitscherlich and Mielke 1978). Beyond those who directly participated were many others, such as the renowned Berlin neuropathologist Professor Julius Hallervorden, who examined the brains of 697 victims of euthanasia. Hallervorden is recorded to have said, "after all, where those brains came from was none of my business." Many professionals continued to use tissue derived from these victims until the 1970s, when such practices came to general attention (Aly 1994; Pross 1992).

The Nuremberg Code (1947) was a set of ten ethical principles for carrying out scientific research, which was published as a result of these medical crimes committed during the period of national socialism. The Code outlines the ethics of medical research and ensures the rights of human subjects. The principles include the requirement that the research be purposeful and necessary for the benefit of society—based on animal studies or other rational justification. There must be informed, voluntary consent and avoidance of and protection from injury. Unnecessary risks of physical and mental suffering to the subject shall not be greater than the humanitarian importance of the problem. Investigators must be scientifically qualified, and the subject may terminate the experiment at any time. The World Medical Association's Declaration of Helsinki (1964) extended such limitations on experimentation.

FAILURE OF SUCH CODES IN TIMES OF PEACE

Despite these charters and codes, American government officials and medical personnel continued the infamous Tuskegee experiments from 1932 until 1972. These trials, conducted by the US Public Health Service on 400 illiterate, black Alabama sharecroppers, were designed to observe the natural history of syphilis. Participants were informed only that they had "bad blood." In the 1930s, accepted treatment was quite toxic, and the fact they were given only low doses of medication may have been justifiable in the first year of the trial. However, the trial continued, and even after penicillin became the standard treatment for syphilis, the subjects of these experiments were treated only with ASA, they were not told of their diagnosis, and their families were actively prevented from learning their cause of death (autopsies were conducted only at special labs). Even though 250 of the sharecroppers registered for the draft as patriotic Americans, and treatment of the disease would have been obligatory, they were given a special "exemption." In the end, 28 died directly of syphilis, 100 from related complications. And because of their unknowingly passing the disease on to spouses, lovers, and indirectly to children, 40 wives and 19 children were infected (Jones 1981, 1993).

Similarly, the US military conducted dozens of secret radioactivity experiments from 1945 to 1975 on test subjects with neither their knowledge nor their consent (McCally, Cassel, and Kimball 1994). Clearly, the presence of conventions requiring informed consent is not in itself sufficient to prevent abuse.

TORTURE AND RELEVANT TENETS OF ETHICS

The Declaration of Geneva (1948) adopted by the World Medical Association includes service to humanity, conscience and dignity in the practice of the art of healing, along with dutiful attention to the health of the patient, to colleagues and to traditions of the art. The primary concern is patient welfare. Practice is supposed to be in accordance with the laws of humanity, regardless of one's individual or societal racial, religious, political, or social prejudices. This would appear to prohibit participation in any form of torture.

Torture has been quite widespread in the world (Amnesty International 2007), but the degree of medical complicity in such actions is unknown. The World Medical Association directly addressed the issue of torture in its Declaration of Tokyo in 1975 (WMA 1975). The Declaration prohibits such complicity in torture, defined both as "the deliberate, systematic or wanton infliction of physical or mental suffering by one or more persons acting alone or on the orders of any authority, to force another person to yield information, to make a confession, or for any other reason" and as action taken "to weaken the physical or mental health of a human being without therapeutic justification."

Considering it to be "the privilege of the medical doctor to practice medicine in the service of humanity, to preserve and restore bodily and mental health without distinction as to persons, to comfort and to ease the suffering of his or her patients," "the doctor shall not countenance, condone, or participate in the practice of torture, or other forms of cruel, inhuman, or degrading procedures, whatever the offense of which the victim of such procedures is suspected, accused or guilty, and whatever the victim's beliefs or motives, and in all situations, including armed conflict and civil strife" (Declaration of Tokyo 1975). The doctor's fundamental role is to alleviate the distress of fellow human beings. No motive, whether personal, collective, or political, shall prevail against this higher purpose.

The UN General Assembly, "alarmed that not infrequently members of the medical profession or other health personnel are engaged in activities which are difficult to reconcile with medical ethics," passed resolution 37/194 without dissent (UN General Assembly 1982), considering it to be a "gross contravention of medical ethics as well as an offense under applicable international instruments, for health personnel, particularly physicians, to engage, actively or passively, in acts which constitute participation in, complicity in, incitement to or attempts to commit torture or other cruel, inhuman or degrading treatment or punishment." Health personnel, particularly physicians, charged with the medical care of prisoners and detainees, have a duty to protect their patients' physical and mental health and treat their diseases with the same attentiveness and care as is afforded to those who are not imprisoned or detained. Detainee medical records are presumed to be confidential.

OBLIGATIONS OF MEDICAL MILITARY PERSONNEL

What are the specific obligations of health professionals working for the military? The Geneva Conventions directly address the "dual loyalty conflict" faced by medical personnel treating prisoners, stating that "although [medical personnel] shall be subject to the internal discipline of the camp . . . such personnel may not be compelled to carry out any work other than that concerned with their medical . . . duties."[1]

Former camp commander Major General Geoffrey Miller introduced the Behavioral Science Consultation Teams (BSCT)—known colloquially as Biscuits—to the Guantánamo facility in late 2002. The "Biscuits" were staffed at various times by psychologists and/or psychiatrists bound by ethical codes (Marks 2005). These professionals adapted techniques designed to protect the mental health of US soldiers facing torture in the hands of uncivilized regimes to develop torture techniques to inflict on inmates. Miller deemed such practices as hooding, prolonged isolation, sleep deprivation, and exposure to loud noise and temperature extremes to be an "essential" part of the interrogation process, maintaining that prisoners had to be subjected to extreme levels of stress in order to erode established patterns of behavior.

Time magazine reported on the case of Guantánamo detainee Moham-med al-Qahtani. In late 2002 and early 2003, Qahtani was questioned for 18 to 20 hours per day for 48 out of 54 consecutive days and subjected to an array of tactics that included exposure to temperature extremes, barking military dogs, strip searches, stress positions, being led around on a leash, and being forced to stand naked in front of women. In addition to these measures, "a medical corpsman forcibly administered three and a half bags of intravenous fluid. Qahtani was refused a promised bath-room break, and when he became desperate, he was told to go in his pants." At one time he needed to be hospitalized because his heart rate dropped to 35 beats per minute. Before this interrogation regime, Qah-tani had been subjected to 160 days of isolation, and according to a let-ter of complaint sent by the FBI to the Pentagon, he was "evidencing behavior consistent with extreme psychological trauma" (Marks 2005). This torture was almost certainly known to clinicians, who should have been bound by ethical codes to act on their observations.

Evidence of further ethical breaches emerged in a complaint lodged by Guantánamo detainees, alleging that physicians under the supervision of Dr. John Edmondson, head of the facility's naval hospital, made medical care contingent on cooperation with interrogators, witnessed and partici-pated in abuse, and shared medical information with interrogators to expose detainees' weaknesses and thus help them develop an interrogation plan.

REACTIONS OF HEALTH PROFESSIONAL BODIES

Although Physicians for Human Rights and Physicians for Social Respon-sibility condemned such practices, the American Medical Association and the American Psychiatric Association were somewhat slower and milder in their criticism. In June 2005, however, the American Psychiatric Associa-tion said it was "troubled by recent reports regarding alleged violations of professional medical ethics by psychiatrists at Guantánamo Bay. Its Presi-dent Scharfstein spoke out against these practices more directly over the next year. In June 2006, the American Medical Association declared that

"Physicians must neither conduct nor directly participate in an interrogation, because a role as physician-interrogator undermines the physician's role as healer and thereby erodes trust in the individual physician-interrogator and in the medical profession."

The American Psychological Association (APA) took a different tack and developed a Presidential Task Force on Psychological Ethics and National Security. PENS concluded that "it is consistent with the APA Ethics Code for psychologists to serve in consultative roles to interrogation and information-gathering processes for national security-related purposes." Its President Gerald Koocher declared, "A number of opportunistic commentators masquerading as scholars have continued to report on alleged abuses by mental health professionals." It was not until August 10, 2006, in response to massive public and professional outcry, that the APA finally reaffirmed its "absolute opposition to all forms of torture and abuse, regardless of the circumstance." The resolution furthermore affirmed United Nations human rights documents and conventions as the basis for APA policy.

There is no evidence for the claims of some health professionals who have attended interrogations that their presence mitigated the effects of ill treatment—and somewhat more evidence that their participation may have legitimated such abuse in the eyes of those directly engaging in it. A threat of losing professional licensure for participating in torture may be a more effective way of discouraging psychologist or physician participation in torture, but this was not proposed (Soldz 2007). Organizations such as Amnesty International's Medical Network and Physicians for Human Rights continue to speak out against such abuses throughout the world.

IRAQ AND AFGHANISTAN

Confirmed or reliably reported abuses of detainees in Iraq and Afghanistan include beatings, burns, shocks, bodily suspensions, asphyxia, threats against detainees and their relatives, sexual humiliation, isolation, prolonged hooding and shackling, and exposure to heat, cold, and loud noise. These include deprivation of sleep, food, clothing, and material for personal hygiene, and denigration of Islam and forced violation of its rites. Abuses of women detainees are less well documented but include credible allegations of sexual humiliation and rape (Miles 2004).

Miles also records falsification of death certificates of detainees in Afghanistan and Iraq—for example, attributing to "natural causes . . . during his sleep" the asphyxiation of a beaten detainee tied to the top of his cell door and gagged. Another Iraqi man who was taken into custody by US soldiers was found months later by his family in an Iraqi hospital, comatose, with three skull fractures, a severe thumb fracture, and burns on the bottoms of his feet. The accompanying US medical report stated that heat stroke had triggered a heart attack that put him in a coma but did not mention the injuries. A US medic inserted a catheter into the corpse of a detainee who died under torture in order to create evidence that he was alive at the hospital.

Such violations were most notorious in Iraq in Abu Ghraib, where a nurse, "when called to attend to a prisoner who was having a panic attack, saw naked Iraqis in a human pyramid with sandbags over their heads but did not report it until an investigation was held several months later." Furthermore, "two doctors who gave a painkiller to a prisoner for a dislocated shoulder and sent him to an outside hospital recognized that the injury was caused by his arms being handcuffed and held over his head for "a long period," but they did not report any suspicions of abuse" (Zernike 2004). Medics stitching or tending to collapsed prisoners but failing to interrupt torture or to report it to higher authorities are guilty of violating standards of medical ethics.

The International Committee of the Red Cross (ICRC) found various violations of the Geneva Conventions—on health inspections and care, failure to treat or report illnesses, and injuries to families or authorities. The military command, including medical personnel, seemed permissive with regard to human rights abuses.

These grave ethical infringements by health professionals are, of course, also human rights abuses. Declaring people as "unlawful" or "enemy" combatants does not excuse mistreatment of anyone. Moreover, in participating in such regimes, health personnel jeopardize their own (relatively) protected status as neutral altruistic parties and the safety of their own country's POWs. And allied regimes whose cooperation is necessary for US security have been less willing to cooperate with what they consider a regime that does not respect norms of conduct. The International Criminal Court (to which most Western countries except the United States are signatories) and some War Crimes Tribunals may represent a way to enforce individual accountability for human rights offenses judicially and to end the impunity of perpetrators of such abuses where regimes in power refuse to take action.

OTHER APPLICATIONS OF MEDICAL ETHICS

For many in the United States, the death penalty represents a serious violation of professional as well as personal ethics (Curran and Cassel 1980).

The American Medical Association, the American College of Physicians, the American Public Health Association, and the American Nurses Association all prohibit the participation of health professionals in legally sanctioned executions.

Physicians harvesting organs from executed prisoners in China and Taiwan and the active participation of health professionals in punitive amputations in some Muslim countries have drawn condemnation from around the world.

CONCLUSIONS

In times of violent conflict, health professionals often face conflicting loyalties. This can lead to serious violations of human dignity and human rights. Following principles of basic medical professionalism, codes of ethics, and laws can guide them through these dilemmas and help them to promote peace and ultimately security. Appealing to these principles and speaking out in favor of basic rights is another way in which health professionals can promote peace and nonviolence.

REFERENCES

Aly, G. 1994. Pure and tainted progress. In *Cleansing of the fatherland: Nazi medicine and racial hygiene,* ed. G. Aly, P. Chroust, and C. Pross. Baltimore: Johns Hopkins University Press. Quoted in Lucas and Pross 1995.

Amnesty International. 2003. Available online at the web.amnesty.org website.

———. 2007. Available online at the web.amnesty.org website.

Beauchamp, T. L., and J. F. Childress. 1979. *Principles of biomedical ethics.* Oxford: Oxford University Press.

CBS. 2003. *Face the Nation,* March 23 interview with Secretary Rumsfeld by Bob Schieffer and David Martin.

Curran, W. J., and W. Cassel. 1980. The ethics of medical participation in capital punishment. *New England Journal of Medicine* 302:226–30.

Jones, James H. 1981 and 1993. *Bad blood: The Tuskegee syphilis experiment.* New York: The Free Press. See also U.S. Public Health Service Syphilis Study at Tuskegee, available online at the www.cdc.gov website.

Lifton, Robert Jay. 2004. Doctors and torture. *New England Journal of Medicine* 351 (July 29): 415–16.

Lucas, Torsten, and Christian Pross. 1995. Caught between conscience and complicity: Human rights violations and the health professions. *Medicine and Global Survival* 2 (2): 106–14.

Marks, Jonathan H. 2005. The silence of the doctors. *The Nation,* December 26. Available online at the www.thenation.com website.

McCally, M, C. Cassel, and D. Kimball. 1994. U.S. government-sponsored radiation research on humans 1945–1975. *Medicine and Global Survival* 1:4–17.

Miles, Steven H. 2004. Abu Ghraib: Its legacy for military medicine. *The Lancet* 364 (9435): 725–29.

Mitscherlich, A., and F. Mielke, eds. 1978. *Medizin ohne menschlichkeit.* Frankfurt: Fischer Taschenbuch Verlag.

Physicians for Human Rights. PHR welcomes American Medical Association's adoption of rules against physician involvement in interrogation; Pentagon must commit to adhere to AMA's guidelines. Available online at the www.physiciansforhumanrights .org website.

Physicians for Human Rights and University of Cape Town Health Sciences Faculty. 2006. International Dual Loyalty Working Group. 2002. Physicians for Human Rights and University of Cape Town Health Sciences Faculty. Dual loyalty and human rights in health professional practice: Proposed guidelines and institutional standards. See http://physiciansforhumanrights.org/library/documents/reports/report-2002-duel loyalty.pdf. **Alternate reference Beyrer, Chris.** 2003. *Dual loyalty and human rights in health professional practice: Proposed guidelines and institutional mechanisms JAMA* 290 (5): 671–72. August 5, 2003. See http://jama.ama-assn.org/cgi/content/full/ 290/5/671

Pross, C. 1992. Nazi doctors, German medicine and historical truth. In *The Nazi doctors and the Nuremberg code—human rights in human experimentation,* ed. G. J. Annas and M. A. Grodin. New York and Oxford: Oxford University Press.

Rumsfeld, D. 2003. Stakeout following CNN interview, March 23.

Soldz, Stephen. 2007. Psychology and coercive interrogations in historical perspective: Aid and comfort for torturers. *Common Dreams,* April 15. Available online at the www.commondreams.org website.

Sudfeld, P. 1990. Psychologists as victims, administrators and designers of torture. In *Psychology and torture,* ed. P. Sudfeld. New York: Hemisphere Publishing. Quoted in Lucas and Pross 1995.

UN General Assembly. 1982. Resolution 37/194 (Principles of medical ethics relevant to the role of health personnel, particularly physicians, in the protection of prisoners and detainees against torture and other cruel, inhuman or degrading treatment or punishment). 111th plenary meeting, December 18.

World Medical Association. 1964. World Medical Association Declaration of Helsinki. Adopted by the 18th World Medical Assembly in Helsinki, Finland.

World Medical Association. 1975. Guidelines for medical doctors concerning torture and other cruel, inhuman or degrading treatment or punishment in relation to detention and imprisonment. Adopted by the twenty-ninth World Medical Assembly, held in Tokyo in October.

Zernike, K. 2004. Only a few spoke up on abuse as many soldiers stayed silent. *New York Times.* May 22, A1. Quoted in Lifton 2004.

NOTE

1. Many of the strategies deployed in the "war on terror" represent grave violations of US or international law, including the Geneva Conventions on the humane treatment of detainees. The Bush administration seemed to argue, for example, that the ban on cruel, inhuman, and degrading treatment did not apply to foreigners outside the United

States and that it did not consider such people to be either prisoners of war or soldiers, but enemy combatants, terrorists, citizens of a failed state, insurgents, or criminals. Therefore, it was permissible to kidnap citizens of other countries and render them to third countries, where they might be tortured, or to places like Guantánamo, where no rights under US or international law applied.

Yet after five US soldiers captured by Iraq during the early part of the 2003 Gulf War were paraded on Iraqi television, US Secretary of Defense Donald Rumsfeld expressed outrage, describing this treatment as degrading and therefore a violation of the Geneva Conventions. "There are international standards that civilized regimes adhere to and then there are regimes like Saddam Hussein['s]." (Rumsfeld 2003). Rumsfeld added that "the Geneva Convention indicates that it's not permitted to photograph and embarrass or humiliate prisoners of war, and if they do happen to be American or coalition ground forces that have been captured, the Geneva Convention indicates how they should be treated" (CBS 2003).

Rumsfeld was right. "Article 13 of the Third Geneva Convention says clearly that prisoners of war must at all times be protected against insult and public curiosity," said Red Cross spokeswoman Nada Doumani. But both the ICRC and Amnesty International (Amnesty 2003) declare that the Geneva Conventions also prohibit "violence to life and person, in particular murder of all kinds, mutilation, cruel treatment and torture; . . . Outrages upon personal dignity, in particular, humiliating and degrading treatment. . . . Prisoners of war who refuse to answer may not be threatened, insulted, or exposed to any unpleasant or disadvantageous treatment of any kind."

Beyond the Geneva Conventions, the United States is signatory to such standards as the Universal Declaration of Human Rights, which states that "no one shall be subjected to torture or to inhuman, cruel, or degrading treatment or punishment," and to the UN Standard Minimum Rules for the Treatment of Prisoners and the Convention Against Torture.

10

Respect for Culture

Maria Kett and *Karen Trollope-Kumar*

CULTURE AND CROSS-CULTURAL COMPETENCY

The ability to effectively take culture into consideration is an essential skill that must be mastered by those who wish to work in cross-cultural settings. Culture influences understandings of health and illness, which in turn influence health-seeking behavior and engagement with health interventions and programs. The purpose of this chapter is to provide the reader with a framework to analyze the importance of culture, both in health-care settings and in situations of violent conflict, by looking at several levels of interaction: individual, community, state, and international. The chapter includes an exploration of the concept of cultural competency and concludes with a discussion of practical ways in which a student or health-care worker may prepare for work in a cross-cultural setting.

Within any given cultural context, there is an array of beliefs and practices, norms and customs. Knowledge of these is acquired through a learning process that begins in childhood, and this knowledge provides meaning, structure, and "ways of being" for members of that culture. A sense of personal identity is often strongly linked to key cultural orientations, and even when the child matures and develops his or her unique identity, the culture of origin still serves as a reference point. Although the many facets of culture have an enduring stability that can be transmitted across generations, they are also dynamic and capable of changing in response to alterations in external circumstances.

Culture includes linguistic, ethnic, and religious components, which are embedded within social, political, historical, and economic contexts. However, we must be careful not to reify culture as a thing in itself (or to associate it merely with superficial customs, etiquette, or superstitions). Nor should we assume that it is homogeneous or that an individual possesses only one culture.[1] Thus there cannot be one "correct" cultural approach to health, and insight into our own and others' cultural values promotes understanding and lowers barriers.

CULTURE, ETHNICITY, AND CONFLICT

Violent conflict is usually deeply rooted in historical and sociopolitical contexts. These roots are sometimes not even apparent to members of the opposing groups. For example, the economy of a country may be undergoing a serious downturn linked to wider sociopolitical forces affecting the global economy. It may not be readily apparent to the citizens of the country that the national economy is being affected by international financial policy. Although the origins of the problem may be obscure, the consequences may be all too apparent, with direct and painful effects on livelihoods. When people feel threatened, the potential for violent conflict is heightened. If the cause of the perceived threat is not readily apparent, people may search for answers in their immediate environment. Two groups living in proximity, and sharing the same resources, may begin to chaff at differences that had previously never been a problem. Perceived cultural differences are often the most obvious and easily identifiable and may be the flashpoint for conflict. Once violent conflict breaks out, the cultural differences tend to be magnified in the eyes of both groups. The difficult work of moving toward common understandings is abandoned as violence escalates. An example of this can be seen in the conflicts across the former Yugoslavia in the 1990s.

Although cultural differences are frequently cited as a source of violent conflict, culture is often a confounding factor in understanding a conflict. Since cultural differences are so apparent, it is far too easy to attribute the conflict to these differences, rather than to look more carefully for the deeper roots of the conflict. This is similar to the process one must undertake when analyzing disparities in health status between cultural groups. It is easier to attribute poor health status to cultural differences than to do the more serious work of analyzing the economic, social, and political inequities that underlie these disparities.[2]

Culture and ethnicity are not synonymous, even though the words are often used interchangeably. Ethnicity has been defined as "a type of cultural collectivity, one that emphasizes the role of myths of descent and historical memories, and that is recognized by one or more cultural differences like religion, customs, language or institutions" (Smith 1991, 20). This definition highlights the subjective nature of ethnicity, in which members of the group consciously identify shared cultural or historical markers in the creation of a collective identity.

At times of conflict, group identity may be strengthened by mobilizing around an awareness of difference. This may be done by telling and retelling the stories of the common myths underlying ethnic identity. Sometimes these stories are deliberately exaggerated (or even fabricated) to foster group solidarity. In an example from the former Yugoslavia, Bowman describes a scene where photographs of skeletons of World War II victims (who actually were from many different ethnic groups) were shown to Slovenes as an example of what "they" (the communists) had done to "them" (the Slovenes). This kind of powerful myth-making led to a rapid strengthening of ethnic identity followed by mobilization toward violent action (Bowman 2001, 41). In Albania, the breakdown of state institutions led to economic disintegration and serious social unrest. In the struggle for power that followed, the dominant ethnic group in the north used "traditionalist" logic to establish its own legitimacy and to justify exclusion of other ethnic groups (Schwandner-Sievers, 2001, 97).

Ethnicity is a social construction, in which there is room for multiple interpretations. In a situation of conflict, ethnic groups may interpret and use their cultures and histories to define themselves and to advance their claims for power and resources. As Eller states, when such groups come into conflict, they are not fighting *about* culture but rather fighting *with* culture (Eller 1999, 48).

STRUCTURAL VIOLENCE AND CULTURE

Violence has not only a direct impact on health and well-being but also indirect and even culturally "acceptable" effects. One way these indirect effects are felt is through structural violence, which occurs whenever people are disadvantaged by political, legal, economic, or cultural traditions. It is often a result of poverty, and it causes suffering and death as often as direct violence does, although the damage is slower, more subtle, more diffuse, more common, and more difficult to repair. Structural violence is nearly always invisible, because it is embedded in ubiquitous social structures and has become normalized by (state) institutions and everyday experience. Because they are long-standing, structural inequities usually seem ordinary—the way things are and always have been.

Because these structures are embedded in social norms, they become accepted as "part of the culture." In what we may call a culture of violence, violence becomes both normative and normal, an expected and culturally sanctioned response to (perceived) threats, and is often inflicted on one another by those suffering most from cultural violence. "Structural

violence—the violence of poverty, hunger, social exclusion and humiliation—inevitably translates into intimate and domestic violence" (Scheper-
Hughes and Bourgois 2004, 1). An example of this comes from the *favelas*
of Brazil, where the poorest people in Brazilian society turn on themselves as much as on those outside of the *favelas* who perpetuate the
inequities that afflict them. In South Africa, the transmission of violence
has been examined from a psychological perspective. Psychologists argue
that violent gang warfare in the townships has been passed on through
succeeding generations of children who have grown up in them (REF).
Psychologists working with the children and their families attempt to reduce this culture of violence.

Others have contended that populations subjected to structural violence are more willing—and more likely—to be manipulated into express-
ing their anger and resentment as murderous rage, as happened in Rwanda
in the 1990s (Uvin 1998). Seen from this perspective, the resulting genocide was linked as much to structural inequalities as to any perceived ethnic (Hutu versus Tutsi) differences, and those perceived differences may
have been emphasised and exaggerated to incite violence.

EXPLORING CULTURAL COMPETENCE

Worldwide, people of diverse cultures meet and interact in ever-increasing
numbers. In health-care settings in Western countries, patients come from
many cultural backgrounds, and health-care providers themselves reflect
diversity. When there is a clash between cultural understandings of health,
serious misunderstandings can arise that may lead to inappropriate diagnosis and treatment. The challenges that occur when a patient and provider come from different cultural background may involve differences
in beliefs, values, and expectations about illness and its treatment. Communication styles vary greatly and can result in significant misinterpretation. Also, the clinical encounter is played out within a cultural context
of disparity in social power, inequity, and racism. These inequalities can
lead to significant health disparity between cultural groups.

The first essential step in the development of culturally appropriate
health care is the awareness that culture counts. The health provider
must understand that cultural differences affect the way health care is
perceived and utilized—and also that the effective provision of health
care across a cultural barrier must take into account the power differences inherent in such encounters. Yet it is not enough simply to be aware
of cultural differences when providing health care. Problem formulation

and management strategies must be culturally congruent to be truly effective. These are the attitudes and skills that underlie the concept of *cultural competence*. One of the first definitions of this term was suggested by mental health researchers, who defined cultural competence as a set of congruent behaviors, attitudes, and policies that come together to work effectively in cross-cultural situations (Cross et al. 1989). Most definitions of cultural competence highlight the importance of valuing diversity, understanding the ways in which cultural differences may affect care, and developing a practical set of skills to maximize the effectiveness of healthcare strategies across a cultural divide. The provider must reflect on his or her own cultural biases and beliefs and must realize that they will affect the cross-cultural encounter.

Cultures and cultural knowledge are dynamic and ever-changing. Just as there is no one single definition of culture, there cannot be an exact definition of cultural competency or any universal guideline on how it should be operationalized in training and best practices (Kleinman and Benson 2006). If cultural competency evolves into a list of "do's and don'ts" for various ethnic groups, then the transactional nature of the clinical encounter may be compromised. Within that encounter, healthcare provider and client need to negotiate a set of common meanings around key health issues. This attention to shared meanings underlies a recent approach for culturally competent care using a "Culture Care Framework" (Srivastava 2007). The health-care provider needs to identify the core values at stake in a given clinical encounter. Provider and patient may then work toward a health-care plan that reflects congruence between the values of the stakeholders.

CROSS-CULTURAL COMMUNICATION

Communicating across a cultural barrier is complex. The most obvious component of communication is language, and when people of two cultures speak different languages, an immediate barrier is created. Interpreters can be of assistance, but there are numerous problems associated with their use.[3] More subtle than language are the barriers created by differences in communication style. Body language is often quite different cross-culturally and can be subject to misinterpretation. Tone of voice and manner of speaking may vary considerably; in one culture loud and rapid speech might indicate interest and engagement in the topic of conversation, whereas in another culture this type of speech might be interpreted as aggressive. Whereas North Americans value direct discussion and questioning for clarification, people from another culture may consider it inappropriate to speak in such a direct manner to someone perceived as an authority. Personal space and the use of touch also vary, and a degree of touching that would be appropriate in one culture may be unacceptable in another.

Culturally sensitive communication is made easier with some preparatory study of the other culture's communication style and a willingness to keep an open mind throughout the communication process. Listening with attention, observing communication patterns, and consulting with a cultural interpreter can all be helpful.

The principles of cross-cultural communication apply both in health work and in the task of peacebuilding. In the health-care setting, provider and client must work toward a common understanding of the illness and a treatment approach that is mutually agreeable. In the process of peacebuilding, particular attention must be paid to the issue of meanings. What values are at stake in the conflict? What might reconciliation look like, for both parties? Working toward common understanding often involves a delicate negotiation of meanings, searching for areas of congruence.

CULTURE, PEACE, AND HEALTH

One premise of Peace through Health work is that health-care workers can be catalysts for peacebuilding work and that this can happen at individual, community, state, and international levels. At the individual level, the health-care worker can attempt to build relationships between two groups in conflict. By becoming familiar with the values, beliefs, and practices of both cultures, the health-care worker is in a good position to build relationships of trust. As she or he opens the lines of communication, conflict between the groups can lessen at the same time that access to health care improves. In Peace through Health initiatives, health-care workers may play key roles in the dual function of conflict reduction and health promotion.

At the community level, health-care workers can be attentive to local forms of conflict resolution. Nearly all cultures have some form of local mechanism for retributive or restorative justice; some have long-held traditions of peacemaking and conflict resolution.[4] Many also have individual and local coping mechanisms and strategies to deal with traumatic events, such as local healing or cleansing rituals. These are an essential part of recovery and rehabilitation, and they are used, for example, when demobilized child soldiers are returned to villages and families in parts of Africa. It is important that health-care workers acknowledge the role these practices play in community and social healing.

Another example is the use of *gacaca* in postconflict Rwanda. These tribunals based on traditional methods of restorative justice were initiated after it became clear that the International Criminal Tribunal for Rwanda[5] would be unable to cope with the sheer volume of cases to be tried. *Gacaca* tribunals are led by *inyangamugayo* ("judges," usually respected men of the community), who chair the debate and decide the sentence if the accused is found guilty (Pham, Weinstein, and Longman 2004).

At the state and international level, there are now a number of approaches looking at peace and health linkages. An interesting initiative designed to integrate cultural sensitivity more effectively into health is the Health and Peace-building Filter developed by a team led by Anthony Zwi at the University of New South Wales (Zwi et al. 2006). Other examples include the World Health Organization's Health as a Bridge to Peace and McMaster University's Peace through Health. The latter is an initiative that is generating interest in the links among culture, peace, and health at both community and international levels.

THE CROSS-CULTURAL ENCOUNTER ABROAD— CULTURE AS CONNECTION

Increasingly, health-care students and providers from the Western world are choosing to travel to remote parts of the world to be involved in study tours or volunteer work. The ability to communicate across a cultural divide can mean the difference between a relevant and useful experience and one that is frustrating for all concerned.

The student or health-care provider who wishes to engage in a meaningful cross-cultural encounter abroad can begin by doing some preparatory work before leaving for the trip. Learning about the culture can perhaps best be done by meeting people from that ethnic background while still in one's country of origin. These people have been acculturated to the West and are in a good position to identify key values and cultural orientations that may affect health services. The traveler will want to learn something about the major health challenges in the country to be visited, as well as to acquire a basic understanding of the country's health system and services. Does biomedicine predominate or is there a pluralistic system of health care? Is health care delivered through private as well as publicly funded services? If the student is traveling to an area of violent conflict, perhaps when working in a Peace through Health initiative, preparation is absolutely essential. Besides learning about the health-care needs of the people, the student must study the conflict situation itself. Learning about the sociopolitical roots of the conflict, and the ways in which various ethnic groups have defined themselves in relation to the violent conflict, will be essential.

Once the health-care worker arrives in the country, the most useful tool he or she can bring is an open and inquiring attitude toward the new environment. More questions arise: Are there health disparities between people of various ethnic groups, and is this contributing to the tensions between the groups? How do communication styles differ? What peacebuilding activities have been tried, and with what success? By asking these questions and working toward mutual understanding, the newcomer can find a path to effective communication.

Cross-cultural encounters are mind-expanding, allowing those who travel to realize that underlying the myriad differences that constitute cultural variation is a common humanity. People all around the world search for love, purpose, meaning, respect, and (perhaps above all) under-standing. This insight is often experienced as a feeling of deep connec-tion to "the other" and can be an extraordinarily powerful moment. Learning to understand is perhaps the most precious gift of international travel and cross-cultural encounters, and it can also lay the foundation for true peacebuilding.

Websites for Cultural Resources

www.ethnicityonline.net/default.htm
A resource from the United Kingdom for building understanding of cross-cultural issues in health care.

www.health.qld.gov.au/multicultural/default.asp
An Australian resource to assist in the development of culturally sensi-tive care in health-care settings.

www.cprn.org/en/diversity.cfm
Presents information on diversity issues from a Canadian perspective.

www.omhrc.gov/clas
Provides information on culturally and linguistically appropriate services (CLAS) in health care (US Department of Health).

REFERENCES

Bowman, G. 2001. The violence in identity. In *Anthropology of violence and conflict*, ed. B. Schmidt. London and New York: Routledge.

Cross, T., B. Bazron, K. Dennis, and M. Isaacs. 1989. Toward a culturally competent system of care. Washington, DC: CAASP Technical Assistance Center, Georgetown University Child Development Center.

Eller, J. R. 1999. *From culture to ethnicity to conflict: An anthropological perspective on international ethnic conflict.* Ann Arbor: University of Michigan Press. Available online at the www.sphcm.med.unsw.edu.au website.

Kleinman, A., and P. Benson. 2006. Anthropology in the clinic: The problem of cultural competency and how to fix it. *PLoS Med* 3 (10): 1673.

Last, J. M. 1997. *Public health and human ecology.* East Norwalk, CT: Appleton & Lange.

Lynch, E., and M. Hanson. 2004. *Developing cross-cultural competence: A guide for working with children and their families.* Baltimore, MD: Paul Brooks Publishing.

Pham, P., H. Weinstein, and T. Longman. 2004. Trauma and PTSD symptoms in Rwanda: Implications for attitudes toward justice and reconciliation. *JAMA* 292 (5): 602–12.

Ramsbotham, O., T. Woodhouse, and H. Miall. 2006. *Contemporary conflict resolution.* 2nd ed. Cambridge: Polity Press.

Scheper-Hughes, N., and P. Bourgois. 2004. Introduction: Making sense of violence. In *Violence in war and peace: An anthology*, ed. Nancy Scheper-Hughes and Philippe Bourgois. Oxford: Blackwell.

Schwandner-Sievers, S. 2001. The enactment of "tradition." In *Anthropology of violence and conflict*, ed. B. Schmidt. London and New York: Routledge.

Smith, A. 1991. *National identity.* Reno: University of Nevada Press.

Srivastava, R., ed. 2007. *The healthcare professional's guide to clinical cultural competence.* Toronto: Mosby Elsevier.

Uvin, P. 1998. *Aiding violence: The development enterprise in Rwanda.* Part III: The condition of structural violence. West Hartford, CT: Kumarian Press.

Wolfe, A. 1994. Contributions of anthropology to conflict resolution. In *Anthropological contributions to conflict resolution*, ed. A. W. Wolfe and H. Yang. Athens and London: The University of Georgia.

Zwi, A., A. Bunde-Birouste, N. Grove, E. Waller, and J. Ritchie. 2006. *The health and peace-building filter and the health and peace-building filter: companion manual.* Sydney: School of Public Health and Community Medicine, University of New South Wales. Available online at the http://healthandconflict.sphcm.med.unsw.edu.au website.

NOTES

1. Avruch (1998), cited in Ramsbotham, Woodhouse, and Miall. 2006.

2. For an excellent analysis of the social determinants of health, see Last 1997.

3. For an excellent discussion of cross-cultural communication issues, see Chapter 3 of Lynch and Hanson 2004.

4. See, for example, Wolfe 1994.

5. The ICTR was established in the aftermath of the brutal conflict that engulfed Rwanda during the early 1990s. It was specifically set up to bring to justice those responsible for breaching international humanitarian law and perpetrating acts of genocide.

11

Speaking Truth to Power: Acting on Values, Ethics, and Rights in South Africa

Wendy Orr

Steve Biko, medical student leader of the South African "Black Consciousness Movement," was arrested on August 6, 1977, and died on September 11 as a result of police beatings. Biko was seen by two district surgeons who were later accused of failing to render adequate attention. At the time these doctors were defended by the Medical Association of South Africa and the South African Medical and Dental Council. One of the two continued to practice as a district surgeon in the Port Elizabeth region until the late 1990s.

More than 70 detainees died in detention between 1960 and 1990, with negligence often an important contributing factor. Believing the nation under attack from communists and radicals, the government continued abusing detainees. A close relationship among the medical association's leadership, the department of health, the security police, and the Medical and Dental Council allowed medical complicity in such acts.

Dr. Wendy Orr graduated from the medical school of the University of Cape Town in 1983. In 1985 she began working as a district surgeon in the medical examiner's office in Port Elizabeth under the direction of Dr. Benjamin Tucker and Dr. Ivor Lang. In July of that year, South Africa declared a state of emergency, and Orr noted that many detainees, credibly and consistently with their physical condition, claimed that they had been tortured. After her superiors failed to take any action despite her repeated reports of severe police abuse of political detainees, Dr. Orr applied to the Supreme Court, ultimately successfully, for a restraining order to protect detainees from police assault. Dr. Orr's testimony was acclaimed worldwide, but at home she suffered anonymous threats and eventually left Port Elizabeth.

In 1995 Orr was appointed by then President Mandela as a Commissioner on the Truth and Reconciliation Commission of South Africa.

She served on the TRC until its dissolution in 1998 and was responsible for its investigating the role of health professionals in human rights abuses. Dr. Orr also assisted with the probe into the participation of military doctors in South Africa's chemical and biological warfare program.

The following is adapted from a speech given by Wendy Orr at McMaster University on April 10, 2002. (Available online at the www.cfpc.ca website.)

—Neil Arya

The South African apartheid health-care system into which I emerged, young, inexperienced, and idealistic, was one in which human rights were denied, ignored, and actively abused—but we never spoke about that in medical school.

We are required to examine prisoners in the presence of a chaperone, supposedly for our own safety, and also to examine prisoners to declare them "fit for punishment." The punishment could be "spare diet" (bread and water), solitary confinement, leg irons, or caning. The first time I have to observe a prisoner being caned, I go directly from the prison to Dr Lang's office.

"I can't do this," I say. "It's absolutely horrific." "Don't expect any special treatment in this department, just because you're a woman," he replies.

I refuse to watch any more canings, and the prison authorities ensure that canings are scheduled for days when I am not on duty.

I fall into bed with a sense of despair and hopelessness. I am twenty-four years old. I have spent seven years studying and training to be a doctor, but what I am doing feels absolutely wrong. It feels like betrayal. But the other doctors I work with seem to find it acceptable. District surgeons all over the country do this every day. Who will understand my discomfort? Who will support me if I decide to abandon my contract?

So, long before I took a stand on the issue of torture and assault of political detainees, I was grappling with perhaps more mundane, less dramatic, but nevertheless deeply troubling infringements of human rights. I was young, I was inexperienced, I felt unsupported, I did not know what to do.

A state of emergency, declared in July 1985, allowed for detention, without charge, of anyone perceived to be a "threat to the safety and security of the State," for an initial period of 14 days, subject to extension. Within a week, hundreds of people had been detained.

As part of my routine prison work, I now had to see hundreds of detainees for routine admission examinations and, if they had a specific complaint, as part of the daily sick parades. From the first day that I started working with detainees, I was overwhelmed by the number who showed me fresh injuries at their admission examinations: bruises, lacerations, sjambok[1] marks, abrasions, ruptured eardrums, and swollen joints and limbs. When I asked them what had happened, they all, without fail, said they had been assaulted by the police either at the time of or immediately after arrest. Others had no complaints on admission but were removed by Security Police to police headquarters for questioning. They returned to prison with horrendous injuries and reported that they had been tortured during interrogation.

I duly recorded the injuries and allegations of assault and torture, prescribed appropriate treatment, and requested that the allegations be investigated. Nothing happened. I reported my concerns to Dr. Lang. His attitude was that it was not our responsibility to do anything other than treat the injuries. I spoke to the head of the prison. His response was a remarkable comment (I paraphrase): "It's the police who are beating these people up, not us; all we have to do is house and feed them."

By the end of August that year it became clear to me that complaints via conventional channels were unlikely to put a stop to the daily parade of pain and injury that I was seeing at the prisons. Looking back, I realize how frighteningly easy it would have been for me to stop there. I had tried, I had spoken to those in positions of authority. What else could I do? Nothing I had been taught had prepared me for this. Surely no one could have condemned me for going no further. If action really was required, why had no other district surgeons, anywhere in South Africa, done anything? Maybe I was being naïve in my belief that it was my duty to do something.

The situation was exacerbated by the fact that, because district surgeons are often marginalized by their medical colleagues (and I certainly felt isolated and marginalized), it was tempting to adopt the culture of those who did affirm and support me: prison and police staff. What made my position even more intolerable was that the detainees saw me as part of "the system" and viewed me with distrust and dislike. Thus, the patients, to whom I owed primary responsibility, displayed distrust and hostility; peers and colleagues to whom I might have turned for support and advice were disparaging. A natural response seemed to be to embrace those who were, in fact, intimately involved in the system that was the source of my clinical conflict: police and prison personnel.

Through a serendipitous confluence of events and associations, however, I was put in touch with a well-known human rights lawyer from Johannesburg. He presented me with two options: I could continue being the "good" doctor, recording and treating injuries but doing nothing to prevent them, or I could do something that no district surgeon had done before (or has done since): take my evidence to the Supreme Court and seek an urgent interdict to prevent police from assaulting and torturing detainees.

Once I had been offered what appeared to be an effective way of ensuring that the assaults and torture would diminish, I really had no choice. I could not abandon my patients to the brutality of the Port Elizabeth Security Police, believing that I had an opportunity to do something that could make a real difference. So, after a few days of reflection, I agreed to go ahead with the Supreme Court interdict. I concluded my affidavit, which was submitted to the Supreme Court on September 24, 1985, with the following.

"As a result of my experience, described above, I have felt morally and professionally bound to bring this application. The main considerations that have prompted me to do so are the following:

There seems to me to be an extensive pattern of police abuse upon detainees held under the emergency regulations. . . .

What disturbs me most is that detainees are being taken out of my care for the purposes of interrogation and, during the course of this interrogation, brutally assaulted. . . .

The medical services of the prisons have been unable to cope with the vast numbers of detainees. They are, in my view, not getting the proper medical care to which they are entitled and which I feel professionally and morally bound to provide them.

It has become clear to me that the complaints of police assaults are not being investigated, as they should be. . . .

I gain the impression that, because the police are acting under the emergency regulations, and because they apparently believe that they enjoy an immunity under those regulations, they or some of them are quite unrestrained in the abuses that they inflict upon detainees. . . .

It ultimately became clear to me that, unless I made a stand and did something about the plight of the detainees, I would be compromising my moral beliefs and my perception of my professional responsibility. My conscience told me that I could no longer stand by and do nothing. . . .

What happened thereafter is now well known: the interdict was granted, assaults and torture in that area were reduced dramatically, and I was completely sidelined and prevented from doing any work that could be interpreted as vaguely politically sensitive. I eventually resigned and moved to Johannesburg.

When I had agreed to participate in the Supreme Court application, I had had no idea of what would ensue. It changed my life forever. Overnight, I became worldwide headline news; a hero and a traitor; an object of praise and of vilification; a recipient of bouquets and of death threats.

Over the last twenty years, the question that I have been asked most frequently is "Why did you finally act? What was it about you or your training that led you to take the steps you did?" That is not an easy question to answer. I suppose the visit from the lawyer was a catalyst. It forced me to confront my understanding of my responsibilities. There was also an element of "this far and no farther." After eight months of witnessing unethical and abusive practice, I could keep silent no longer. Undoubtedly my upbringing played an important role. I was raised in a fairly average white middle-class family, but one in which prejudice and discrimination were constantly challenged; where we had a strong sense of right and wrong, a conception of justice and injustice; and the firm knowledge that apartheid was unjust and immoral. I cannot say that my medical education at the University of Cape Town had much to do with it—and that is a terrible indictment. Ultimately, though, I came terrifyingly close to not doing anything—and that thought still haunts me.

On the wall of my study, I have a copy (stamped Top Secret) of a report completed by a doctor who visited Steve Biko while he was in detention. These weekly visits were required by law for all Section 29 detainees. After the visit, a report was sent to the regional police commissioner and the Department of

Justice. What purpose this served, I have no idea. Certainly government offi-cials used the existence of this statutory requirement to maintain that detainees were well looked after. The standard reporting form has a section headed: "Die aangehoudende het die volgende klagtes geopper" (The detainee made the following complaints). In this particular report, Steve Biko is quoted as saying, "I ask for water to wash myself with and also soap, a washing cloth and a comb. I want to be allowed to buy food. I live on bread only here. Is it compulsory for me to be naked? I am naked since I came here."

Long before Steve Biko was tortured and assaulted and killed by security police, his fundamental human rights were violated, his humanity denied. The doctor who saw him did nothing, although all that was required was to order that he be allowed to wash, dress, and eat.

And, ironically, it was this same Steve Biko, not long before his final deten-tion, who had spoken of his vision for South Africa: "In time, we shall be in a position to bestow on South Africa the greatest possible gift: a more human face." If Steve Biko's doctors had shown him that human face, he would prob-ably be alive today. We too can always hold in the forefront of our minds the need for that human face, for human dignity, to triumph.

NOTE

1. A sjambok is a rubber whip, thick at the bottom and thinner at the top. It was com-monly used by police at that time for crowd control.

PART IV

Preparing to Act on
Peace through Health

12

Analyzing a
Peace through Health Problem

Joanna Santa Barbara

Imagine you are facing a problem with both peace and health dimensions, such as the three scenarios presented in Chapter 1. Perhaps you are the health worker facing high youth suicide in an aboriginal community that has a conflictual relationship with the dominant culture, or the physician noting high levels of gun violence in emergency admissions, or a member of the team helping to reconstruct a health system after deadly interethnic conflict. Where do you start?

DIAGNOSIS, PROGNOSIS, THERAPY

We referred in Chapter 1 to three terms familiar in health care and equally applicable to peacework (Galtung 2000, 118). You need a dual **diagnosis,** both of the health issues you propose to address and of the conflict situation. The latter will be provided by the conflict analysis. The **prognosis** in this context is the likely course of events with no intervention. The possibility of recovery of good function with no outside interference should be considered. However, in most violent situations, this seems unlikely. The **"therapy"** is the formula for improving the current situation in both health and peace, at whatever stage of conflict is current. The task of the peace-health worker or team is to consider how input on health problems may simultaneously contribute to moving the social dynamic in the direction of peace. It is fairly obvious that improvement in peace will improve health.

HEALTH NEEDS ANALYSIS

It makes sense to begin with an understanding of the health deficits of the region you are focusing on. Once you have an overview of its deficits and needs, you may engage with a particular kind of health problem: tuberculosis, hearing problems, diabetes, gunshot wounds, mental health problems, low rates of child immunization, the aftermath of war-related rape, and AIDS are the bases of various Peace through Health projects. Other projects have to do with the large-scale rebuilding of health-care systems as a whole, in the aftermath of war.

A decision about where to invest efforts and resources should be made only after extensive input from partners of the region, even if you yourself are native to the region. We shall say more about partnership shortly.

There are various methodologies of health needs analysis. The area has been well developed over many decades, and this text will not expand on the subject.

It is highly likely that the violence in the situation has had an impact on the health problems you are examining. It will be helpful to try to trace the linkage. Very often, war worsens poverty in an area. It reduces resources spent by governments on health care, and it reduces family incomes available to be spent on nutrition, sanitation, and health care. It may be that clinics were destroyed, health workers have fled, and health supplies cannot get through to the area. Structural violence too reduces the access of groups and populations to basic requirements for health. In fact, population differences in health indices such as infant mortality may be telling indicators of structural violence.

ANALYSIS OF PEACE DEFICITS

You now need to do an analysis of peace deficits. Let us return to the definition of peace introduced earlier. Peace is an attribute of a relationship between two or more entities in which, at least, no harm is being done to any party, and conflicts are resolved nonviolently. At most, it is a harmonious relationship of mutual benefit and cooperation. We can now consider the peace deficits. What relationships are falling short of mutual benefit and cooperation? Who is doing harm to whom?

For example, in the scenarios in the first chapter, we can identify which relationships involve harm. In the first scenario, the relationship between the aboriginals and the dominant society is characterized by a long history in which aboriginals have seen themselves as harmed by the others. We will look for racism against the aboriginals in the dominant society as an aspect of cultural violence which fosters the structural and the occasional direct violence.

The second scenario is more complex. The war in the Central American country ended six years ago, but the structural inequities that were part of its cause have not been addressed. Conflict between elements of society continues, and firearms are easily available to translate these conflicts into violence.

In the third scenario, although the direct violence is at an end, there has been no reconciliation. There is still overt hatred of the other ethnic groups. There is certainly no relationship of mutual benefit and cooperation.

You will be aware of deficits in peaceful relationships if you are working in a war zone, and very likely if you are working in an immediate postwar situation with incomplete resolution of the original conflict and incomplete reconciliation. In situations of impending violence and of structural violence, you may need to look harder to see where the peace deficits lie.

Your next task is to delineate the violence in the situation.

VIOLENCE ANALYSIS

We have already distinguished among direct, structural, and cultural violence. Let us now attempt a finer-grained analysis, which could be applied to the above scenarios.

Direct violence will be measured in terms of deaths (both military and civilian), of injuries, and of disabilities. The injuries and disabilities may be physical or mental. The latter may involve mental illness (such as depression or posttraumatic stress disorder) or sadness and loss of confidence after seeing the destruction of all that was meaningful in life.

Direct violence also includes damage to the health-sustaining infrastructure of a society, such as housing, roads, water and sewage systems, energy for heating and lighting, health clinics, hospitals, and schools. Damage to capacity to sustain immunization programs causes large increases in childhood deaths during war.

Direct violence may be done to health-sustaining ecosystems, as in the defoliation of forests and the pollution of land and water with toxic war materiel, and of air when factories with toxic products are bombed.

Direct violence may also be spread over time, with land mines and cluster munitions remaining to kill and injure years later, when children play in the area or farmers till the fields.

Structural violence, the oppression, exploitation, or exclusion of a portion of a population, may have something to do with causing the direct violence, as in the aboriginal land claims scenario and the small arms violence scenario. It may be systemic in a "war economy," a situation in which an armed faction (government or rebel) maintains control over a valuable natural resource, such as gold or timber, and uses the wealth produced to fund an army in order to hold on to that control. The rest of the population, which ought to benefit from the natural resource, is impoverished.

During and after wars, displaced people and refugees are often vulnerable, disadvantaged populations. Their state of oppression and powerlessness makes them targets for direct violence.

Cultural violence is likely to be a major issue fueling a current conflict, with dehumanization of the "other," dulling the conscience of those engaged in killing and injuring men, women, and children. Culture also is a determinant in the tendency of some states to believe that "strength" (seen as a highly desirable quality) is shown in aggressive actions in response to conflict, as opposed to dialogue, or concessions to relieve legitimate grievances.

Harm can be done *to* culture in the course of war. Ethical standards may decay in quickly escalating privation, where people are desperate. They may steal from each other, from the state, or from common property in ways that would never occur in peace time. A culture that had previously embodied acceptance of various ethnicities may harden into one with barriers between the ethnic groups. This is, at least for now, the fate of Sarajevo, once a famously multiethnic city, now a place of insecure ethnic ghettos.

AGE OF CONFLICT

Behind violence, whether past, present, or future, there is likely to be conflict. Let's begin by seeking to understand what phase of conflict we are dealing with.

Conflicts begin in greed or grievances. There is a phase in which the grievance comes to the surface of shared awareness and is expressed as discontent. Grievances may involve disputes over territory or resources, over identity (a wish to secede from another country), over poor governance (a wish to get rid of a ruler or government), or over revenge for perceived harm. Greed may be over acquisition of more land or over control of a valuable resource.

This stage, of course, is the time at which conflict could be dealt with peacefully. Often this is exactly what happens, but in some cases it does not. Sometimes this is due to a lack of democratic process or to a militaristic culture unfamiliar with nonviolent ways to deal with conflict. Sometimes it is because those whose interests are served by war are the same people who have the power to decide on war. Arms manufacturers

Figure 12.1 Cycle of Violent Conflict

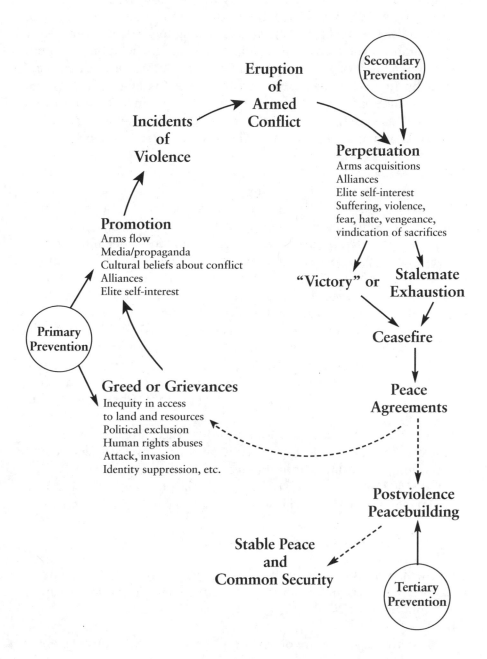

and traders, or politicians whose popularity will increase with population fears during war, for example, may benefit from war.

There are well-known ways of fomenting war. Having influential people spread dehumanizing propaganda devaluing the "enemy" is a widely used technique. The media are an important tool for whipping up public opinion in favor of war. Patriotic rallies and marches may be arranged. Eventually an incident of violence breaks out, providing a pretext to go to war. In some cases an incident or circumstance is invented to provide this pretext, as in the supposed presence of nuclear weapons in Iraq prior to the 2003 attack on that country. The next step is full-blown war, with all its complexity and horrors.

There are many factors that perpetuate wars—arms supplies, allies to reinforce fighting forces, the feeling that the fighting must continue in order to vindicate the deaths that have already occurred, the aversion of politicians to admitting they made a mistake.

Eventually war ends, although modern wars tend to be more drawn out than previously, lasting eight years on average (Collier et al. 2003, 82). War may end in a stalemate or in victory for one side, but it is most unlikely to have resolved the conflict that started it in the first place. There will be peace talks about how this resolution is to be reached and what institutional arrangements it might entail. A ceasefire and peace talks should be regarded as only the beginning of peace. The hard work is yet to be done: forging the peace, building the institutions of peace, reconciling the damaged relationships, rebuilding the destroyed infrastructure both physical (for example, hospitals) and institutional (for example, judicial system).

If this is done well, the area will enter stable peace; if badly, a recurrence of war can be expected. In fact, there is an over 40 percent chance of a country going back into war in the five years following a ceasefire (Collier et al. 2003, 83). Figure 12.1 also depicts the points at which primary, secondary, and tertiary prevention, as explained in Chapter 1, apply.

CONFLICT ANALYSIS

After identifying the stage of the conflict, the analysis will examine its dynamics. There are many schemes of conflict analysis. Here is a simple one (Santa Barbara 2004).

> **Who** are the parties involved? Look beyond the obvious players to see who might be pulling strings behind the scenes.

What is it about, for each of the principal parties? Again, look deeply. Leaders frequently present a pretext for war when the real reasons are hidden. What are their real goals? Which goals are **legitimate** and which are not? There may be legitimate goals on all sides, as well as illegitimate ones.

Why is violence or war happening? What is the history of the conflict?

What has made it worse? What efforts have been made to mitigate it? What **attitudes** and assumptions are part of the conflict?

How is this conflict handled? What harm are the parties inflicting on one another?

What are the **power dynamics** in this conflict? Who has **coercive** power, **reward** power, **persuasive** power, the power to **impede**?

What next? What will happen if nothing is done? What are the strengths and possibilities of this situation? Are there opportunities arising in the situation? What might help?

For example, in one of the scenarios in Chapter 1, a health worker is engaged in humanitarian assistance to earthquake victims in a region torn by civil war. It will be most important for the worker to acquire understanding of the parties to this conflict and of the goals that fueled the violence. The worker will need to probe for the history of the conflict and for the attitudes and cultural elements that underlie it. Where were arms coming from? What are the power dynamics? How has the earthquake changed these dynamics? Who was trying to move in peaceful directions? It will be important to arrange the humanitarian aid in ways that are not seen as favoring one group over another. Better still, there may be ways of bringing people together in the emergency situation to work for the superordinate goal of saving lives on all sides. Something like this happened in Aceh after the tsunami of 2004. In the aftermath, a civil war ended (Renner and Chafe 2007).

THE LINK BETWEEN WAR AND HEALTH PROBLEMS

Peace through Health work can be done during all conflict stages. Sometimes health problems, when examined from a population health perspective, may indicate the marginalization of a population group—their consignment to lower levels of human rights. This dynamic may be part of a set of grievances leading toward violent conflicts. Health professionals might therefore work to reduce health inequalities.

At other times, health workers are engaged in alleviating the impacts of direct violence on a population caught in war, or in dealing with the impacts of war on health infrastructure—for example, water-borne diseases. Peace through Health work is also done in the stage of reconstruction of health and other social systems in the postwar phase, after the worst of the direct violence has ended.

WORKING IN A TEAM

Teams working on Peace through Health problems are often made up of those with a passion to make some difference to a situation of suffering. As you begin to create ideas around the sort of work you might do together, you will identify whom you need to complement your team, in terms of health, cultural, and peace expertise. If possible, include students on your team. Such work makes wonderful learning opportunities for suitable students—and for you at the same time.

The team will need to consider its vision, mission, and objectives and reflect on how to balance skill-sets in distributing the workload and determining roles (Wikipedia 2006a). In many situations, the first team task is to develop a proposal to try to get funding.

It is wise to attend to the process of team functioning. Many teams operate best with **consensus decision making** (Kaner 1996). In this process, every voice is heard and respected, including those of students. Decisions, except for emergencies, are worked on until consensus is reached. Each team meeting may benefit from a facilitator and someone to take minutes. Complex teams need more structure than this, including a coordinator—someone who makes sure everyone is doing their agreed-upon tasks in a timely way and who is receiving all the relevant information. Large teams need project managers with organizational expertise. Good communication among all team members is vital.

Whether small or large, a team needs at least one person who monitors the emotional tone of the team, either informally or formally. Some groups designate a "vibe-watcher" for this purpose. A team also will do well to agree on a way to deal with conflicts as they arise. The work done by groups in the area of Peace through Health is often highly stressful. The potential effects of this should be anticipated and planned for. Building trust between team members through accumulated experience of good functioning is extremely important, and will be crucial to a team's ability to deal with stresses.

FORMING YOUR PARTNERSHIPS

If you are working in any situation other than your home turf (where there may indeed be Peace through Health problems), you will need to form partnerships with groups who share your goals. This is normally done in one or more "site visits," in which the potential for collaboration is explored. Some of the same considerations that are relevant to maintaining a good team apply equally to building good partnerships. Equality is an important dimension of partnerships, especially in relating to partners in low-income regions, where resources for action and salaries of workers may be low. Building trust through trustworthy behavior is critical. Some of these qualities are dealt with well in the Peacebuilding Filter discussed in the next chapter.

SWOT ANALYSIS

SWOT analysis is a widely used tool for teams of all kinds, from business to sports (Wikipedia 2006b). It is a simple team exercise. The acronym stands for Strengths, Weaknesses, Opportunities, and Threats. After clarifying objectives as far as is possible at this early stage in the work, the team assesses its **strengths** in terms of assets of various kinds in its members. In this case those assets will be knowledge, skills, and values. It may seem obvious to assess strengths in knowledge and skills. The team needs to have these dimensions matched against the sort of work it envisions itself doing. Values may be unspoken, but they will be what drives the team, what unifies it, and what holds it together under stress. It may be useful to make them explicit. In this work, the values that motivate team members are often compassion for suffering, justice for those unfairly treated, a belief in the intrinsic and equal dignity of all humans, a belief in the right to health, and the principle of nonviolence.

The team identifies **weaknesses** in knowledge and skills and considers whether to address these deficits by training or by recruiting new members. Some teams may need more knowledge of peace processes. This weakness is being ameliorated by the development of Peace through Health education, and teams may be much enhanced by having a team member who is expert in the area.

Having looked inward for this audit, the team then looks outward to the environment in which it works. It identifies **opportunities.** Perhaps the team has been invited to work by a body capable of facilitating its goals. Perhaps funding has become available for the kind of work the team aspires to do.

The team must assess **threats**. In Peace through Health work, threats to the security of team members are prominent, since some of the work takes place in war zones, or zones of recent war, where arms are still widely distributed.

DEVELOPING YOUR PROGRAM IDEA

It is obvious that each situation is unique and that human creativity is limitless. You may benefit from knowledge of the several case histories of Peace through Health work throughout this book. In a situation of rapidly changing dynamics such as a postwar zone, unforeseen opportunities may arise during the course of the project. The team will have the task of assessing each opportunity as it comes up, looking for the "peace potential" inherent in it, and considering whether the team is equal to the challenges likely to be involved.

APPLYING ACCUMULATED UNDERSTANDING TO PEACE THROUGH HEALTH WORK

At an early stage in developing program or project ideas, the team would do well to conduct a proper assessment of the context and possible impacts. Previous work, especially in zones of violent conflict, has led to significant understanding of how to work well—and how to avoid mistakes. Three tools for analysis are presented in the next chapter: the Peace and Conflict Impact Analysis (PCIA), the Do No Harm instrument, and the Peacebuilding Filter.

REFERENCES

Collier, Paul, V. L. Elliott, Havard Hegre, Anke Hoeffler, Marta Reynal-Querol, and Nicholas Sambanis. 2003. *Breaking the conflict trap: Civil war and development policy*. Copublication of the World Bank and Oxford University Press.

Galtung, Johan. 2000. *Conflict transformation by peaceful means*. United Nations Disaster Management Program.

Kaner, Sam. 1996. *Facilitator's guide to participatory decision-making*. Gabriola Island, British Columbia: New Society Publishers.

Renner, Michael, and Zoe Chafe. 2007. *Beyond disasters: Creating opportunities for peace*. Washington, DC: Worldwatch Institute.

Santa Barbara, Joanna. 2004. Conflict analysis. In *Making peace: A peace education manual for Afghanistan,* ed. G. MacQueen. Available online at the www.humanities.mcmaster.ca website.

Wikipedia. 2006a. Team building. Available online at the en.wikipedia.org website.

———. 2006b. SWOT analysis. *Note:* Nearly all descriptions of the SWOT analysis tool have to do with applying it in the business sphere. The Wikipedia treatment is the most generic. Available online at the en.wikipedia.org website.

13

Tools for Peace through Health Work

As described in the last chapter, those working in the field of peace and development have developed several tools that can be most useful in Peace through Health projects. These are the **Peace and Conflict Impact Assessment,** the **Do No Harm** instrument and the **Peacebuilding Filter.** There is some overlap between these tools, but valuable differences occur in each. The PCIA focuses particularly on the environment in which the work will occur, examining the impact of the project on the environment and the impact of the environment on the project. It asks whether the time and place and circumstances are appropriate, and it systematically examines the impact of the work on various aspects of the society in which it will take place (political, military, socioeconomic) and the impact on partners. It looks for risks and opportunities, especially opportunities for building peace.

The Do No Harm tool also closely examines the impact of the project on local conflict dynamics and sharpens alertness for peace potential. The Do No Harm material draws on a wealth of case studies illustrating positive and negative impacts of various projects on conflict situations.

The Peacebuilding Filter directs attention to the qualities the team brings to the work, in terms of cultural sensitivity and good governance within the project. It then directs attention to the interface of the project with its environment in terms of sensitivity to the conflict and to issues of social justice and social cohesion.

It is useful for team members to have background knowledge of the literature on PCIA, Do No Harm, and the Peacebuilding Filter and to apply these tools before, during (at intervals), and after the project or program.

Peace and Conflict Impact Assessment ■ Kenneth Bush

PEACE AND CONFLICT IMPACT ASSESSMENT (PCIA) is a means of anticipating, monitoring, assessing, and managing the ways in which an intervention may affect, or has affected, the dynamics of peace or conflict in a region prone to violent conflict. Space restrictions limit our ability to delve substantively into the details of this particular approach to the integration of peace and conflict considerations into our work. However, the reader is encouraged to sift through the Dialogue Series on PCIA located on the website for the Berghof Research Center for Constructive Conflict Management.[1]

THE POLITICS OF METHOD

When it comes to evaluation tools and methodologies, there is a tendency for discussion to free-fall into the technical and descriptive. The question of "How" smothers the question of "Why." And in this process, issues of politics—that is, issues of power, control, interests, and money—disappear from sight. One of the consequences of not being sensitive to the fundamentally political underpinnings of mechanistically rendered evaluation tools is the unwitting support for structures and processes that one would cringe to be associated with in the hard light of day—in particular, the use of evaluation as a means of disempowering (and overpowering) partners in the Global South and communities in the areas where we work.

The greatest challenge to the genuine and systematic incorporation of peace and conflict impact assessment into our work is not technical or methodological but overwhelmingly *political*. It is about who will control an initiative.[2] It is about who decides: the questions that will get asked (or not); the stakeholders who will be included or excluded; the uses to which an evaluation will be put; and, of course, who gets paid, how much they are paid, and what they get paid for. In order to sensitize practitioners to political realities of the development industry, I will frame the issue in terms that are overstated and dichotomous: the answers to these questions will determine whether the results of an assessment will benefit those who have implemented an initiative or those upon whom an initiative has been implemented.

Formal and informal expertise in interpreting and understanding peace and conflict impacts rests (currently and ultimately) with those closest to the ground in the Global South. However, even the most cursory google for PCIA-related information illustrates the ways in which claims of professionalized expertise by Northern actors (consultants, private sector companies, bilateral development workers, NGOs, researchers, evaluators, and so on) marginalize and, indeed, appropriate the authentic expertise that resides in those living and dying in violent conflict zones around the world.

PCIA is not rocket science. It is based on observations of the ways in which partners in the Global South work within violence-prone, militarized conflict zones. Building on these field-based observations, simple ideas can be applied in fluid and complex settings, from the corridors of power within bilateral and multilateral organizations, to the footpaths and fields within which community-based organizations work.

Since every intervention in a conflict-prone area will *inevitably* affect the dynamics of peace and conflict, some kind of PCIA will be required every time. The factor that determines whether or not to "do" a PCIA is whether or not the host environment is prone to violent conflict. It is not determined by the type of project. That is, it is just as important for an irrigation project in Eastern Sri Lanka as it is for a "peacebuilding project" in Guatemala.

COMPONENTS OF PCIA

PCIA is composed of three parts: (1) peace and conflict stakeholder mapping, (2) assessment of the impact of the peace and conflict environments on an initiative, and (3) the impact of an initiative on the structures and processes in a conflict.

Peace and Conflict Mapping

This exercise helps develop an understanding of the complex and fluid structures and processes of conflict in the environment surrounding an initiative (from micro to macro levels). In addition to developing a baseline understanding of levels of conflict, this exercise always points to the multiplicity of conflicts: social, political, militarized, economic, historical, interpersonal, intergroup, inter- and intra-organizational, and so on. Sometimes they intersect, sometimes not. Sometimes they involve violence, sometimes not. One particularly important dimension of this mapping exercise is that it opens up the possibility of understanding and anticipating when, why, and how nonviolent conflict *turns* violent. This is essential if efforts are to be made to avoid (that is, to increase the chances of avoiding) conflict-aggravating components of an intervention. The complementary process of mapping peace stakeholders allows the possibility of doing more than not exacerbating a conflict. It opens up possibilities for contributing actively to the nurturing of peace. If nothing else, this exercise cautions against a one-dimensional understanding of conflicts. Such a limited perspective ignores the panoply of actors, the many fluid and varied ways they sustain peace or conflict structures and processes, and the fundamental importance of understanding the thick details of inter- and intragroup relationships.

Risk and Opportunity Assessment (ROA): Impact of the Peace and Conflict Environment on an Initiative

ROA is a process of reviewing the ways in which the peace and conflict environments may affect—or may have affected—an intervention positively and negatively. This is more than standard risk assessment, which asks, "What are the risks to an intervention that would inhibit it from achieving its stated objectives?" In such conventional assessments, the central reference is the a priori objectives of the initiative, not peace or conflict impacts. See Table 13.1.

Peace and Conflict Impact Assessment: Impact of an Initiative on the Peace and Conflict Environment

The final component is "PCIA proper": the process of assessing the ways in which an initiative may affect—or may have affected—the dynamics of peace or violence (potentially, from micro to macro levels). Table 13.2 offers one structure for conceptualizing this process.

How do you know whether an initiative is having positive peace-building impacts? To ensure that an initiative will have a positive peace-building and developmental impact, it should be possible to answer "yes" to the following two questions:

1. Is the initiative increasing the capacities of participants—particularly Southerners—to (a) identify the real and potential peace and violence impacts of an intervention; and (b) formulate and implement their own solutions nonviolently and effectively?
2. Is the initiative built on a partnership that leads toward genuine ownership by Southern partners?

In the field, one quickly realizes that there is no silver bullet—no one blanket solution to address all problems—and that these deceptively simple

Table 13.1 Risk and Opportunity Assessment

		Direction of Impact: Impact of Peace and Conflict Environment on Initiative		
How might conflict escalation or positive peacebuilding efforts (social, political, economic, military, interorganizational) hinder or promote an initiative?				
Risk Level (Low, Medium, or High)	Risks	Issue Area/ Key Factors	Opportunities	Opportunity Level (Low, Medium, or High)
		Location		
		Timing		
		Political Context		
		Military Context		
		Sociocultural Context		
		Economic Context		
		Partners/ Stakeholders		
		Other		
How might these factors threaten the effectiveness/ and/or efficiency of the initiative?			*How might these factors open opportunities to increase the effectiveness and/or efficiency of the initiative?*	
Violence Mitigation/ Management Strategies • What can you do to avoid/ reduce/plan for negative conflict impacts on the initiative? • Rank these risks.			Opportunity Optimization • How can you take advantage of peace opportunities? • What changes are needed before starting or continuing? • Is more information needed? How can you get it?	

questions can be answered "yes" requires an examination of a broad and complex set of issues that are guaranteed to slow initiatives down, increase ambiguity about the process and outcomes of an initiative, and raise awkward political questions of control. But if these are the costs of undertaking PCIA, the costs of not undertaking it are even higher.

Table 13.2 Peace and Conflict Impact Assessment

Direction of Impact: Impact of Initiative on Peace and Conflict Environment				
How might an initiative hinder or promote conflict escalation or positive peacebuilding efforts (social, political, economic, military, interorganizational)?				
Indicators and Impact Level (Low, Medium, or High)	Conflict Impacts	Impact Areas	Peace Impacts	Indicators and Impact Level (Low, Medium, or High)
How might an initiative affect surrounding conflicts in the following impact areas?		Violence Management Capacities	*How might an initiative affect the opportunities for peace/violence management in the following impact areas?*	
		Physical and Human Security	Opportunity Optimization	
		Political Structures and Processes	• How can you take advantage of peace opportunities? • What changes are needed before starting or continuing? • Is more information needed? How can you get it?	
		Economic Structures and Processes		
		Social Impacts/ Empowerment		
Violence Mitigation/ Management Strategies • What can you do to avoid/ reduce/plan for negative conflict impacts *created or worsened by* the initiative? • Rank these risks.			Opportunity Optimization • How can you optimize peace opportunities of the initiative? • What changes are needed before starting or continuing? • Is more information needed? How can you get it?	

NOTES

1. Particularily useful for those interested in linking ideas to practice is the "Hands-On Manual" for conducting PCIAs, which is available on the website as an appendix to my contribution entitled: "FIELD NOTES: Fighting Commodification and Disempowerment in the Development Industry: Things I Learned about Peace and Conflict Impact Assessment (PCIA) in Habarana and Mindanao," in *The Berghof Handbook for Conflict Transformation*, ed. David Bloomfield, Martina Fischer, and Beatrix Schmelzle

(Berlin: Berghof Research Center for Constructive Conflict Management, 2005). See the berghof-center.org website.

2. This is addressed in my contributions to both rounds of the Berghof PCIA debates/dialogues cited above.

Do No Harm[1] ▪ Marshall Wallace

THE DO NO HARM PROJECT was begun in 1994 by the Collaborative for Development Action (as the Local Capacities for Peace Project) to help agencies working in areas of violent conflict learn how to provide humanitarian or development assistance in ways that would avoid exacerbating violence and heightening tensions and, instead, help people find ways to transform conflict. The Project is a collaborative effort, involving NGOs (international and local, UN agencies, and donor countries).

The Do No Harm Project has learned a number of lessons about how assistance interacts with conflict and has developed an analytical framework to assist people in thinking through their impacts on conflict.

1. When assistance is brought into a context of conflict, the assistance becomes a part of that context and a part of the conflict. Even though assistance agencies strive to remain neutral as to the outcome of the conflict, the impact of their aid in that context is never neutral.

Assistance workers have found it useful to keep this reality in mind in order to make sure they design and implement programs that not only are impartial, but also are seen as impartial. They have found it important to remember that local actors do not always see assistance agencies in the same way the agencies see themselves.

When war erupted in Bosnia, international NGOs partnered with already existing local NGOs. Many of the local NGOs were faith-based, and some international NGOs that wanted to appear "even-handed" earmarked their donations specifically to serve the ethnicity associated with these local NGOs. (That is, they gave to the Catholic NGO for Croatians, the Orthodox NGO for Serbs, the Muslim NGO for Muslims, and the Jewish NGO for Jews). In later discussions, leaders of the local NGOs said these donations had forced them to appear too partisan in a situation where they wanted to reaffirm solidarity and a broad humanitarianism.

2. Conflicts are characterized by two sets of factors:

Dividers/Tensions. Conflicts are always characterized by intergroup divisions and tensions that provide reasons for and provoke violence. *Connectors/Local Capacities for Peace.* Conflicts are also characterized by links between people and groups and by efforts to move away from violence.[2]

Assistance workers have found it useful to analyze the contexts in which they work, identifying the dividers and connectors in order to see how their programs interact with the context. In addition, assistance workers have found it useful to remember that violence is not normal and that the vast majority of people in conflict situations are not participating in the violence.

Health services often represent a connector or potential connector. In war situations, many people believe that all sides should have access to health care. Working with this connector, UNICEF has often been able to arrange ceasefires during which health service agencies can inoculate children.

3. Assistance, through the way it is provided, has an impact on both dividers and connectors. That impact can be negative, reinforcing divisions or undermining connections. Or it can be positive, providing opportunities to reduce divisions and support connections.

Assistance workers have found it useful to think about how their work directly relates to and interacts with dividers and connectors.

In Southern Sudan, when the rebel movement split into two factions in the early 1990s, an aid agency that wanted to appear unbiased redesigned its health training program to include two training centers.

> *We rewarded the split by doubling the resources we provided! Because we know health is the one sector where international agencies were allowed to operate across lines, I believe we did not have to do this. I wonder what would have happened if we had continued with our original plan of one center. I suspect we would have recruited from both sides, and this could have represented one place in the society where they could have legitimately met and worked together.*

4. The resources transferred by assistance agencies into a conflict area affect the conflict in predictable ways.

Assistance workers have found it useful to track the way their resources have an impact on the conflict through effects on local wages, profits, and prices; through being distributed along the lines of conflict; through substituting for local government; through either providing legitimacy for local actors or undermining it; and through the theft or diversion of those resources.

An agency working around the Horn of Africa was put under severe pressure, in part because of a large and very visible program stocking clinics with high-quality drugs.

We find that it is our local staff who are pressured to provide aid resources to the local militias and, when they refuse to do so—as is our policy—they are often threatened. Recently one of our health staff was killed and another injured by soldiers demanding drugs from our clinics.

5. Agencies transfer "messages" as well as resources. Staff behavior and interaction with local communities, hiring practices, how security is arranged, and the like all convey messages that can reinforce the modes and mindsets of people in conflict, or that can promote a mindset and modes of interaction not predisposed to war.

Assistance workers have found it useful to observe their own behavior and how it reinforces conflict mindsets through the use of armed guards, through treating local people or their staff or even other NGOs with disrespect or mistrust, through bursts of anger and suspicion, through emphasizing their own powerlessness, through lack of accountability with regard to using the agency's resources, through demonstrating that some lives are less valuable than others, and through the way agencies portray the conflict in their publicity.

NGOs trying to support and not undermine local health-care systems in the Balkans during and after the war were sometimes seen by locals as taking sides as a result of the way programs were designed.

Aspects of our health interventions create the impression that we favor one community involved in the conflict. To respond to the health needs of the displaced, several NGOs established clinics with free services and medicines in the areas where the IDPs (internally displaced persons) had congregated. In other areas, the existing health system continued to function without NGO support. Clients in the state-run clinics were required to pay a fee for medical services and they felt angry about this.

6. These impacts result from specific details of the design and implementation of an assistance program. How agencies choose their beneficiaries, how they hire local and international staff, how they choose their partners, how they work with local authorities, and what they decide to deliver have impacts on dividers and connectors.

Assistance workers have found it useful to remember that their programs are intended and designed to help people. When a program has a negative impact, it may not be appropriate to abandon the whole program, the good along with the bad. Every aspect of a program design involves a specific choice that can be altered to have positive impacts when assistance workers have done a Do No Harm analysis of the situation.

The recognition that our assistance is promoting competition between the two groups is not, in the eyes of most of our staff, an argument for abandoning the principle that aid should go to those most in need. We can find operational strategies to provide health services to those who need them and still lessen the sense of exclusion among others.

7. There are always options for providing assistance in ways that reduce dividers and that support and strengthen connectors.

Assistance workers have found it useful to analyze the context where they work through the "dividers and connectors" lens. They have found that it is always possible to improve some aspects of their programs in order to take into account the context of conflict where they work.

NOTES

1. Because they are working in ongoing conflicts, the agencies referred to in this text have requested anonymity.

2. It should be noted that the terms *dividers* and *connectors* do not refer to individuals or groups. Rather, they refer to the things people say and do.

The Peacebuilding Filter
■ **Anne Bunde-Birouste and Anthony Zwi**

BACKGROUND

For the last two decades many international aid agencies have focused attention on improving security and stability, as well as devoting attention to "good governance" and poverty reduction. Concerned Australian academics and development practitioners lobbied to keep health on the development agenda. The Australian Agency for International Development (AusAID) supported a team based at the School of Public Health and Community Medicine (SPHCM) at the University of New South Wales (UNSW) in Sydney, Australia, to explore how health sector action might contribute to the broader objectives of peacebuilding in fragile postconflict settings.

BEHIND THE DEVELOPMENT
OF THE PEACEBUILDING FILTER

Although various conflict impact assessments and sensitivity tools had become popular with international donor agencies in the 1990s, few of these explicitly addressed health or health sector work as part of their analyses. The extent to which health initiatives might contribute to preventing violent conflict or promoting peacebuilding in postconflict settings remained anecdotal (Anderson 1999; Bush 1998, 2003; MacQueen and Santa Barbara 2000; Silove 2000; Gaigals and Leonhardt 2001).

The UNSW team hypothesized that combining a conflict impact assessment with a health assessment could generate a more informed understanding of how health initiatives could be designed and/or monitored to enhance their contributions to peacebuilding in precarious, unstable settings (Bunde-Birouste et al. 2004).

An ideal tool would be multipurpose, allowing (1) assessment and monitoring of existing health service and health promotion activities in terms of their violence prevention and peacebuilding potential, and (2) early guidance in new program design and development to ensure the incorporation of peacebuilding elements.

DEVELOPMENT AND TRIALING

A variety of methods were used to move from a developing framework to a tool that could be trialed "in vivo" (Zheng et al. 2002). An initial survey of practitioners and academics was followed by key informant interviews, conference workshops, and focus group sessions. These led to the Peacebuilding Filter being assessed in three fragile states with which the UNSW Health and Conflict Team had ongoing links: Sri Lanka, East Timor, and the Solomon Islands.

The Peacebuilding Filter was initially designed for use by the in-country staff of the donor organization. The field trials included piloting the Peacebuilding Filter with the primary intended users (AusAID staff) as well as a group of secondary users, mostly project managers and key staff within civil society organizations and NGOs. Information gained from these interviews was also triangulated with data and insights derived from the in-country field research by the team. The focus was on the characteristics of projects and programs that would contribute most to peacebuilding. Data were collected through focus group discussions, interviews of key informants involved in project delivery, and direct observation at the community level. This made possible an informed discussion about the project in relation to peacebuilding principles.

THE PEACEBUILDING FILTER AND COMPANION MANUAL

What started out as an idea to develop a simple framework to guide and assess the peacebuilding potential for health sector initiatives resulted in the development of a set of interrelated products. These are all available on the team website (http://healthandconflict.sphcm.med.unsw.edu.au).

The final version of the Peacebuilding Filter is divided into five color-coded sections that reflect core principles underlying a peacebuilding approach to health (see Box 1):

Section 1   Cultural Sensitivity
Section 2   Conflict Sensitivity
Section 3   Social Justice
Section 4   Social Cohesion
Section 5   Good Governance

The Peacebuilding Filter is presented in tabular format, consisting of four columns:

1. Peace-promoting principles
2. Indicators, implementing a peacebuilding component
3. Activity and reflections corresponding to the indicator
4. Space for noting relevant comments, queries, or explanations to stimulate reflection on the project's strengths or weaknesses in relation to the indicator statement

A final section provides space for development of an action plan, which highlights project strengths and opportunities to encourage further development of these activities. This section may also identify risk areas where the project may be directly or indirectly reinforcing divisions or grievances that feed into conflict or disputes. Action may be required to avoid harm being done and improve project practice. Where insights into project activities are shallow, a key action point may be to obtain more detailed and refined information.

Box 1 Cultural Sensitivity

A culturally sensitive approach recognizes and respects cultural diversity and demonstrates awareness of the range of beliefs, customs, rituals, and religious practices of groups and communities. It recognizes indigenous perspectives and seeks to work with them. It sees issues such as language as potentially divisive and therefore requiring considerable attention. Cultural sensitivity is particularly important in areas where conflict has been about political independence, self-determination, and the maintenance of particular cultures and tradition.

Conflict Sensitivity

A number of possible factors can propel conflict toward violent confrontation: ethnic, religious, or other disputes over resources may have provided the basis for instability and social fragmentation. Greed and grievance both warrant attention and response. Appreciating the history and contributors to intercommunity tensions and violence, and understanding how they manifest themselves in the community, is important when considering intervention options and the implications of acting, or not acting, in a particular way, with particular partners, at a particular point in time.

Social Justice

In the context of this work, social justice includes consideration of human rights and dignity, responding to inequalities (in service access, delivery, and staffing), discrimination on the basis of gender, race, ethnicity, political affiliation, and/or any other social or economic characteristics. In the planning and implementing of projects with intent to contribute to peacebuilding, consideration to addressing inequalities and inequities, and to providing transparent and fair grievance procedures in services and systems, should apply both across and within the communities engaged in conflicts.

Social Cohesion

Social cohesion reflects the quality of social relationships and the existence of trust, mutual obligations, and respect within communities and the wider society. At a societal level, violent conflict disrupts social networks and destabilizes the political, social, and economic life of a community. Considering how the disputes and violence might have disturbed or harmed relationships, and understanding what could help rebuild these relationships, is important in project or service design and delivery.

Good Governance

Governance consists of the processes and means by which groups and organizations manage their resources and run their programs. Good governance includes key factors such as a commitment to enhancing local capacities, to operating in a transparent and open way, and to broadening accountability to communities.

The Companion Manual provides further information to clarify principles and indicators within the Peacebuilding Filter, as well as offering examples, resources, and opportunities for further action. The Companion Manual also provides a set of simple ways to promote, or put into action, the key principles in the Peacebuilding Filter.

Together, the Peacebuilding Filter and the Companion Manual are designed to ensure careful and purposeful design, planning, and implementation of projects and programs in order to avoid provoking further grievances or worsening existing tensions.

REFLECTIONS ON THE DEVELOPMENT AND TRIALING OF THE PEACEBUILDING FILTER

The length of this chapter does not permit extensive discussion of the many things learned from the development and trialing of the Peacebuilding Filter. However, brief points related to its principles and use follow.

Peacebuilding Filter Principles

The Peacebuilding Filter does not prioritize any principles above any others. All the five principles are considered integral, and indeed they overlap and are often cross-referenced. The field trials reflected broad agreement about the relevance of the underlying principles. The emphasis and priorities given to individual items differed, however, depending on conflict context and origin, the actors involved, and the phase of the conflict, whether escalating violence or postviolence stabilization. In the Solomon Islands, where simmering ethnic tensions persist, health workers identified cultural sensitivity and respect as particularly important. In Sri Lanka, where the twenty-plus-year war rages on with periodic escalations and intensification, conflict sensitivity includes awareness of background social, economic, and political factors that have contributed to conflict and tensions and threaten fragile ceasefires. In Timor-Leste, where efforts were focused on the job of building one of the world's newest nations, issues of good governance and accountability to the community were considered central to health and peacework.

A trend observed throughout the piloting process was that regardless of origin (local, national, or international), community-level staff typically placed emphasis on cultural sensitivity, social justice, and cohesion issues, whereas donor agency staff tended to emphasize good project governance.

Peacebuilding Filter Use

The Peacebuilding Filter does not aim to offer a "blueprint" for health and peacebuilding work, nor is it intended to score or grade projects; it should not, on its own, be used to evaluate the success or failure of a project. It does, however, help personnel to describe and reflect on what the project is, or is not, achieving. The Filter can assist in transforming concepts such as "good governance," which are usually focused at the national level, into concrete points of engagement at a local project level.

Designed to promote discussion about "sensitivities" within a project, the Peacebuilding Filter can make explicit what is often implicit, and it can allow issues such as cultural sensitivity or trust to be explored alongside the more technical concerns that otherwise dominate monitoring and evaluation efforts. The Peacebuilding Filter complements the traditional logframe, a development tool used by many development agencies in their planning, implementation, and evaluation activities. The Peacebuilding Filter highlights issues that are more concerned with relationships, as well as being more process- and value-focused (Grove and Zwi in press).

The research process indicated that the Peacebuilding Filter provided a particularly useful platform for dialogue. Thus, it may be especially helpful to view the Filter as part of a discussion with those planning to deliver services. Its utility is in highlighting the challenges inherent in conflict-affected settings and in drawing attention to developing strategies to ensure that services and programs do no harm, and indeed it can play a positive part in building and sustaining peace where the political environment is conducive to its doing so.

The five guiding principles should be considered generic concepts for good development practice and can be applied across other sectors apart from health. It is important to note that although each principle is important in its own right, it is their collective integration into a project that will provide an environment more conducive to peacebuilding (Zwi et al. 2006).

REFERENCES

Anderson, Mary B. 1999. *Do no harm: How aid can support peace—or war.* Boulder, CO: Lynne Rienner Publishers.

Bush, K. 1998. Peace and conflict impact assessment (PCIA) of development projects in conflict zones. Working Paper No. 1. The Peacebuilding and Reconstruction Program Initiative and the Evaluation Unit, IDRC: International Development Research Center. Available online at the www.idrc.ca website.

———. 2003. PCIA five years on: The commodification of an idea. In *Berghof handbook conflict and dialogue, Dialogue Series No. 1. Peace and conflict impact assessment*

(PCIA), ed. A. Austin, M. Fischer, & O. Wils. Berghof Research Center for Constructive Conflict Management. Available online at the www.berghof-handbook .net website.

Bunde-Birouste, A., M. Eisenbruch, N. Grove, M. Humphrey, D. Silove, E. Waller, and A. Zwi. 2004. *Background Paper I: Health and peacebuilding: Securing the future.* The School of Public Health and Community Medicine, University of New South Wales, Sydney. Available online at the www.healthandconflict.sphcm.med.unsw.edu .au website.

Gaigals, C., with Manuela Leonhardt. 2001. Conflict-sensitive approaches to development: A review of practice. London: *International Alert, Saferworld, IDRC.* Available online at www.bellanet.org/pcia/documents/docs/conflict-sensitive-develop.pdf

Grove, N. J. and A. B. Zwi. In press. Beyond the logframe: A new tool for examining health and peacebuilding initiatives. *Development in Practice.*

MacQueen, G., and J. Santa Barbara. 2000. Peacebuilding through health initiatives. *British Medical Journal* 321:293–6.

Silove, D. 2000. A conceptual framework for mass trauma: Implications for adaptation, intervention and debriefing. In *Psychological debriefing, theory, practice and evidence,* ed. B. Raphael and J. P. Wilson, 337–51. Cambridge: Cambridge University Press.

Zheng, B., M. Hall, E. Dugan, K. Kidd, and D. Levine. 2002. Development of a scale to measure patients' trust in health insurers. *HSR-Health Services Research* 37:1, 187–202.

Zwi, A., A. Bunde-Birouste, N. Grove, Waller E, and J. Ritchie. 2006. *The Peacebuilding Filter* and *The Peacebuilding Filter: Companion Manual.* Sydney: School of Public Health and Community Medicine, University of New South Wales. Available online at the www.healthandconflict.sphcm.med.unsw.edu.au website.

NOTE

The Peacebuilding Filter has been carefully piloted, and the vast majority of interviewees considered the products relevant, user-friendly, and insightful. Additional assessment of the practical use of these materials is being generated. We encourage interested groups to work with the authors in using these materials and in assessing their value within programming, design, and planning activities.

Authors

Anne W. Bunde-Birouste
Senior Lecturer
Convenor, Health Promotion Program
Convenor, Refugee Soccer Program,
Coordinator, Health and Conflict Research Project
School of Public Health and Community Medicine,
The University of New South Wales
Sydney, NSW 2052 Australia
CRICOS Provider No: 00098G

Tel: +61(2) 9358 2591; 2517
Fax: +61(2) 9385 1526
E-mail: ab.birouste@unsw.edu.au
web: www.soccer.sphcm.med.unsw.edu.au/
www.healthandconflict.sphcm.med.unsw.edu.au

Professor Anthony Zwi
Professor of Public Health and Community Medicine
    and Associate Dean (International)
School of Public Health and Community Medicine
Faculty of Medicine
The University of New South Wales
Sydney, NSW 2052 Australia
Phone: +61(2) 9385 2445
Fax: +61(2) 9313 6185
E-mail: a.zwi@unsw.edu.au

ACKNOWLEDGMENT

Natalie Grove, Emily Waller, and Jan Ritchie were, with the authors, central to the design and development of the Peacebuilding Filter. Particular recognition and appreciation go to them. In addition, the authors would like to express their appreciation to the other UNSW Health and Conflict team members and to all those who provided invaluable assistance to this work. Too numerous to list here, they are recognized in the various documents available on the project website at http://www.healthandconflict.sphcm.med.unsw.edu.au.

This work was funded by the Australian Agency for International Development (AusAID).

14

Dealing with Conflict[1]

Joanna Santa Barbara

Conflict occurs when two or more entities pursue incompatible goals. It is a natural part of human interaction and will always be with us. But not all ways of handling conflict are productive. Health, happiness, and social progress are routinely squandered in conflicts that are unnecessary and that persist because of habit and culture, conflicts that are violent when they do not need to be, or conflicts that involve the oppression of one group by another. In the course of the career of any health worker, myriad conflicts will present themselves: interpersonal conflicts with colleagues or patients and conflicts with players in the structure of organizations, such as hospitals and universities. Health workers engaged in arenas of violent conflict may find themselves challenged by conflicts with other organizations working in the field, with political actors, or even with armed groups challenging their impartial care. Occasionally health workers have the opportunity to try to influence the course of large-scale conflict. The health worker needs fundamental knowledge of ways of dealing with conflict. This chapter will outline basic concepts.

The goal of dealing with conflict is to improve the situation for all parties and, ideally, to have all parties fulfill their legitimate goals. In general, when people have a variety of ways of dealing with conflict, they are less apt to resort to violence or other ways of hurting those whose goals seem to conflict with their own. Under the best of circumstances, conflict may be creative, not destructive, stimulating the invention of a better state of affairs than before.

POSSIBLE OUTCOMES OF CONFLICT

In considering the various approaches to conflicts, it is useful to begin with Johan Galtung's (2000, 21) delineation of the possible outcomes of a conflict between two parties. We can think of the parties as A and B.

They hold goals that appear to be incompatible. Their conflict has the following possible outcomes:

1. The parties can fight out the conflict by one means or another, each hoping to achieve victory for themselves and defeat for their opponent. A might win and achieve all of their goals; B will get none of theirs. Or B will achieve all of their goals and A none of theirs.
2. Both parties might withdraw from the conflict, and neither will get what they want.
3. The two parties might compromise; each will get part of what they want.
4. The parties might enter into a creative process of working through the conflict, at the end of which each gets what they want—and possibly even more than they originally desired. This is sometimes called a "transcending" solution because it goes beyond, or transcends, what seemed possible before. This kind of solution cannot be achieved for all conflicts, but it can for some. It is certainly worth attempting.

Example: There is one orange and there are two sisters, Aisha and Jameela. Each sister shouts that she wants the orange. Now, if they continue fighting over it, Jameela might win and get the orange; then Aisha would get nothing. Or Aisha might win the orange and Jameela would get nothing. Perhaps they might decide that fighting is undignified and leave the orange alone (withdrawal); neither would get anything. They might cut the orange in half and share it (compromise). Or they might calm down and ask the other what she wants to do with the orange. Aha! Aisha wants to make orange juice, and Jameela wants the rind to flavor a cake! So each of them can get what she wants. Furthermore, each can enjoy a delicious drink of orange juice and a piece of orange cake.

This is a transcending solution: each gets more than she originally asked for.

LEGITIMACY OF CONFLICT GOALS

Usually each party to a conflict has at least some legitimate goals. However, this is not always the case. Occasionally, it may be reasonable to regard the goals of one party as largely illegitimate. In such conflicts, one party utterly violates the human rights of another party or denies others the means to fulfill their basic human needs. In such cases, it may be more appropriate to urge the waging of nonviolent struggle by the oppressed party and others sympathetic to its position. It is important to note that even conflict parties widely vilified by the public on one side of the conflict may have some legitimate goals; examples include the Taliban in Afghanistan and terrorists in several parts of the world. Legitimacy of goals is appraised by matching goals with universal principles, such as the Universal Declaration of Human Rights.

POWER IN CONFLICT

It is common to find a serious power imbalance between parties, so that any negotiated settlement reached is apt to greatly favor the powerful party and to violate principles of justice. A mediator must make an effort to compensate for power differences. Such situations may also call for the nonviolent use of power by the oppressed party and others sympathetic to it. For the purposes of the remainder of this chapter, we shall assume that we are dealing with conflicts in which there are some legitimate goals on both sides, even if there are power imbalances and even if the goals of one or both sides coexist with illegitimate goals or are currently being pursued with violent or otherwise harmful behavior.

WAYS TO DEAL WITH CONFLICT

We shall discuss the following four ways of dealing with conflicts: collaborative problem solving, mediated conflict resolution, arbitration and adjudication, and conflict transformation. Before we attend to these methods, however, we need to address three important aspects of how skilled people deal with conflict: dialogue, creativity, and cooperative orientation.

Dialogue

A carefully conducted conversation between conflict parties is one of the keys to the proper handling of conflict. If the conflict is between two friends or colleagues, they can simply have a face-to-face conversation about the problem. If levels of anger and mistrust are high, or if one party might try to overpower another, a mediator needs to control and facilitate this dialogue.

Where mistrust or tension is sufficiently high that the parties cannot work well together in a face-to-face encounter—at least in the early stages of handling the conflict—the mediator needs to speak separately with each party. Johan Galtung points out that many high-level attempts at mediation fail because of a single-minded insistence on "getting everyone to the negotiating table" at the beginning of peace dialogues. Sitting together at the same table may actually increase stereotypical behavior, rhetoric, and grand-standing. He recommends that at any point in the conflict—even while bombing and shooting are still going on—the mediator try to talk to the parties in conflict, one at a time, and find out what they want and need.

Whether dialogue is taking place between the mediator and a conflict party or directly between conflict parties, four skills are especially important for good communication.

Active listening involves listening attentively to a person's statement of her or his position without interrupting with argumentative or judgmental comments. If this is a two-party dialogue, you may disagree or think the other person is lying, but all the same, you listen to this statement. You listen even if negative things are said about you. You can and should politely ask questions that bring out more of the story (this asking of questions is part of what it means to be *actively* listening), but you must be genuinely seeking information or clarification, not covertly criticizing. For example, you might ask, "Can you say more about that?" "What happened when your offer was refused?" "Could you give me an example of something I did that offended you?" Here, on the other hand, are some questions that include judgments and therefore should not be asked: "Why do you always blame other people for your problems?" "Have you always been so oversensitive?"

When actively listening in a conflict situation, a mediator will generally ask key questions such as "What is your biggest worry in all this?" and "What would you like to have happen?"

Speaking constructively of our own needs in a conflict situation requires, according to Marshall Rosenberg (1999), clear statements on

- What we observe (for example, "A rural medical clinic, clearly marked so as to be visible from the air, was destroyed by one of your helicopter gunships last night.")
- How we feel about this ("We are deeply distressed by the loss of life involved and very disturbed by the loss of medical services to the surrounding population.")
- What we need ("We need assurance that you will comply with international humanitarian law with respect to protection of medical facilities in violent combat.")

In addition to these three crucial elements, we may sometimes want to add a fourth:

- A request ("We suggest our envoys meet with a UN mediator to ensure that there are no further occurrences.")

You will not always want to add the fourth step because there may be other solutions to this problem, and you may want to give the other person an opportunity to suggest them. But the first three elements—observation, feelings, and needs—are key elements of speaking constructively in a conflict situation. Try not to judge, criticize, or moralize (even though the example given is a very grave one). There is also plenty of room for creativity and respect in interactions. You do not have to follow these three stages in a mechanical way. In less grave circumstances, friendly rituals (commenting on the weather, inquiring about the welfare of the other person's family, or interjecting mild humor) are often invaluable in the healthy handling of conflict.

Empathy—the capacity to put yourself "in someone else's shoes" in order to see the world from another's perspective—is crucial to good dialogue and to good handling of conflict. It is difficult to have empathy for a person or group that has been hurting you or your group. It can even be difficult for an outsider who knows that one party has committed serious violence against others. But there is no substitute for empathy if we want lasting, just solutions to conflict. You are probably aware of conflicts that continue to damage and destroy over long periods because of serious failures of the parties to understand each other's needs and attitudes.

The fourth skill crucial to developing good communication skills is the **ability to distinguish interests from positions** and, in a conflict situation, to state your interests rather than your position. A position is what a person has decided is the right solution to a conflict. Remember that in the story about the sisters and the orange, it was only after the sisters stopped shouting that they wanted the orange (this was their *position*) that they calmed down and stated their *interests* in using the orange. Then they realized that the interests of both could be accommodated.

Creative solutions can be arrived at if people state their interests or their needs in a situation. If they state fixed positions, creativity may be blocked.

Creativity

Individuals and communities in conflict can get stuck in particular positions. These positions may persist for generations, being solidified through songs and poems, rituals and heroic stories. The more blood is shed to maintain a position, the more inflexible it may become. It may even be considered sacred and immutable, even though it is outmoded, nonsensical, or self-destructive. In these situations, the parties to a conflict urgently need to get a new perspective. This is where creativity—the ability to look beyond old positions and see new possibilities—enters the picture. Creativity is not merely desirable in the handling of conflict; it is essential. It can bring hope where there is none. It can unblock years of fruitless impasse and destruction.

The negotiations typically used to deal with large-scale conflicts, such as those between conflicting states, seldom maximize the parties' creativity. Often these negotiations are formal; are carried out with the antagonistic parties in tense, face-to-face conversation; are accompanied by a good deal of publicity; and are managed by negotiators with little training in creative problem solving. These are conditions that smother creativity. It is important that conflict workers try to find ways to do better.

A person does not have to be outstandingly creative—an artist or writer, for example—in order to promote creativity in themselves and others. There are ways of problem solving that have been designed to enhance the creativity of groups of people. These should be learned and used. Later, we will briefly describe one of these, "brainstorming."

> *Example: Consider one of the scenarios in Chapter 1: A health team is attempting to reconstruct health infrastructure after the devastation of an earthquake. However, the conflicting ethnic groups had previously had a dual health-care system—a clinic in each area, the clinics being quite close to each other. Each group demands that the new health facilities be built in their area. The team bears in mind potential for peace as well as reconstructing health care. The team suggests entering into a discussion with both factions about the possibility of constructing shared facilities. If the groups could find a way of sharing, there would be resources for both a clinic and a pathology laboratory in the area, expanding standards of care and reducing the need to travel for certain health needs.*

Cooperative Orientation

The best solutions emerge when parties in conflict are working together to solve a problem rather than fighting each other to achieve a victory. This does not mean that a party must be weak or passive; weakness is an entirely different thing from a cooperative attitude. Weakness involves a failure to state needs clearly and to strive hard to satisfy them. In cooperative problem solving there may be times when a party will have to strive very hard to make sure that its needs are met. But while striving hard, this party does not deny the needs of other parties and does not seek to achieve victory over them or to destroy them.

What can one party do when another party has a competitive orientation to conflict—that is, when the other party is convinced that the only way to deal with a conflict is to fight by fair or unfair means to achieve victory? Research on conflict has yielded an interesting finding: parties in conflict tend to mirror each other. If one party behaves in a cooperative way, uses only fair means, remains polite, tries to empathize, and states needs rather than hard positions, it is more likely that the other party will do the same (Deutsch 2000).

APPROACHES TO CONFLICT

Now we will turn to a number of different approaches to dealing with conflict. They vary in how formal or informal they are, in how much outside intervention they involve, and in how much coercion is involved in enforcing the solution.

Collaborative Problem solving	Mediation	Arbitration/Adjudication
Least formal		Most formal
Least outsider intervention		Most outsider intervention
Least coercion		Most coercion

Collaborative Problem Solving

In collaborative problem solving, parties meet face-to-face and try to work together to resolve a conflict. If they use active listening, constructive communication, empathy, creativity, and a cooperative orientation to conflict, their chances of success are increased.

Mediation

In mediation, an impartial outside person assists the parties in dealing with a conflict. Mediation is used when feelings are too high to contain them easily, when there is a significant power imbalance in the conflict, and when the parties are stuck and have lost their creativity. Mediators should have some skill in working to help people in conflict. There are training programs for mediators that help them develop these skills. In some situations it may not be necessary for the mediator to have a great deal of formal training. Children, for example, can be taught to be mediators for conflicts in school settings; they are quite capable of grasping many of the important aspects of mediation. On the other hand, there are good reasons to ensure that mediators for very difficult, complex, intractable, potentially violent conflicts have a high level of skill and a good deal of experience with many different strategies adapted to various situations.

A mediator is not a judge of who is right or of what is the correct solution to a conflict, nor does a mediator impose a solution. A mediator's job is to help the people in conflict communicate with each other in order to resolve it. In some styles of mediation, the mediator helps the conflict parties to develop their own ideas but does not contribute his or her own ideas toward a solution. Other styles of mediation encourage the mediator to contribute creative suggestions to the pool of ideas about possible solutions. This will be successful only if the mediator remains detached from the ideas he or she throws in and exerts no pressure on others to adopt these particular ideas. Since people in conflict often become stuck and fall into rigid patterns of thinking, it makes sense in most cases for the mediator to be willing to contribute concrete ideas for solving the conflict. But this is not the mediator's main role. The mediator is a helper, a facilitator, who assists the parties in working through their difficulties.

Here is a form of mediation that is easy to learn. It assumes that the parties are able to work productively together, in face-to-face dialogue, on the conflict. Later, we shall suggest an alternative method to use when face-to-face meeting is impossible or unwise.

1. *Introduce the process.* Explain your role. Explain that you are not a judge in this dispute, but that you will help each party speak and listen to the other and will then help them to reach a solution. Get clear agreement from all parties that they wish to participate in this process. You may want to say something about the importance of a cooperative orientation. In some situations it could also be helpful to refer to the conflict outcomes schema at the beginning of the chapter to show that you will be aiming for a solution that gives everyone what they need. Some people call this a "win-win" solution in contrast to a "win-lose" solution.

Next, set the ground-rules for a helpful session:

- One person at a time speaks, and the others listen. You will try to ensure that everyone has a fair amount of "air time."

- Participants share all relevant information truthfully.
- The person speaking should focus on what the situation is like for himself or herself, rather than blaming the other party.

State how long this session will last and what will happen if you need another session. Explain that you will help the disputants observe the rules of active listening and constructive communication. Explain that you may have to interrupt if you find that there is blaming or insulting.

2. *Identify the issues.* At this point you will give both parties an opportunity to state their problems. You may need to control for interruption or attempts to argue while this is happening. If the parties present themselves in terms of their *positions*, you may need to ask questions to try to get them to state their *needs and interests* instead.

3. *Explore assumptions, values, hopes, and fears.* This part of the process requires skilled questioning by the mediator. It is an opportunity for the parties to understand each other in new ways and to identify common ground. Misunderstandings may be corrected, and in some happy circumstances, this may resolve the conflict. A useful question when people are reluctant to move from entrenched positions is to ask what they think will happen if they both keep on going in the same way they are now. At the end of this phase, summarize the common ground that has been identified and the areas of difference that have been clarified.

4. *Generate solutions.* A brainstorming session often works well for this phase. The participants are encouraged to come up with as many different solutions as they can, without initially stopping to evaluate them critically. The ideas are written up for all to see on a flip chart or blackboard while they are being produced. This is the point at which the mediator may wish to throw in his or her own creative ideas. (See the accompanying box for more information about brainstorming.)

5. *Reach agreement.* First, the brainstormed ideas need to be discussed and evaluated. Many ideas may look impractical, but sometimes they will contribute to a good solution. Inevitably, some ideas will favor the interests of one side, and some those of the other. Often, during this discussion, new combinations of ideas will arise, which build on the brainstorming and which can satisfy the needs of both sides. At the end of this phase, you will get an agreement from both parties.

6. *Plan steps to implement agreement.* This can be quite difficult, and it tests the commitment of the parties. If they set up roadblocks, you may have to go back to the stage of generating more solutions. Try to achieve a concrete plan with a time line and with clear duties and tasks

for each party. If you end this process with an agreement and a plan to implement it, you can all feel very pleased with yourselves. You should celebrate!

Brainstorming

Brainstorming is the name given to a process meant to stimulate creativity in a group. It is based on the idea that we often judge our own ideas and the ideas of others prematurely and in this way smother our creativity before it has a chance to flower. Brainstorming is easy to do and is often fun. You should not do it with a serious face; humor is part of the creative process!

Here are steps and rules for a facilitator running a brainstorming session that is intended to lead to a solution and group decision. They are presented in a generic format applicable to nonconflictual problem solving as well as to resolving a conflict.

Beginning Phase

- Explain what brainstorming is and how it works. Do not assume that everyone knows! Encourage everyone in the group to participate, but do not force anyone to.
- State clearly the problem that the brainstorming is supposed to address. You want the group to generate lots of ideas, quickly and without discussion.
- Set a time limit (for example, ten minutes) right at the outset, and stick to it.

Middle Phase

- Encourage the group to generate as many ideas as it can as rapidly as possible.
- Encourage people to build on each other's ideas.
- No criticism, discussion, or evaluation of ideas is permitted in this phase.
- No idea is too silly or "way out."
- Write the ideas where they are visible to everyone as they are being generated.

End Phase

The task of the group is to now move from its wildly creative phase to a more sober, evaluative phase without throwing out all the new or slightly peculiar ideas. Begin by sorting the ideas into groups. Then discuss each group of ideas one at a time.

You will often find that an idea that seems crazy can be transformed by the group into a practical idea. Give the group the time it needs to test each idea for practicality and to see whether it can be changed in ways that make it better.

Frequently, in this phase a solution acceptable to most people in the group will emerge. If this does not happen, or if different groups of people favor different ideas, you will need to implement decision making according to some method acceptable to the group—for example, consensus decision making or voting.

Mediation Engaging the Parties One at a Time

When people are engaged in violent conflict, when they are deeply mistrustful of each other, or when they hate each other intensely, it will be better to begin by having the mediator talk with each party separately. This is often useful even in less severe cases. In this way the mediator can develop rapport with the parties and build up trust in a relaxed environment; has an opportunity learn about the background of the conflict and the concerns, wants, needs, and interests of each party; and has a chance to discover what is making the conflict difficult to solve. After such a meeting or meetings, the mediator can determine whether the parties are ready for a face-to-face meeting.

As in all mediation, the mediator needs to be someone trusted by both parties, and the process needs to be open and transparent. Confidentiality is also an important issue; the mediator needs to come to an understanding with all parties about what information can and cannot be divulged to the other parties.

Here are some of the questions that Johan Galtung suggests may be covered in such a meeting:

> "Describe for me a future in which all parties can live happily."
> "Given the current situation, what do you think will happen if things continue as they have?"
> "Are you sure the other party is standing in your way (obstructing your goals)?"
> "What is it in the other party that you are actually afraid of?"
> "Do you see anything positive in the other party?"
> "Do they see anything positive in you?"
> "What are your dreams and hopes?" "How can they be materialized?" "What are the obstacles?"

Arbitration and Adjudication

These forms of dealing with conflict are mentioned here briefly for the sake of completeness. They usually involve specialized roles and training. Arbitration is a strategy to resolve conflict whereby both or all sides agree to submit their conflict to an impartial and knowledgeable person, the arbitrator. They agree that the arbitrator's decision will be binding; they will abide by the decision even if they do not agree with it. The arbitrator formally hears the case of each side and invites them to present suggestions to resolve the problems. The arbitrator then hands down a decision. This form of dealing with conflict is often used in labor disputes between a union and management in a work situation.

Adjudication is even more formal. This term most commonly applies to formal judicial arrangements. A dispute comes before a judge who hears the cases for both sides. The judge then issues a ruling, and it is binding on all parties. This ruling will be backed by force: a person who does not abide by it may be arrested and jailed. War crimes tribunals are an example of adjudicated resolution of conflict resulting from a war.

Conflict Transformation

This term has come into use in recent years in recognition of the fact that some conflicts will not be resolved quickly—and, in some cases, may never be resolved. In these cases, methods are needed for *changing the form of these conflicts* from destructive to nondestructive, from violent to nonviolent, in order that fewer people suffer. For the conflict to be "transformed" in these ways, there may need to be changes in the built-in social arrangements by which things are done (structure). There may also need to be changes in values, beliefs, and attitudes in a society (culture).

REFERENCES

Deutsch, Morton. 2000. Cooperation and competition. In *The handbook of conflict resolution,* ed. Morton Deutsch and Peter T. Coleman. San Francisco, CA: Jossey-Bass.
Fisher, R. and W. Ury. 1998. *Getting to yes: Negotiating agreement without giving in.* Baltimore, MD: Penguin Books.
Galtung, J. 2000. *Conflict transformation by peaceful means.* United Nations Disaster Management Training Program. This can also be downloaded from TRANSCEND at the www.transcend.org website.
Rosenberg, M. 1999. *Nonviolent communication: A language of compassion.* Encinitas, CA: Puddledancer Press.
Tillett, G. 1999. *Resolving conflict: A practical approach.* 2nd ed. Melbourne, Australia: Oxford University Press.

NOTE

This chapter is adapted with permission from a similar one by the same author in *Making peace: A peace education manual for Afghanistan,* ed. Graeme MacQueen. Available online at the www.humanities.mcmaster.ca website.

15

Epidemiology as a Tool for Interdisciplinary Peace and Health Studies

Rob Chase and Neil Arya

WAR AND VIOLENCE:
THE EPIDEMIOLOGY OF A NEGLECTED "DISEASE"?

In 1854 London physician John Snow mapped cases of deaths and diarrhea in relation to the local water source during a disease outbreak. Snow's empirical evidence convinced authorities to remove the handle of the suspected water pump, and new cases dropped dramatically. His statistical analysis countered the theory of "miasma in the atmosphere" accepted at the time as explaining disease, decades before bacteriologist Robert Koch discovered the bacteria that caused cholera. Koch later formulated rules (Koch's postulates) whereby controlled, objective scientific experiment proves that a microbial agent causes disease—the foundation of modern microbiology and scientific experimental method (Summers 1989, 113–7).

Epidemiology—the study of how often diseases occur in different groups of people and why (Coggon, Rose, and Barker 1997)—is the foundation of logic underlying public health and preventive medicine and of research on effective prevention, treatment measures, and evidence-based practice in control of disease outbreak, immunization, and drug therapeutics.

Epidemiologic measurement of disease outcomes are expressed in relation to *populations at risk*, not individual cases. Consider these findings:

- *Cause-specific death rates in general population:* Over the centuries, worldwide population-based rates for military deaths vaulted from 16 per million in the seventeenth, eighteenth, and nineteenth centuries to 183 per million in the twentieth century, an 11-fold rise (Taipale 2001).
- *Proportional mortality:* During the twentieth century, the proportion of civilian deaths from armed conflict rose from 10 percent in

World War I to half the war casualties of World War II (including Nazi death camps) to current levels of up to 90 percent, the ironic result of the century's technological progress in the science and delivery of war (Garfield and Neugut 1997).[1]

- *Global disease burden:* Violence from all causes is a major determinant of health. Each year over 1.6 million people worldwide die by direct violence, accounting for 14 percent of deaths among males and 7 percent among females aged 15–44 years (Krug et al. 2002).

In contrast to dramatic reductions through modern medicine and public health in infectious and preventable diseases, the epidemic of public, "man-made" death has gone unchecked and understudied by medicine and public health. Although war can be likened to a disease outbreak, there is no isolatable, physical causal agent. Instead, the primary cause is the conscious intention to kill or inflict harm, leading to violent actions and to an interrelated web of individual and collective consequences.

How does epidemiology, with its tools and statistical methods, contribute to the interdisciplinary study of peace and health? This chapter will present illustrative examples of the application of epidemiology to weapons systems and war and will briefly discuss key concepts, conceptual and practical gaps, opportunities, and challenges. Not included are the important contributions of environmental and mental health epidemiology.

TYPES OF EPIDEMIOLOGIC STUDY

Epidemiologic study is of two general types:

1. Descriptive, analytic methods used by social sciences to measure associations, assess bias, and study relationships between exposures and outcomes.
2. Experimental methods, as in community or clinical interventions.

In the study of war and violence, researchers are mostly constrained to observational study, which we will discuss first with the following examples. More incisive experimental study designs (discussed later) may apply to community interventions before, during, or after conflict.

Example 1: Atomic Bomb Survivors of Hiroshima and Nagasaki

In the first days after the Hiroshima and Nagasaki atomic explosions, Japanese medical and scientific teams were collecting clinical data. Within days of Japan declaring defeat, the Joint Commission for the Investigation of the Effects of the Atomic Bombs, under the U.S. National Academy of Sciences, engaged 60 American military and civilian scientists and 90 Japanese physicians and scientists in the Atomic Bomb Casualty Commission (ABCC). Later, the Radiation Effects Research Foundation had 1000 employees; it is presently the world's longest continuing health survey (Putnam 1998). Objectives included scientific research on the medical and genetic aftereffects of radiation, American military interests in the offensive and defensive implications of atomic radiation, and Japanese expectations of medical care.

As a "clinical population trial," the A-bomb experiment would have violated bioethical codes developed after World War II, including the Nuremburg Code (1947) and the Helsinki Declaration (1964) (Berdon 2005). In terms of study design, Hiroshima and Nagasaki would be considered prospective, observational studies, with unexposed, control populations. The Life Span Study of 93,000 survivors and 27,000 unexposed individuals used longitudinal cohort and case-control designs to study the life-long health risks of cancer and radiation effects (www.rerf.org.jp/). Objective, quantifiable exposures to the singular, localized event were measured by radiation dosages, distance from the epicenter, or absorbed body burden counts. Acute and long-term health outcomes—cancers in particular—were meticulously tracked, as were immune conditions, pregnancy terminations, and chromosomal effects in offspring. Nonexposed civilian control groups made possible reliable calculations of population risk that were generalizable to human populations elsewhere.

Leading US medical voices used A-bomb epidemiology to bring home to the American public that there could be no meaningful medical response to a nuclear attack. In 1962, Physicians for Social Responsibility projected Hiroshima's devastation and health effects to Boston, Massachusetts, estimating the impact of the firestorm, blast wave, and gale causing projectile debris in terms of mortality, physical trauma, and short-term and long-term radiation effects. Among the projections: 98 percent of medical personnel would die within the central city; the entire United States would not have enough burn beds to deal with this one city's victims; and environmental radiation would cause cancers years after an attack (Sidel, Geiger, and Lown 1962).

Example 2: Landmines

In contrast to the A-bomb studies, assembling data on landmines is a multinational initiative, driven by the efforts of humanitarian, medical, and refugee organizations and agencies in the field. In the late 1990s the worldwide civilian toll of landmines was tabulated at 10,000 deaths annually; every 22 minutes someone was killed or maimed somewhere in the world (Stover, Cobey, and Fine 1997). Focusing on the effects of a specific technology, the consistency of this civilian cost across the nations studied strengthened the argument for banning the production and use of landmines. Multisite evidence was backed by persuasive analysis demonstrating that landmines do indiscriminate damage affecting civilian noncombatants vastly out of proportion to the landmines' military utility.

Epidemiologically, casualties of landmines and unexploded ordnance who are admitted to hospitals are expedient sources of data, but this approach fails to register those who do not get treatment or who enter the morgue. Thus it has low sensitivity and may often underestimate the true incidence within the population at risk. Community-based sampling (such as household survey questionnaires) may better estimate incidence and the size of the population at risk, to calculate rates. Evaluation can involve qualitative rapid appraisal methods to gather data from key informants, institutional reviews, and focus groups of survivors of landmines (Andersson 1995). Important outcome measures include the incidence of mine injuries and deaths, the prevalence of landmine disability; the physical, psychological, social, and economic costs of acute care and rehabilitation; and the effects of landmines on food security, residence and refugee resettlement, livestock, and land use (Stover et al. 1994).

The International Campaign to Ban Landmines (ICBL) (www.icbl .org/) was founded in 1992 by six nongovernmental organizations as a flexible network calling for an international ban on the use, production, stockpiling, and transfer of antipersonnel landmines, and for increased international resources for humanitarian mine clearance and mine victim assistance programs. The ICBL movement rapidly grew to include dozens of national campaigns, along with documentation of mortality, morbidity, and costs of rehabilitation—physical and psychological, and it galvanized a civil society effort to ban these weapons. Multidimensional analysis of the impact of landmines was strategically prepared for governments and stakeholders at both regional and international levels. As a result, political, industrial, and military support for continued use of landmines dwindled, leading to the Mine Ban Treaty (the Ottawa Convention) in 1997, which now has more than 150 signatory states. The ICBL was awarded the Nobel Prize the same year.

Example 3: Small Arms and Light Weapons

Compared to landmine mortality and morbidity, small arms and light weapons (SALWs) constitute a far greater global public health hazard, killing an estimated 500,000 annually: 300,000 in armed conflict and 200,000 in peace (Cukier 2001). Indeed, more injuries, deaths, displacements, rapes, kidnappings, and acts of torture are inflicted or perpetrated with small arms than with any other type of weapon (Hillier and Wood 2003). There is an international Control Arms campaign (see www .controlarms.org/ and www.iansa.org), but several factors make small arms less amenable to categorical control than landmines. These include greater and more diverse production and distribution; varied use, some of which is beneficial to human livelihood (hunting for food, control of pests, and sport); legally sanctioned use by some (such as law enforcement agencies and state armies); and the difficulty of regulating trade and trafficking of illegal small arms.

In the United States, roughly 30,000 people are killed each year with firearms, which are second only to motor vehicles as the most frequent cause of injury death overall (Stiebal 2000). One innovative study design compares geographically and demographically similar cities that differ in the prevalence of gun ownership: Seattle, Washington (41 percent) vs. Vancouver, Canada (12 percent). During the study period, robbery, home burglary, and aggravated assault rates were near comparable, within 15 percent of each other, but rates of assault with firearms was 7.7 times higher, and homicides involving firearms 4.8 times higher, in Seattle. Rates remained significantly higher when "legally justifiable" and self-defense cases were excluded (Sloan et al. 1988).

Epidemiologists have compared rates between countries using national health statistics based on International Classification of Diseases (ICD-9) codes on firearm-related homicides, suicides, unintentional deaths, and deaths of undetermined intent. A study of 46 high-income (HI) and upper-middle-income (UMI) countries found age-adjusted annual firearm mortality rates to be five to six times higher in countries in the Americas (12.72 per 100,000) than in Europe (2.17) or Oceania (2.57), and 95 times higher than in Asia (0.13). The rate of firearm deaths in the United States (14.24 per 100,000) exceeded that of its economic counterparts (1.76) eightfold and that of UMI countries (9.69) by a factor of 1.5. (Krug, Powell, and Dahlberg 1998). This is an example of an ecological study, in which the unit of study being compared is a population (in this case, routinely collected national firearm mortality), not data gathered by the researcher's own methods.

However, most developing countries affected by small-arms violence and armed conflict lack reliable national mortality data and were excluded from analysis, a selection bias partly controlled by limiting the study to high-income and upper-middle-income countries. National health databases classifying mortality and morbidity are often unavailable or unreliable in developing countries, which significantly limits research designs commonly used in industrialized countries. In most settings of armed conflict, data collection by the researchers, NGOs, or international agencies requires considerable human, logistical, and technical resources (Arya and Cukier 2005).

Death registration systems such as ICD-9 use a dual code for "accident" or "injury": the *manner* of death (accidental, self-inflicted, homicide or assault, intention not able to be determined, legal intervention, act of war); and *mechanism* (such as firearm injury, poisoning, vehicle crash). However, this fails to record the *source* or context (such as domestic, criminal, political, suicide following torture or rape), and this limits their usefulness for causal analysis. This information gap is highlighted by recent revisions by the United States to ICD-9 classification to include "acts of terrorism" as a recordable "manner of death," in congruence with institutionalizing the War on Terror (Centers for Disease Control, 2005).

No international agency is mandated to collect data on trends in political violence (Human Security Centre 2005). This is in stark contrast to the wealth of official data tracking global and regional trends in the AIDS pandemic and mobilization toward the Millennium Development Goals. This dearth of data on political violence is ironic, given the founding principles of the UN and its international health agencies, but it is indicative of the relative paralysis in the UN system vis-à-vis armed conflict and political violence.

Example 4: Public Health Impact of War and Conflict: Iraq Case Study

Since the beginning of the Iraq conflict, estimations of casualties have been the subject of greater scrutiny and controversy than in most previous war theaters. Operation Desert Storm began on January 16, 1991, with the invasion to liberate Kuwait and bombardment in Iraq; the campaign lasted 43 days. Daponte presented a summary analysis of the range of estimates from various sources. An estimated 20,000–25,000 Iraqi soldiers died from air attacks in Kuwait, 12,000–15,000 died from air attacks in Iraq, and 17,000–23,000 died during the final ground war. An estimated 3500 civilian were killed from direct war effects. Driven out of Kuwait, Iraqi troops returned to subjugate Kurdish and Shia uprisings, resulting in a further 30,000 civilian deaths, occasioning 5000 military deaths, and causing massive population displacements, including 2 million Kurds in the northern areas who moved across the Iranian and Turkish borders. Overall, from a population of 18.4 million, an estimated 205,500 Iraqis died from effects of the 1991 Gulf War or postwar turmoil (Daponte 1993).

However, surveillance from casualty reports in war conditions are known to underreport war deaths several-fold. For this reason, epidemiologic determination of population death rates, when based on unbiased sampling and appropriate cluster designs, are understood to yield more valid estimates of mortality. Unique to modern war history, the Iraq conflict has been studied epidemiologically with noteworthy results.

In August 1991, the International Study Team conducted independent research to objectively document the impact on civilian population. This effort was organized by graduate students from Harvard University Schools of Law and Public Health and health professionals and academics in the Gulf Peace Team (Burrowes 1991). Eighty-seven researchers with Jordanian translators negotiated access to all Iraqi cities and provinces and noninterference in their efforts to conduct comprehensive field investigations on health-care facilities, water and sewage systems, electrical facilities, women's issues, child psychology, and malnutrition (International Study Team 1991).

The major component was a population-based study of mortality rates among infants and children under five years old. A nationwide multistage, stratified cluster sampling of Iraqi households (6000 households in 271 randomly selected clusters proportional to the population distribution) collected data on 16,172 live births and 803 deaths for 1991 and the four prior years. Infant mortality rose from 17.0 per 1000 person-years to 70.1, an increase in relative mortality of 4.1 (95% confidence interval 3.5–5.2); mortality for children under five years old increased by a factor of 3.8 (95% CI 2.6–5.4). Analysis of cause of death found the increase due to infectious disease and collapsed public health services more than physical injuries from the conflict: proportional death by cause for diarrhea rose from 21% before the war to 38%, whereas death by physical injury declined 8.8% to 7.2% (Ascherio et al. 1992).

Three notable epidemiologic studies conducted after the 2003 Iraq invasion highlight important differences between epidemiologic mortality estimates and reported counts by hospitals and officials to estimate civilian death toll in war. The Iraq Body Count project (www.iraqbody count.org) provides a cumulative database of civilian deaths from military actions, as reported by journalists, military spokespersons, and hospital and government sources. The comprehensive Iraq Living Conditions Survey 2004 by UNDP surveyed the mortality experience of 21,668 households; their estimations of population mortality differed from estimates based on morgues' and hospitals' death data by less than a factor of 2 (UNDP, 2004). Johns Hopkins University researchers conducted cross-sectional cluster sample surveys of mortality in Iraq (all ages) in 2004 and 2006 (Roberts et al. 2004; Burnham et al. 2006). The first of these showed a threefold difference. In the second study, researchers accompanied Iraqi doctors to 1849 homes in 47 randomly selected community clusters, documenting 629 deaths among 12,801 household members over a 3.4-year period. Annual crude mortality rates (all ages) rose from 5.5 per 1000 to 13.2; violent deaths rose from pre-2003-war levels of 2 percent to 60 percent; and 78 percent of these deaths occurred among adult males aged 15–59 years. The population risk calculations arrived at an excess mortality of 650,000 Iraqi casualties in the 40 months after the invasion, more than 10 times higher than the cumulative report of civilian casualty figures (Iraq Body Count 2006). Keiger (2007) provides an excellent narrative description of the study rationale and methods.

The validity of epidemiologic research depends on several factors, including the unbiased selection of households, the pre-wartime period for risk comparison, and corroboration of deaths with valid death certificates. The controversial findings of the 2006 study received widespread attention by media and policy circles, including critical analysis by the research community (Dardagan, Sloboda, and Dougherty 2006). Others affirmed the underestimation of mortality by prior studies and body count estimations (Media Lens 2006).

OPPORTUNITIES AND CHALLENGES FOR
EPIDEMIOLOGY IN WAR AND ARMED CONFLICT

Rhodes (1988) wrote that "the scale of man-made death is the central moral as well as material fact of our time" and asserted that "death from war, political violence, and their attendant privations, should be monitored, nation by nation, to expose to public view national responsibility for a major loss of human life and thereby encourage its reduction."

Historically, however, the social and health sciences have underplayed the issues of politics, warfare, and armed violence.

Health research is the systematic investigation designed to develop or contribute to generalizable knowledge about major health issues. As a major resource of public health research, epidemiology is a tool to amass "burden of proof"—that is, corroboration from a variety of study designs and statistical methods—of population health risk. To be valid scientifically, epidemiologic findings must be unprejudiced, reproducible and conducted according to rules and conventions of hypothesis testing, study design, sampling methods and accounting for bias, and statistical analysis. Only recently have best-practice epidemiologic studies in contemporary war zones come under scrutiny by political, international law, and human rights arenas and the media. Downstream from study design and field work are the challenges of disseminating knowledge, advocacy, tailoring public health messages, and exerting pressure on implicated public, corporate, and sociopolitical organizations.

In a broad sense the major barrier to war and conflict epidemiology remains that social and political violence is not seen as a health determinant in public health sciences. Compared to the vast scope of health research, epidemiologic methods are much underutilized in the field of war and violence. Frontline documentation the fate of civilians affected by armed conflict by health workers is vital. Excess mortality is the most useful measure collected through population-based surveys (Checchi and Roberts 2005), along with other indicators and methods to monitor the impact of humanitarian relief and programs, mobilize resources, and influence policy (Brennan and Nandy 2001).

Problems with security and access can make consistent collection of accurate data difficult, but political obstacles can pose greater problems. Situational factors directly affect the choice of study design and methods of fieldwork, often demanding innovation and adaptation. Research under such conditions requires dedicated effort and careful adherence to scientific and ethical principles. Health research in violent settings poses considerable ethical challenges, such as imperiling the safety of personnel, study participants, or the local community (Zwi et al. 2006).

Although this is changing, many humanitarian assistance NGOs limit their use of information to project management functions and are reluctant to collaborate in operational research, to share data, or to publish studies (Mills 2005). Methodologically stronger designs that include control groups and follow cohorts (rather than just cross-sectional surveys) involve rigor and resources for research that compete with other priorities of frontline organizations and health workers (Toole, Waldman, and Zwi 2006). Developing for field use practical, user-friendly "toolkits" for health data gathering and analysis—validated instruments applicable to both violent conflict settings and nonviolent conflict (control) settings—would be an important step forward.

Beyond descriptive analysis of the impact of violent conflict are the experimental study designs, a higher level of evidence to make causal inferences. Ideal study designs to evaluate humanitarian (or Peace through Health) interventions would use population-based sampling methods, include control groups (e.g., from unaffected communities) and study timeframes that span conflict phases.

REFERENCES

Ahlström, C. 1991. *Casualties of conflict: Report for the World Campaign for the Protection of Victims of War.* Uppsala, Sweden: Uppsala University.

Andersson, N. 1995. Social cost of land mines in four countries: Afghanistan, Bosnia, Cambodia, and Mozambique. *British Medical Journal* 311 (7007): 718–21.

Arya, N., and W. Cukier. 2005. The international small arms situation: A public health approach. In *Ballistic trauma: A practical guide,* ed. Peter F. Mahoney, William C. Schwab, Adam J. Brooks, and James Ryan. London: Springer-Verlag, 3–30.

Ascherio, A., R. Chase, T. Cote, G. Dehaes, E. Hoskins, J. Laaouj, M. Passey, S. Qaderi, S. Shuqaidef, M. Smith, and S. Zaidi. 1992. Effect of the Gulf War on infant and child mortality in Iraq. *New England Journal of Medicine* 327:931–36.

Berdon, V. 2005. Codes of medical and human experimentation ethics. Poynter Center for the Study of Ethics and American Institutions, University of Indiana. Available online at the www.wisdomtools.com website.

Brennan, R. J., and R. Nandy. 2001. Complex humanitarian emergencies: A major global health challenge. *Emergency Medicine* 13:147–56.

Burnham, G., R. Lasta, S. Doocy, and L. Roberts. 2006. Mortality after the 2003 invasion of Iraq: A cross-sectional cluster sample survey. *The Lancet* 368:1421–28.

Burrowes, Robert. 1991. The Gulf War and the Gulf peace team. *Social Alternatives,* 20 (2): 35–39.

Centers for Disease Control. 2005. Classification of death and injury from terrorism. National Center for Health Statistics. Available online at the www.cdc.gov website.

Checchi, F., and L. Roberts. 2005. Interpreting and using mortality data in humanitarian emergencies: A primer for non-epidemiologists. Humanitarian Practice Network, Paper 52, September. Available online at the www.odihpn.org website.

Coggon, D., G. Rose, and D. J. P. Barker. 1997. Epidemiology for the uninitiated. *British Medical Journal.* Available online at the www.bmj.com website.

Cukier, W. 2001. Small arms: A major public health hazard. *Medicine and Global Survival* 7 (1): 3–30. Available online at the www.ryerson.ca website.

Daponte, B. O. 1993. A case study in estimating casualties from war and its aftermath: The 1991 Persian Gulf War. *PSR Quarterly* 3 (2): 57–66. Available online at the www .ippnw.org website.

Dardagan, H., J. Sloboda, and J. Dougherty. 2006. Reality checks: Some responses to the latest *Lancet* estimates. Iraq Body Count Press release, October 16. Available online at the www.iraqbodycount.org website.

Garfield, R. M., and A. I. Neugut. 1997. The human consequences of war. In *War and public health,* ed. B. S. Levy and V. W. Sidel, 27–38. Oxford: Oxford University Press.

Hillier, D., and B. Wood. 2003. Shattered lives report. Oxfam International and Amnesty International. Available online at the www.controlarms.org website.

Human Security Centre, *Human Security Report 2005: War and peace in the 21st century.* New York: Oxford University Press. Available online at the www.humansecurity .report.info website.

International Study Team. 1991. Health and welfare in Iraq after the Gulf crisis: An in-depth assessment. Available online at the www.warchild.ca website.

Iraq Body Count. 2006. Available online at the www.iraqbodycount.org website.

Keiger, D. 2007. The number. *Johns Hopkins Magazine,* February. Available online at the www.jhu.edu website.

Krug, E. G., et al., eds. 2002. World report on violence and health. Geneva: World Health Organization. Available online at the www.who.int website.

Krug, E. G., K. E. Powell, and L. L. Dahlberg. 1998. Firearm-related deaths in the United States and 35 other high- and upper-middle-income countries. *Int J Epidemiol* 27 (2): 214–21.

Media Lens. 2006. *Lancet* report co-author responds to questions, Znet November 2. Available online at the www.zmag.com website.

Mills, E. 2005. Sharing evidence on humanitarian relief. *British Medical Journal* 331: 1485–6.

Putnam, F. 1998. The Atomic Bomb Casualty Commission in retrospect. *Proceedings of the National Academy of Sciences* 95 (10): 5426–31.

Rhodes, R. 1988. Man-made death: A neglected mortality. *JAMA* 260 (5): 686–7.

Roberts, L., R. Lafta, R. Garfield, J. Khudhairi, and G. Burnham. 2004. Mortality before and after the 2003 invasion in Iraq: Cluster sample survey. *Lancet* 364:1857–64.

Sidel, V. W., H. J. Geiger, and B. Lown. 1962. The medical consequences of thermonu-clear war II: The physician's role in the post-attack period. *New England Journal of Medicine* 266:1137–45.

Siebal, B. J. 2000. The case against the gun industry. *Public Health Rep.* 2000 Sep.–Oct. 115 (5): 410–18.

Sloan, J., A. Kellermann, et al. 1988. Handgun regulations, crime, assaults and homicide: A tale of two cities. *New England Journal of Medicine* 319 (19): 1256–62.

Stover, E., J. C. Cobey, and J. Fine. 1997. The public health effects of land mines: Long-term consequences for civilians. In *War and public health,* ed. B. S. Levy and V. W. Sidel, 137–46. Oxford: Oxford University Press.

Stover, E., A. S. Keller, J. Cobey, and S. Sopheap. 1994. The medical and social conse-quences of land mines in Cambodia. *JAMA* 272:331–6.

Summers, J. 1989. *Soho—a history of London's most colourful neighborhood.* London: Bloomsbury. Available online at the www.ph.ucla.edu website.

Taipale, I., et al., eds. 2001. *War or health? A reader.* London: Zed Books.

Toole, M., R. Waldman, and A. Zwi. 2006. Complex emergencies. In *International public health: Disease, programs, systems and policies,* ed. M. Merson, R. Black, and A. J. Mills. Sudbury: Jones and Bartlett.

United Nations Development Program (UNDP). 2004. The Iraq living conditions survey. Available online at the www.iq.undp.org website.

Zwi, A. B., N. J. Grove, C. MacKenzie, E. Pittaway, D. Zion, D. Silove, and D. Tarantola. 2006. Placing ethics in the centre: Negotiating new spaces for ethical research in conflict situations. *Global Public Health* 1 (3): 264–77.

NOTE

1. This figure has been questioned. It may include both morbidity and mortality. Ahlström's *Casualties of Conflict* (1991) is often considered a primary source for this figure but Ahlström reports that, of 36 major armed conflicts going on in 1988–1989, "Three out of four deaths are civilian in the conflict locations where distribution of civilian and military deaths is listed (i.e., 13 locations, covering about 50% of all deaths). For the other 23 locations with no available figures, a "conservative" assumption (lower than in the 13 locations) of an equal distribution between civilian and military deaths can be made.

This gives the result that nine out of ten of all victims (dead and uprooted) are civilian" (p. 19).

PART V

Case Studies

THE FOLLOWING CASE STUDIES illustrate many principles and modes of acting on Peace through Health. These will be categorized in a health preventive framework, as described in Chapter 1. Included in this framework are the categories of primary prevention (before extensive direct violence), secondary prevention (during violent conflict), and tertiary prevention (rebuilding and prevention of renewal of conflict).

Primary prevention activities include the weapons limitations advocated by IPPNW and the HELP Network; the actions of individuals such as Helen Caldicott, who was immortalized in the Academy Award winning film *If You Love This Planet;* the courageous Nepali doctors who, in performing their professional duties, managed to help bring down an oppressive government; and peace education efforts such as those of the McMaster group in Croatia and Afghanistan.

Secondary prevention activities during "hot war" include humanitarian ceasefires and the three contrasting approaches that have arisen from the Israel–Palestine conflict. These are the medical magazine *bridges;* Healing Across the Divides, an American physician–led project in which Israeli and Palestinian professionals collaborate to improve the health of their respective populations; and the Canadian–Palestinian PACT project, which focuses on psychosocial healing of Palestinians on the West Bank. In Iraq, Iraq Body Count, an initiative to measure the damage of war, demonstrates the power of citizen engagement. Even prior to this hot war, various health professionals went to visit Iraq to bear witness during the period of sanctions in the 1990s, which killed more people than the war has up to the time of this writing.

Tertiary prevention includes the roles of psychosocial healing and community-based rehabilitation; the World Health Organization's joint reconstruction efforts to integrate health systems and personnel throughout the world; and the Butterfly Peace Garden, a unique initiative that enlists primarily artists, rather than medical personnel, to promote healing.

16

Primary Prevention

Preventing War by Weapons Limitation ▪ Ian Maddocks

PRIMARY PREVENTION OF WAR between nation-states requires the building of supportive structures that maintain harmony and peaceful cooperation between them and facilitate relationships that recognize equality of status and mutual respect. Such a goal will not be easily achieved through the example of a single leader or the efforts of hard-working diplomats; it will require an understanding and a will that extends through all levels of society. Global history offers few pertinent examples of such harmony; instead, most periods of relative peace have been achieved through the dominance of one major power over others, as in the "Pax Romana" (Roman peace). That dominance is eventually followed by the emergence of competing alternative powers, resulting in conflict and war. The current efforts of the states of Europe to form a single federation hold the promise of an end to the repetitive rounds of wars that have marked thousands of years of European history, but only time will tell whether that sad history can be relegated to the past. In the meantime, controlling the means to wage war may contribute to primary prevention.

ATTEMPTS TO CONTROL WEAPONS OF WAR: INTERNATIONAL TREATIES AND CONVENTIONS

The Lieber Code, framed by an international lawyer of German origin, was a set of rules on land warfare promulgated as *Instructions to Armies in the Field* by President Lincoln at the time of the American Civil War. It provided norms for the behavior of troops toward civilians, prisoners of war, and wounded individuals. In 1868, an International Military Commission met in St. Petersburg and framed a declaration renouncing the use of explosive projectiles under 400 grams in weight (which were regarded as causing unacceptable injury to individuals). This was followed, in 1899, by a call from Czar Nicholas of Russia to recognized nation-states to meet and consider the wasteful expenditure by all governments on ever more destructive and expensive armaments. He proposed agreement to refrain from developing more powerful arms and to eliminate those that threatened the greatest human suffering. The czar's initiative resulted in the Hague Peace Conference, the first of many international meetings that have addressed prevention of military conflict and have sought to limit its adverse effects.

Of particular concern at that time were "dumdum" bullets that spread on impact, armaments launched from balloons, and poison-gas shells. To an age that has seen the use of napalm, nuclear weapons, and intercontinental missile systems, such concern over relatively small items seems almost trivial. Yet it reflects the two major areas within which efforts at prevention continue to be proposed: the infliction of unnecessary suffering on combatants, and indiscriminate injury and harm to noncombatants (Coupland 1999, 583; Kalshoven 1991, 175).

Numerous international meetings over the years have explored ways to reduce or remove from use a wide spectrum of instruments of war, particularly when they can be depicted as indiscriminate (affecting civilian as well as military personnel) or as causes of unnecessary suffering to those affected by them. The following list of such weapons includes sources of information about proposals to limit or end their use.

- Poison gas and other chemical agents, which cause skin eruptions, asphyxia, or paralysis (OPCW 2005)
- Biological weapons initiating fatal infection or prolonged morbidity (Department of Peace Studies, University of Bradford 2006)
- Small arms, available in their thousands, which enable even children to be turned into combatants (Cukier 2002)
- Landmines, which target victims indiscriminately and cause unacceptable mutilation (ICBL 2004)
- Laser weapons that inflict permanent blindness (Doswald-Beck 1993)
- Electric shock weapons, used as stun guns for crowd control, but more often for torture (Martin and Wright 2003)
- Nuclear weapons, which are capable of causing massive destruction and death or injury to entire populations (Report of the Canberra Commission 1996)

A majority of nations have the ability to manufacture any of the weapons listed above except nuclear weapons. Sophisticated industrial capacity is necessary to produce and accumulate a sufficient quantity of the nuclear materials required. Only a few major powers are able to deploy these most destructive and indiscriminate of all weapons of war. Nations that have eschewed possession of nuclear weapons or have been prevented from developing them, and many nongovernmental organizations, continue to protest their production and deployment.

DIFFICULTIES IN OBTAINING AGREEMENT

The instructions given to United States delegates who attended the Hague Conference (US Department of State 1899) reflected suspicion and skepticism about the usefulness of international agreements and foreshadowed comments repeated in virtually all arms limitations conferences through the ensuing century. US representatives were enjoined "not to give the weight of their influence to the promotion of projects the realization of which is so uncertain." They were to be guided by the following opinions:

1. "[The proposals] *seem lacking in practicability, and the discussion of these propositions would probably prove provocative of divergence rather than unanimity of views."*
2. *"It is doubtful if wars are to be diminished by rendering them less destructive, for it is the plain lesson of history that the periods of peace have been longer protracted as the cost and destructiveness of war have increased."*
3. *"The expediency of restraining the inventive genius of our people in the direction of devising means of defense is by no means clear, and, considering the temptations to which men and nations may be exposed in a time of conflict, it is doubtful if an international agreement to this end would prove effective."*
4. *"The dissent of a single powerful nation might render it altogether nugatory [(of no consequence)]."*

These comments bring to mind several thoughts. The concept of deterrence—that the threat of use of very terrible weapons will keep nations from engaging in war—has been repeatedly endorsed over the years, most recently by nuclear-weapons states to justify retention of their considerable arsenals. Many modern efforts in the United Nations to achieve meaningful limitations on weapons of war have been "rendered nugatory" by such dissent, and the effectiveness of any treaty is eroded when even one major power remains a nonsignatory. Both the need to allow scientific research to proceed without constraint, and the wish to have some technical advantage available when conflict threatens, persist in modern discussions. These principles make it next to impossible to achieve substantial multilateral agreement on any issue of controlling arms. International institutions designed to dispel enmity and foster peace between nations (from the Hague Conference through the League of Nations and the United Nations) have been able to claim only limited success.

One recurring theme since the 1899 Hague meeting—a theme that continues to hold out a better promise of agreement—is the more restricted aim of arms limitations or the outlawing of particular weapons systems. In addition to the reasons that the United States proposed for withholding its agreement in 1899, issues of verification and of commercial confidentiality consistently constrain agreement within the United Nations. For example, a system for the inspection of production facilities was put in place to monitor whether chemical weapons were being produced clandestinely (OPCW 2005), but a similar system proved impossible to use for biological weapons because major multinational companies objected, citing the risk that their commercial secrets would be exposed (Department of Peace Studies, University of Bradford 2006).

Can health professionals make some difference in the achievement of agreement concerned with war prevention?

IPPNW

International Physicians for the Prevention of Nuclear War was founded in 1981 with the particular aim of opposing any use of nuclear weapons and advocating an early end to their production, testing, and deployment (Maddocks 1995). A major point of IPPNW's argument was that the explosion of even a single nuclear weapon in a population center had been shown to cause such massive destruction and human injury that no adequate medical response was possible. Hence prevention must be the only feasible medical policy. Nuclear weapons should never again be used and therefore must be abolished. Analysis of the potential effects of a nuclear strike on any big city—and their graphic demonstration—allowed this message to be delivered effectively to medical and lay audiences, and to highlight to governments the futility of building nuclear shelters.

Did this advocacy make a difference? When officers of IPPNW were invited to meet with President Gorbachev in 1987, he claimed to have heard IPPNW's message and to have been influenced by it. The Soviet Union had ceased building nuclear shelters. Perhaps the main positive outcome, however, was a sense of encouragement within public opinion globally: if doctors from both sides of the Cold War divide were speaking out, they should surely be heard. That was emphasized in the 1985 awarding of the Nobel Prize for Peace to the global medical movement.

IPPNW's focus on nuclear weapons came at a time when two superpowers were building huge arsenals of nuclear warheads and delivery systems. This gave its message relevance and clarity, and the abolition of nuclear weapons remained the central tenet of its mission through succeeding decades. Over time, however, with the ending of the Cold War, and with the increased risk of nuclear technologies being directed toward weapons production by other nations, the message proclaimed by IPPNW became more complex. IPPNW felt a need to extend its mission to include the elimination of other weapons, such as landmines, that caused large-scale or indiscriminate destruction of human life or major injury. IPPNW also became a major participant in the International Campaign to Ban Landmines.

INTERNATIONAL CAMPAIGN TO BAN LANDMINES

The International Campaign to Ban Landmines (ICBL) was founded in 1993. Health organizations were a major part of the founding group. The ICBL argued that antipersonnel landmines inflicted horrific injuries, mainly on civilians and often on young children—injuries that were impossible to repair (amputation of limbs, blindness) and resulted in major disability for life (ICBL 2004). With supporters such as Princess Diana, the Campaign gained momentum. A bold proposal by the government of Canada, supporting a global campaign of publicity by a coalition of nongovernment organizations in the International Campaign to Ban Landmines highlighting the terrible injuries incurred by military and civilian victims of these weapons, led to the so-called Ottawa Treaty, which encouraged worldwide cessation of the use of landmines, even by those countries that did not sign and ratify the treaty.

SMALL ARMS

Concerning small arms, it has been said that "legislation not only has a practical effect on limiting supply, but may also shape values and limit demand" (Cukier 2002). In many situations, however, that may be no more than a pious hope. In the United States, gun ownership is for many a matter of patriotic pride (even though it is clearly associated with high levels of gun violence and suicide). In Papua New Guinea, tribal conflicts have become increasingly dangerous through the availability to warriors of huge numbers of handguns and automatic rifles stolen from or sold by police and army personnel. Most of these weapons arrived from Australia via legitimate government-to-government transfers under supposedly strict controls (Roberts 2006).

As well as being a member of the ICBL, IPPNW gave strong support to the campaign of the International Action Network on Small Arms (IANSA) to demonstrate that major injury may follow the firing of a single bullet and may require the victim to undergo expensive surgical repair and prolonged hospitalization (Cukier 2002). Prevention remains the obvious and appropriate medical response to the use of all such weapons.

IS THERE A WAY FORWARD?

No single strategy offers hope of significantly reducing the weapons of war. But to fail to protest their continued presence and proliferation is to abandon societies all around the world to increasing mayhem and injury.

Although the United Nations continues to encourage nation-states to achieve effective treaties, no comparable forum exists to address the use of weapons by nonstate parties. Most modern conflicts now occur *within* states, and nonstate actors engaged in military conflict refuse to be bound by agreements entered into by governments they are trying to depose.

It is only by establishing universal norms agreed to among states concerning legitimate systems of weaponry—together with agreements by nation-states to limit the production, transfer, and use of weapons deemed unacceptable—that progress can be envisaged among nonstates parties. Health professionals, by focusing on the health effects of unacceptable weapons, may continue to help establish these norms. A global movement of revulsion against landmines inspired the Ottawa process; similar global awareness among ordinary citizens may build a similar commitment to discredit nuclear and biological weapons as legitimate instruments of war and to control the availability of small arms.

At its initial meeting in London in 1981, the Medical Association for Prevention of War, a pioneer medical organization dedicated to the promotion of peace, agreed on aims that reflect the ideals of primary prevention:

- Study of the causes and results of war
- Examination of the psychological mechanisms by which people are conditioned to accept war as a necessity

- Advocacy to direct monies spent in preparation for war toward the fight against disease and malnutrition

A message from Lord Boyd-Orr to that meeting noted that "war is the worst of the psychological diseases of human society and its prevention might well be regarded as the most important part of preventive medicine" (Poteliakoff 2006).

In his introduction to the volume *War or Health?* (Taipale 2002), United Nations Secretary-General Kofi Annan applauds the many physicians and groups of physicians who have actively spoken out to save human lives endangered by violence. He notes that "the health profession shows its expertise in a responsible way." But peace is an issue for *all* professions and all individuals to address in a responsible way. Annan continues: "[C]onflict prevention . . . will not be achieved by grand gestures or by short-term thinking. It requires us to change deeply ingrained attitudes." Continued reliance on weapons, large and small, for resolving conflict is deeply ingrained, and even major changes in attitudes will not lead to the elimination of all weapons, but only of those that can be stigmatized as unacceptable in special ways. Poison gas was one such weapon; antipersonnel landmines were another. The elimination of nuclear weapons awaits global agreement—something to be devotedly sought and tirelessly pursued.

REFERENCES

Christoffel, K. Kaufer, Firearm injuries: Epidemic then, endemic now. *American Journal of Public Health* 2007, 97:626–629.

Coupland, R. A. H. 1999. *Review of the legality of weapons: A new approach—the SIrUS project.* In *ICRC No. 835*. Geneva: ICRC.

Cukier, W. 2002. More guns, more deaths. *Medicine, Conflict and Survival* 18 (4): 367–79.

Department of Peace Studies, University of Bradford. 2006. *Convention on the prohibition of the development, production and stockpiling of bacteriological (biological) and toxin weapons and on their destruction.*

Doswald-Beck, L. E. 1993. *Blinding weapons. Reports of the meetings of experts convened by the International Committee of the Red Cross on battlefield laser weapons 1989–1991.* Geneva: International Committee of the Red Cross.

ICBL. 2004. *Landmine monitor report 2004.* Landmine Monitor Core Group: Human Rights Watch, Handicap International, Kenya Coalition against Landmines, Mines Action Canada, Norwegian People's Aid.

Kalshoven, F. 1991. *Constraints on the waging of war.* Geneva: International Committee of the Red Cross.

Maddocks, I. 1995. Evolution of the physicians' peace movement: A historical perspective. *Health and Human Rights* 2 (1): 88–109.

Martin, B., and S. Wright. 2003. Countershock: Mobilizing resistance to electroshock weapons. *Medicine, Conflict and Global Survival* 19 (3): 205–22.

OPCW. 2005. *Report of the OPCW on the implementation of the convention on the prohibition of the development, production, stockpiling and use of chemical weapons and on their destruction in 2004.* In OPCW Conference of the States Parties.

Poteliakoff, A. 2006. A commitment to peace: A doctor's tale. *Medicine, Conflict and Global Survival* 22 (Supplement 1): S1–S55.

Report of the Canberra Commission on the elimination of nuclear weapons. 1996, Department of Foreign Affairs, Commonwealth of Australia: Canberra.

Roberts, G. 2006. Canberra-supplied guns rife in Pacific. In *The Australian* (August 7).

Taipale, I. 2002. *War or health? A reader.* London: Zed Books.

US Department of State, 1899. *Instructions from the Department of State to delegates on the part of the president of the United States to the peace conference at the Hague, 1899, Washington, April 18.* Available online at the www.yale.edu website.

Opposing Gun Violence in the United States
■ Katherine Kaufer Christoffel

BACKGROUND: GUNS IN THE UNITED STATES

THE ROLE OF GUNS IN US SOCIETY has been an issue since the nation was founded. The ongoing debate affects many aspects of life, including work in the health-care sector.

In recent years, gun ownership and gun deaths in the United States have been higher than in other developed nations (Small Arms Survey 2001; World Health Organization 2001). The toll has waxed and waned and is related to both social conditions and handgun production (Reich et al. 2002; Wintemute 1987). At times, the nation has passed new laws to control civilian access to guns (Legal Community Against Violence 2006; Vernick and Mair 2002). Policies have been guided both by the criminal justice perspective (particularly regarding homicides) and by the health sector perspective (including suicides, which account for a majority of US gun deaths).

HEALTH PERSPECTIVES ON US GUN DEATHS
IN THE LATE TWENTIETH CENTURY

Because the epidemic surge in US gun deaths from the mid-1980s to the mid-1990s (Christoffel 2007) particularly affected youth, US pediatricians led work to reduce the toll. The American Academy of Pediatrics (AAP, www.aap.org) called for clinical counseling on the dangers of guns to children and youth and for a ban on civilian possession of handguns (Committee on Injury and Poison Prevention 2000). Health providers in other specialties involved their societies as well (Longjohn, Christoffel 2004). The HELP Network (www.helpnetwork.org) was founded in 1993 to unite involved health organizations. With the support of the Joyce Foundation (www.joycefdn.org) and other philanthropies, HELP became an information hub on the health toll of guns. Over several years, Physicians for Social Responsibility (PSR, www.psr.org) and Doctors Against Handgun Injury (DAHI, www.doctorsagainsthandguninjury.org) developed gun injury prevention agendas.

Less clinical parts of the health sector were also involved. The National Center for Health Statistics and the National Center for Injury Prevention and Control (NCIPC) increased surveillance of violent deaths and injuries, including those involving guns (National Violent Death Reporting System, www.cdc.gov/ncipc/wisqars). NCIPC-funded research in the early 1990s led to groundbreaking policy-relevant research, such as establishing the relationship between guns in the home and suicide (Kellermann, Rivara, and Somes 1992). The health perspective was put forward, during legislative battles, by various organizations, such as the Violence Policy Center (www.vpc.org), which has emphasized guns as consumer products that warrant safety regulation. The policy implications of this approach were explored by leading health sector scholars (Teret and Lewin 2003). Public education campaigns raised awareness of the risk of private gun ownership.

Gun deaths and gun ownership rates in the United States fell substantially in the mid-1990s. A new plateau in deaths was reached at approximately 30,000 per year, compared to a peak of almost 40,000. The health sector probably contributed to this improvement via public and clinical education on the medical risks of gun ownership, safer storage options, and the vulnerability of children to guns in their environment. Altered crime conditions, such as the waning of crack cocaine sales in large cities, surely contributed as well (Blumstein et al. 1995; Christoffel 2005). Increasingly productive efforts were predicted by these successes, by accumulated information on the epidemiology of gun deaths and injuries, and by emerging information on intervention approaches that might work to reduce gun misuse.

HEALTH SECTOR WORK ON US GUN DEATHS AND INJURIES IN THE TWENTY-FIRST CENTURY

It has not worked out that way. Several factors induced physicians and scholars to turn their attention to other areas of work.

The ebb began in the mid- to late 1990s, when health sector work on gun deaths was consistently attacked by the National Rifle Association (NRA) and its allies, who argued that guns are a crime issue and that most health-based research is pseudo-science. A few NRA-allied physicians pressed this case directly to journal editors and funding agencies, urging the rejection of research reports and proposals. Harassing calls and e-mails were aimed at physicians and scholars actively involved in gun injury prevention. Despite popular support for efforts to reduce gun deaths, a federal law was passed that sharply limited CDC research related to gun deaths and injuries. With the arrival of the Bush administration in 2001, the NRA perspective came to guide federal actions.

Once US gun death rates fell from their peak, the media tended to minimize the ongoing toll; this led to reduced salience of the toll in the public eye. A recession shrank the assets of the foundations that were supporting health-based work on gun deaths and injuries, reducing funding for gun injury prevention. The events of September 11, 2001, led funders to give priority to other health aspects of violence, as attention shifted from the large number of actual gun deaths to the unknown risks posed by bioterrorism.

As a result of these changes, the health sector networks that focus on the prevention of gun injuries and deaths have ended their organizational work. Individuals are now working to create a Web-based training program about gun injuries that will help to weave the lessons of the 1990s work into the fabric of health-care delivery in the current era.

The knowledge and experience gained during health sector work in the 1990s on gun injury prevention will be of use in other nations and during future outbreaks in the United States. Such outbreaks are likely to lead to renewed work by the health sector to prevent and manage gun death and injury. Work can be done during the current endemic period to create structures and processes that will be useful during epidemic periods (World Health Organization 2001).

REFERENCES

Blumstein, A., and R. Rosenfeld. 1995. Explaining recent trends in US homicide rates.
· *Journal of Criminal Law* 86:1036.
Christoffel, K. Kaufer. 2005. Evaluating Gun Policy. *Injury Prevention* 11:126–127.
Christoffel, K Kaufer. 2007. Firearm injuries: Epidemic then, endemic now. *American Journal of Public Health* 97:626–629.
Committee on Injury and Poison Prevention, American Academy of Pediatrics. 2000. Firearm-related injuries affecting the pediatric population. *Pediatrics* 105:888–95.

Gotsch, K. E., J. L. Annest, J. A. Mercy, and G. W. Ryan. 2001. Surveillance for fatal and non-fatal firearm-related injuries, United States 1993–1998. 1–32. Available online at the www.cdc.gov website.

Guns at home equal higher suicide risk: Study. 2007. *Health Science & Technology* 12 (2). Available online at the www.thenewamerican.com website.

Kellermann, A. L., F. P. Rivara, and G. Somes. 1992. Suicide in the home in relation to gun ownership. *New England Journal of Medicine* 13:467–72.

Legal Community Against Violence. 2006. *Regulating guns in America.* San Francisco: LCAV.

Longjohn, M., and K. Kaufer Christoffel. 2004. Are medical societies developing a standard for gun injury prevention? *Injury Prevention* 10 (3): 169–73.

National Violent Death Reporting System. *The public health problem.* Available online at the www.cdc.gov website.

Reich, K., P. L. Culcross, and R. E. Behrman. 2002. Children, youth, and gun violence. *The Future of Children* 12 (2). Available online at www.futureofchildren.org/pubs-info 2825/pubs-info_show.htm?doc_id=154414, accessed Feb 12. 2008.

Small Arms Survey. 2001. *Profiling the problem.* Oxford: Oxford University Press.

Teret, S. P., and N. L. Lewin. 2003. Policy and technology for safer guns: An update. *Annals of Emergency Medicine* 41:32–34.

Vernick, J. S., and J. S. Mair. 2002. How the law affects gun policy in the United States: Law as intervention or obstacle to prevention. *Journal of Law Medicine Ethics* 30 (2): 692–704.

Wintemute, G. 1987. Firearms as a cause of death in the United States, 1920–1982. *Journal of Trauma* 27:532–36.

World Health Organization. 2001. *Small arms and global health.* Available online at the www.whqlibdoc.who.int website.

The Health Professional as Activist ▪ Helen Caldicott

I FIRST BECAME CONCERNED about the consequences of nuclear war at age 15 when I read *On the Beach,* by Neville Shute. In this book, a nuclear war triggered by accident in the Northern Hemisphere kills all people except those in Melbourne. Eventually they too died, and all human life is extinguished.

In 1956, just seventeen years old and in the first year of medical school, I learned of Muller's radiation-induced mutations in *Drosophila* (fruit flies) that were passed on through generations. At that time, atmospheric nuclear testing conducted by the Soviet Union, the United States, and China generated radioactive fallout that was polluting human habitats and biological systems in the Northern Hemisphere.

Years later, in 1971, after discovering that French atmospheric nuclear testing in the South Pacific was polluting Australia, I initiated a public educational campaign to teach about the medical dangers of radioactive fallout. Then a massive grassroots movement arose over a period of nine months, causing the Australian and New Zealand governments to take France to the International Court of Justice and force it to abandon above-ground testing.

Two years later I launched another medical campaign—this one against uranium mining in Australia—teaching the Australian union movement about the dangers of mining uranium and the nuclear fuel cycle. Both of these educational campaigns were based purely on grassroots education on the medical dangers of radiation.

The Jefferson ethic had prevailed: "An informed democracy will behave in a responsible fashion."

In 1978, while working at Harvard Medical School specializing in cystic fibrosis, I was asked by Arnold Relman, editor of the *New England Journal of Medicine,* to write an article on the medical dangers of nuclear power. A young intern from the Cambridge City Hospital, Ira Helfand, required some medical data on nuclear power to support an antinuclear referendum in the city of Cambridge. As we talked, I said, "This is a medical topic, Ira. Let's start a medical organization to combat nuclear power."

The first small meeting, held in my sitting room a week later, was attended by several doctors. Thus began the second version of Physicians for Social Responsibility (PSR). (The first PSR was founded in 1961 and died a natural death in 1971.) Serendipitously, we placed a full-page ad in the *New England Journal of Medicine* on the medical dangers of nuclear power one day after Three Mile Island melted down. Five hundred physicians immediately joined PSR.

Soon thereafter, our first symposium at Harvard on the medical effects of nuclear war received enormous media attention. A large grant was then allocated for further symposia, so we took the show on the road, holding what were referred to as "bombing runs" in many major US cities.

Simultaneously I traveled around the United States and the world giving grand rounds and recruiting doctors to PSR and the global medical movement. Over five years we recruited 23,000 US physicians to PSR, forming a total of 153 chapters. Similar medical movements were commenced in numerous other countries.

During the years 1978 to 1985, I encountered no problems recruiting physicians to the movement, but the animosity surrounding the Cold War among the US general public was sometimes difficult to resolve.

However, the strictly medical model usually disarmed all dissenters. The global medical movement received the Nobel Peace Prize in 1985.

Acting on Human Rights in Nepal
■ **Khagendra Dahal[1] and Sonal Singh[2]**

THE SMALL HIMALAYAN KINGDOM OF NEPAL has witnessed rapid political changes during the last few years, including an end to the violent conflict between the Maoist rebels and the Royal Nepalese Army (now known as the Nepal Army) that claimed more than 13,000 lives (Singh 2004, 1499–1501) and the beginnings of peace transformation in the aftermath of war. Both parties to the conflict engaged in widespread human rights abuses during the violent conflict (Singh, Dahal, and Mills 2005, 9). Health professionals, including doctors, not only bore witness to this historic transformation in Nepal but also have contributed in the struggle to ensure health as a human right within the broader macroeconomic and political picture (Maskey 2004, 122–30). Dedicated health professionals helped spark the activities of the 1990 revolution, which ushered in multiparty democracy in Nepal (Adams 1998). The doctors used human rights arguments to justify their participation in the movement, which was necessary for the eradication of poverty and repression (Adams 1998). They have continued to participate in the human rights movement in the last decade by speaking out against torture, documenting human rights abuses by both parties to the violent conflict, and refusing to succumb to draconian measures that would significantly limit the capacity of health professionals to treat victims of violence.

In a major political change in April 2006, the autocratic regime of King Gyanendra was ousted and replaced by a representative government in response to widespread protests around the country (Pandey 2006a, 1052). Doctors, lawyers, journalists, engineers, professors, teachers, and businesspeople were actively involved in this movement. The Nepal Medical Association (NMA), along with the Nepal Nursing Association, the Nepal Paramedic Association, and the Nepal Ayurvedic Doctors Association, called for the impartial treatment of victims of violence, and the health professionals acted promptly, providing such treatment at the Tribhuvan University Teaching Hospital, Kathmandu Model Hospital, Binayak Hospital, and many other hospitals in the capital, Kathmandu. Several doctors were detained, medical students were violently beaten, and some foreign physicians were even deported for treating the victims of violence. Health professionals associated with Physicians for Social Responsibility, Nepal (PSRN), the Nepali affiliate of IPPNW (International Physicians for the Prevention of Nuclear War), and several other health professionals throughout the country participated in the movement for restoration of peace and democratic rights in Nepal. Through mobilization of IPPNW and medical human rights networks, physicians from all around the world came out in support of their imprisoned Nepalese colleagues through an open letter and petition distributed on the Web (Singh et al. 2006, 1730). This received important press coverage (Pandey 2006b, 931). Such actions contributed to the global movement, which not only protected health personnel and others from reprisals in prison, but also put pressure on the government for some semblance of democratic transformation. Physician leaders in Nepal are still at the forefront of this ongoing transformation, as the Maoist rebels and the political parties work toward a new constitution and system of government in Nepal.

The success of this nonviolent revolution in Nepal points, however, to a dilemma well beyond its borders. How far should health workers engage in politics? Perhaps one may question the role of physicians in a political movement, but can health professionals in a poor, undemocratic country like Nepal steer clear of politics? Can a person treat illness without taking into account the social context in which it occurs? As Vincanne Adams (1998) puts it, "[C]an medicine be politicized and still be an objective science?" These are questions that physicians in all humanitarian situations around the world need to grapple with.

REFERENCES

Adams, V. 1998. *Doctors for democracy: Health professionals in the Nepal revolution.* Cambridge: Cambridge University Press.
Maskey, M. 2004. Practicing politics as medicine writ large in Nepal. *Development* 47 (2): 122–30.
Pandey, K. 2006a. Protests and bombing disrupt health care in Nepal. *BMJ (Clinical Research Edition)* 332 (7549): 1052.
———. 2006b. Doctors in Nepal take part in democracy protests. *BMJ (Clinical Research Edition)* 332 (7547): 931.
Singh, S. 2004. Impact of long-term political conflict on population health in Nepal. *Canadian Medical Association Journal* 171 (12): 1499–1501.
Singh, S., N. Arya, E. Mills, T. Holtz, and G. Westberg. 2006. Free doctors and medical students detained in Nepal. *The Lancet* 367 (9524): 1730.
Singh, S., K. Dahal, and E. Mills. 2005. Nepal's war on human rights: A summit higher than Everest. *International Journal for Equity in Health* 4 (June 28): 9.

NOTES

1. International Physicians for the Prevention of Nuclear War (IPPNW), Kathmandu, Nepal.
2. Department of Medicine, Wake Forest University, Winston-Salem, NC 27157.

Peace Education as Primary Prevention ■ Joanna Santa Barbara

WE HAVE NO DIFFICULTY UNDERSTANDING that a society's stock of knowledge on health issues—pathological processes disrupting health, management of disease processes, public health maintenance—is related to the level of health that society can sustain. Health education therefore is an important area of intervention. The same applies to the level of peace a society can sustain. A society's understanding of processes likely to disturb peace, how to handle these processes nonviolently, and how to institutionalize practices that maintain peace will have much to do with that society's level of peace. Learning these processes constitutes peace education.

Levels of understanding of peace appear to differ in different societies. Many indigenous societies have had strong and effective peace systems that functioned until they encountered outside interference. For example, many Australian aboriginal groups had elaborate systems of conflict resolution, and wars did not occur (Fry 2006). Other societies have a much greater tendency to resort to violence in the face of conflicts. Knowledge of modes of peace maintenance may be present but may conflict with other cultural themes, making violence a preferred modality. The highlighting of these methods of peace may be important at a time when the society is struggling to rebuild peace.

Social evolution continues. Although nonviolent struggle has appeared again and again as a way of dealing with unjust situations, since Gandhi's thoughtful and dramatic use of it on a large scale, it has become better understood, and knowledge of it has dispersed more widely over the last half-century. People have even learned of its dynamics from the famous Richard Attenborough film *Gandhi* and have used this knowledge to stage their own nonviolent revolutions. This specific linkage has been noted in Chile and the Philippines (Ackerman and Duvall 2000, 291–375) and in Poland (Spencer 2006, 22–24). Yet the highly effective methods of nonviolence are still not fully understood by many people. There is much more peace education to be done.

We continue to learn from ongoing social experiments in reconciliation processes, such as the innovative South African Truth and Reconciliation Commission processes (Govier, 2006). Nonviolent ways of transforming conflict continue to develop, as it becomes clear that such transformative ways can be found in all societies alongside violent methods.

There is an argument, then, for strengthening a society's knowledge of its own peace processes, which may have become buried in episodes of violence, and for introducing promising methods from other societies for consideration. There is a particular argument for introducing peace education to children. This applies to all children, but especially to those in societies vulnerable to repeated episodes of violence. Increasing the stock of knowledge of peace, sometimes referred to as *peace literacy,* may serve to immunize against further outbreaks of violence.

War-affected people—children and adults—suffer severely from the psychological aftermath of the terrible events of war. In addressing their anger, sadness, confusion, fear, and intrusive memories, the adults, in particular, have wanted to understand why this happened to their society. How can they achieve a working understanding to grasp the disaster that has affected their lives? From about 1999, the McMaster Peace through Health group was actively involved in Afghanistan working on peace education, initially with Afghan nongovernmental organizations. A method of conflict analysis evolving out of repeated conversations with people who view the conflict from many different perspectives has been developed out of this project (Weera 2002). People in workshop situations begin to achieve an understanding of the multiple parties and their multiple goals, the history behind the present state of affairs, the ways people have hurt each other (and that other groups besides their own were severely hurt), and how power is disposed. Once a group conflict analysis is accomplished, they can begin to see where the strengths and possibilities for ending the violence may lie. They can see the need for reconciliation. This is a consequence of peace education.

The methodology applied by the McMaster group working in Afghanistan was derived partly from the peace education methods of Johan Galtung of TRANSCEND (Galtung 2000) and adapted by one of the group's members, Afghan-Canadian physician Seddiq Weera, who understood the local context. At times, principles would be conveyed through examples far distant from the realities of Afghanistan so that concepts could be learned with less controversial cases. When the concepts were understood, they would be applied to the immediate situation, usually very creatively.

Alongside this, a school-based program of peace education, combined with ways of addressing mental health problems, was developed for children. This was done in a series of stories based on the saga of a family affected by the war (McMaster Afghanistan Working Group 2005). Themes of conflict resolution, reconciliation, ethnic tolerance, rebuilding a peaceful society, and resistance to joining a militia appear in the stories. Teachers who were trained in the delivery of this program reported that they themselves found it a transforming experience and benefited from applying the ideas in their family life. This program and others developed for younger children have since been incorporated into the standard curriculum for Afghan children. All schools in Afghanistan have been supplied with the storybooks, puppets to animate the stories, and a teacher's guide for the curriculum. Teacher training in child-centered methods to teach this material is now in progress.

In addition to the program for children, we created a manual with the same themes for teachers and parents. Later, when there was a demand for the training of peace educators, we developed a manual of elementary peace studies (MacQueen 2004). Several of those who went through this program are now ministers in the Afghan government.

The program for children was based on prior work in Croatia, which employed a similar combination of mental health issues and major themes in peace and human rights education. This program was delivered in elementary schools. We evaluated its effectiveness and found modest positive effects, compared with controls, in both mental health and reduction of ethnic antipathy. These effects lasted at least a year after the end of the study (Woodside, Santa Barbara, and Benner 1999).

The fitting together of these two levels of healing—individual and social—has a strong rationale. The appalling events of war have caused the psychological distress experienced by many or most in a war context. It would seem strange to seek to relieve the impact of war on human minds without strengthening people's capacity to keep the cause of their problems at bay. Strengthening their capacity with knowledge is a form of primary prevention. The period immediately after violent conflict is an especially risky one for the recurrence of violence. Many decisions are made above the heads of ordinary folk; however, peace education includes empowerment to act. A corollary of peace education is the cultivation of a culture of peace—the strengthening of values of peace—as promoted by United Nations Educational and Scientific Organization (UNESCO).

If peace education is to be linked to certain health interventions, who is to do this? In some cases, health workers have trained themselves in peace education, and in other cases, peace scholars have been part of a working team.

We see increasing the knowledge of peace in order to accomplish social healing of fractured societies as a peace intervention in its own right. People build their own peace; the more options they have to accomplish this, the better.

REFERENCES

Ackerman, P., and J. Duvall. 2000. *A force more powerful: A century of nonviolent conflict.* New York: St. Martin's Press.

Blumstein, A., and R. Rosenfeld. 1995. Explaining recent trends in US homicide rates. *Journal of Criminal Law* 86:10–36.

Christoffel, K., and K. Kaufer. 2005. Evaluating gun policy. *Injury Prevention* 11:126–27.

Fry, D. 2006. *The human potential for peace: An anthropological challenge to assumptions about war and violence.* New York and Oxford: Oxford University Press.

Galtung, J. 2000. *Conflict transformation by peaceful means: The Transcend Method.* United Nations. Available online at the www.transcend.org website.

Govier, T.. 2006. *Taking wrongs seriously: Acknowledgment, reconciliation and the politics of sustainable peace.* 283–95. Amherst, New York: Humanity Books.

MacQueen, G. ed. Revised 2004. *Making peace: A peace education manual for Afghanistan.* Available online at the www.humanities.mcmaster.ca website.

McMaster Afghanistan Working Group. 2005. *A journey of peace.* Available online at the www.journeyofpeace.ca website.

Spencer, M. 2006. *Two aspirins and a comedy: How television can enhance health and society.* Boulder and London: Paradigm Publishers.

UNESCO. Culture of peace. Available online at the www3.unesco.org/iycp website.

Weera, S. 2002. Afghanistan conflict analysis (1). Available online at the www.humanities.mcmaster.ca website.

Woodside, D., J. Santa Barbara, and D. Benner. 1999. Psychological trauma and social healing in Croatia. *Medicine, Conflict and Survival* 15:355–67.

17

Secondary Prevention

Humanitarian Ceasefires ■ Neil Arya

INTRODUCTION

DURING THE EARLY 1980S, Central America was plagued with civil war, and children were dying in great numbers, not because of direct violence but primarily because of poor sanitation services and low rates of immunization. From 1981 to 1985 infant mortality rates in El Salvador, Guatemala, Honduras, and Nicaragua (countries that suffered from the effects of war) were about 80 per 1000, while Panama, Costa Rica, and Belize (their neighbors that were not engaged in war) had levels just below 25 per 1000 live births (Rodriguez-Garcia et al. 2001). In the case of El Salvador, UNICEF under Executive Director James Grant, the Pan American Health Organization (PAHO), and the Roman Catholic Church brought these facts to the attention of the Duarte government and the Frente Farabundo Martí para la Liberación Nacional (FMLN) rebels in El Salvador and brokered a series of ceasefires beginning at Christmas 1985, allowing children throughout the country to be immunized.

Soon numerous other national and international organizations, including Rotary International and the International Committee of the Red Cross, joined in the planning and implementation of the ceasefires, and the "days of tranquility" were expanded to three times a year. Almost 300,000 children were immunized annually at several thousand sites until peace accords were signed in 1992. The incidence of measles and tetanus dropped dramatically, and polio was eradicated. The ceasefires were a major success as a health venture, and this effort is also thought of as a peace venture, which facilitated an atmosphere of trust and made possible the identification of common goals, setting the stage for the peace accords.

With the help of intermediaries such as the International Committee of the Red Cross (ICRC) and WHO, similar efforts were made in Lebanon in 1987, in the Philippines from 1988 to1993, in Afghanistan from 1994 to 1997 and again in 2000–2001, in the Democratic Republic of Congo in 1999 and 2000, and in Iraq/Kurdistan from 1996 onward. Temporary pauses in fighting have been arranged in at least nineteen countries since 1985, and humanitarian ceasefires, days of tranquility and "corridors of peace" meet significant health needs. But it is also important to consider how they can be part of larger peacebuilding processes.

Ceasefires offer a tranquil reminder of what peace is really like and can inspire hope and strengthen people's commitment to work for peace. Negotiations for ceasefires and corridors of peace also help make communities aware of their basic human rights to receive food and medical care. They can draw a wide range of parties at the local, national, and international levels into dialogue and can help to shed light, both nationally and internationally, on the effects of the war on all people, especially children. They might develop new channels of communication and foster confidence in negotiations to end the armed conflict.

In Sudan in 1989, UNICEF's James Grant again achieved an agreement with the Sudanese government and the Sudan People's Liberation Army (SPLA) to establish corridors of peace to deliver relief supplies to the desperate people of southern Sudan. This Operation Lifeline Sudan has been credited with increased commercial activities in these regions, resulting in a more stable environment and a zone of "almost peace," even without a real ceasefire occurring.

However, ceasefires also facilitated rearming, repositioning of forces, and smuggling in of weapons. NGOs that delivered aid were forced to sign agreements with the government or rebels, which limited their independence so severely that the ICRC refused to participate (Hendrickson 1998; Macrae 1998). What makes the difference between efforts that pave the way to lasting peace and those that merely provide a temporary lull in fighting? Mary Anne Peters (1996) examined this question.

WHAT ARE THE CHARACTERISTICS OF HUMANITARIAN CEASEFIRES WITH POSITIVE PEACE IMPACTS?

The ability to establish *common ground* between warring factions is critical. Intervenors have to help parties identify a concern or goal that is of value to all sides. The well-being of children is an ideal superordinate goal transcending conflict. Another might be dignity and respect for human life. The benefits of the humanitarian operation must be delivered *impartially and transparently,* with assistance focused on the civilian population. There must be *agreement on standards and monitoring;* that is, time limits have to be defined, the parties must establish a minimum code of conduct, and there must be a way to apply pressure to induce all parties to adhere to these rules. For example, clearly identifying vehicles used and offering assurance that no arms will be transported, or military information passed, may be helpful.

The choice of **intermediaries** is important. *International governments* can apply pressure, and *international nongovernmental organizations,* with their capacity for neutrality and their ability to act without the constraints of governments and official agencies, are often helpful. For the sake of sustainablility of a peace process, **community participation** is essential, with the *voices of women and children* being strongly represented. If possible, *local NGOs* of the country or region, with understanding of and respect for indigenous cultures and political realities, are the best vehicles for providing aid. Training of *community health-care workers* can strengthen the outcomes of these initiatives, but health workers must make use of the peacebuilding potential through building partnerships with many outside of the health sector. *Local human rights and legal organizations* can make clear reference to international agreements and laws to safeguard the peace. The *media* can also play a vital role in communication and peace education. Distance education through radio teaching or correspondence courses can complement standard education. The *military and militias* must be made part of the solution, and any attempt to address political and strategic questions must recognize that members of the military and militias and their families are often also victims of war.

CONCLUSIONS

Humanitarian ceasefires are one tool of secondary prevention in which the health sector can play a crucial role. Care must be taken to understand the conflict and develop partnerships to make such ventures a success.

Source material for this section and good references for learning about humanitarian ceasefires include Galli 2001, Guerra de Macedo 1994, Hess and Pfeiffer 1997, Large 1997, Manenti 2001, Peters 1996, Rodriguez-Garcia et al. 2001, UNICEF 1996, and WHO 1997. This material has previously been used by the author in Arya 2007.

REFERENCES

Arya, N. 2007. Peace through Health. In *Handbook of peace studies,* ed. CharlesWebel and Johan Galtung. London: Routledge.

Galli, G. 2001. Humanitarian cease-fires in contemporary armed conflicts: Potentially effective tools for peacebuilding. Master's thesis, University of York.

Guerra de Macedo, C. 1994. Health, development and peacemaking: Health as a bridge for peace. Speech made at the international symposium on Health, Development, Conflict Resolution and Peacemaking, Copenhagen, Denmark, June.

Hendrickson, D. 1998. Humanitarian action in protracted crisis: An overview of the debates and dilemmas. *Disasters* 22 (4): 283–7.

Hess, Gregory, and Michaela Pfeiffer. 1997. Comparative analysis of WHO "Health as a Bridge for Peace" case studies. Available online at the www.who.int website.

Large, J. 1997. Considering conflict: Concept paper for first "health as a bridge for peace" consultative meeting, Les Pensières, Annecy, October 30–31. World Health Organization. Available online at the www.who.int website.

Macrae, J. 1998. The death of humanitarianism? Anatomy of the attack. *Disasters* 21 (3): 309–17

Manenti, A. 2001. Health as a potential contribution to peace: Realities from the field. World Health Organization, Health and Conflict, Department of Emergency and Humanitarian Action. Available online at the www.humanities.mcmaster.ca/peace-health/Conf2001/maneti.htm website.

Peters, M. A. 1996. A Health-to-Peace Handbook. *Journal of Humanitarian Assistance.* Available online at the www.humanities.mcmaster.ca website.

Rodriguez-Garcia, R., J. Macinko, F. X. Solórzano, and M. Schlesser. 2001. *How can health serve as a bridge for peace?* Washington, DC: School of Public Health and Health Services, The George Washington University.

UNICEF. 1996. *Children as zones of peace.* Available online at the www.unicef.org website.

World Health Organization. 1997. *Report on the first WHO consultative meeting on health as a bridge for peace.* Les Pensières, Annecy, October 30–31. Available online at the www.who.int website.

The Role of Medical Journal bridges, an Israeli–Palestinian Public Health Magazine

■ Ambrogio Manenti

"THERE ARE TWO WAYS TO SURVIVE the hell of living. The first is easier for many people: to accept the hell and become a part of it until they no longer see it anymore. The second one is risky and requires continuous attention and study: to seek and to be able to recognize who and what, in the middle of hell, is not hell and make it last and give it space to grow." This is what the Italian writer Italo Calvino wrote in his novel *The Invisible Cities,* in 1972.

CONTRIBUTION OF MEDICAL JOURNALS

In recent years, several medical journals have made specific contributions to understanding of the effects of war on health. *The Lancet,* the *British Medical Journal,* the *New England Journal of Medicine,* and the *Croatian Medical Journal,* among others, have published articles related to these issues.

> Medical journals can provide several contributions to promoting peace. First, they can provide a space where detailed research findings about health problems in conflict areas can be published. This is a very important area of research that is too often neglected. . . . For example, there can be various views of the number of casualties in war or violent conflict areas. The answer to this, rather than who is right or wrong, becomes how can we get better information and data about casualty numbers—and this involves science. This means we need to search for better evidence. And that is tremendously powerful. Secondly, such journals provide a neutral forum for discussion and debate. Civilized differences can be played out and individuals can be held accountable for their point of view (Horton 2005).

The efforts produced by the medical journals are just an example of a more general commitment that the health sciences should develop for the analysis of violent conflict, the complex relationship of such conflict to health, and the mechanisms whereby health workers can make their unique contributions to the prevention, termination, and mitigation of war (Santa Barbara and MacQueen 2004).

This paper describes a medical journal that aims to contribute to conditions for dialogue in the Middle East. In the Middle East, there has been no tangible progress toward resuming the peace process, and this has had severe consequences for the health and well-being of both Palestinians and Israelis. The recent war in Lebanon has worsened the impact of the violent conflict in the region. In the occupied Palestinian territory, violence continues to claim innocent lives, and military occupation continues to have severe negative effects on the daily lives of the people.

In recent years, war has been framed as a public health problem. Indeed, war (including long-term "low-intensity" violent conflict[1]) affects human health both directly, through the violence of bombs and bullets, and indirectly, by disrupting economic and social systems that address health needs. This highlights the role of health workers in preventing violent conflict and limiting its destructiveness, and it raises questions surrounding the challenges they face (MacQueen and Santa Barbara) 2001).

The journal to be described was founded under the auspices of the World Health Organization. WHO has developed the Health as a Bridge for Peace (HBP) approach, which is intended to promote both health and peace.

"Joint action in a technical space" is an expression referring to HBP initiatives in which health personnel coming from different parties in conflict work jointly in the areas of health policy, training, service delivery, and health information. Field experience shows that health-related goals may be shared among parties involved in conflict, providing them the necessary basis for cooperation. This may create an opportunity to build a framework for negotiation, to counteract stereotyping and dehumanization of the other, and even to demonstrate the possibility of ending violence and oppression.

Advocating for health- and peace-related values is another HBP strategy. Armed conflicts (including the Israeli–Palestinian conflict) exhibit common features, such as increasing isolation, polarization, stereotyping, lack of empathy, use of selective communication, discrimination, racism, and violence. In such a context, promoting health means also promoting principles, values, and attitudes that support peace and discourage war, such as dialogue, inclusion, tolerance, multiculturalism, humanization of the enemy, and peaceful coexistence.

A PUBLIC HEALTH MAGAZINE AS A TOOL

In the Israeli–Palestinian context, there is a need for greater understanding between the Palestinian and Israeli public health communities. This has been enhanced through *bridges,* a health magazine that was first published in December 2004 and has been published bimonthly until the present time.

Bridges is an Israeli–Palestinian public health magazine that is written, produced, and managed by Palestinian and Israeli health professionals and academics under the sponsorship of the World Health Organization. It has been covering public health topics of importance to both populations, seeking to analyze the impact of the conflict on the health and well-being of both societies, and bringing readers information in various health and social fields.

So far, eleven issues of *bridges* have been published and have discussed the following main topics: poverty, disabilities, nutrition, women's health, quality of care, mental health, health behavior, nursing, chronic diseases, crisis in the Palestinian health system, and infectious diseases.

Three thousand five hundred copies of each issue have been distributed to Palestinian and Israeli health professionals, medical centers, policymakers and authorities, national and international NGOs, and different stakeholders, with particular focus on the diplomatic/development cooperation community, locally and worldwide. An electronic version is available online at the www.bridgesmagazine.org website.

Bridges is unique—it is the first such magazine to be shared between Israeli and Palestinian people—and very promising for the prospects of further collaboration between the two sides.

LIMITS AND CHALLENGES

Through an evaluation recently implemented,[2] however, remarks critical to *bridges* have emerged, including the following claims:

1. It is politically biased or not well balanced (this criticism comes mainly from the Israeli side).
2. It does not adequately reflect the reality of the violent conflict and occupation (this criticism comes from the Palestinian side).
3. The overall content provides too much room for Israeli contributions because of the larger size of Israel's scientific community.
4. It does not lead to enough genuine collaborations between Israelis and Palestinians, whereas it should be an ongoing forum that sets up initiatives related to public health—a platform to call for new projects that would promote cooperation between the two communities.
5. Some articles require a more scientific presentation, perhaps in the form of peer-reviewed papers.
6. It should have more down-to-earth content and deal more with issues that arise in the everyday lives of health professionals on both sides.

An internal analysis examined the content of *bridges* and considered, among other things, how much content addresses violence-related issues and cooperative efforts, because striking a balance between these two variables is an essential aspect of the goals of *bridges*.

The conclusion was that *bridges* is highly aware of the complex context in which it acts and of the disparities on the ground and that it seeks to highlight aspects important to both Israelis and Palestinians, trying to maintain balance in its presentation of the situation. The analysis made it clear, as well, Israeli and Palestinian authors and interviewees emphasize conflict-related issues and cooperative efforts differently.[3]

The magazine also carried feature articles dealing with WHO activities and with international scientific debate. This, together with thematic features and several other contributions, gives *bridges* a certain value as a scientific magazine and demonstrates its ambition to disseminate international health policy and strategic information relevant to the local and subregional context. But the magazine seems also to have provided a variety of more down-to-earth items, including the real-life perspective given through *A Day in the Life* features and those included in the *How . . . to* section, as well as others appearing in the *Readers' Forum* and the news.

The magazine has also modeled Palestinian–Israeli cooperation by featuring some articles of joint Palestinian–Israeli authorship—an approach that will be further developed in upcoming issues, because it has proved to be a remarkable tool of communication and advocacy. This could be a first step toward the establishment of links between the two communities. In fact, two Palestinian–Israeli working groups, generated from *bridges* joint articles, are currently working on disability, nursing, and infectious diseases.[4]

CONCLUSIONS

Because it is the first joint Israeli–Palestinian public health magazine, we must keep the uniqueness of *bridges* in mind when evaluating it. *Bridges* is an ongoing project; the magazine itself relies on building cooperation and partnership between Israeli and Palestinian health professionals and communities. Extra effort should be invested to consolidate the current experience.

Bridges should strive to represent a platform of debate and information. It should further encourage involvement of the scientific community, at both the local and the international levels, as well as creation of long-lasting collaborations, and should commit itself to nurturing those partnerships generated from its activity. *Bridges* should continue fine-tuning its work, taking into account the comments and contributions that readers and members of the Advisory Board provide to the Editorial Board. Its members should keep on investing their passion and knowledge, in the hope that these efforts can contribute to mutual understanding, dialogue, and the promotion of both health and peace.

Bridges will "seek and . . . recognize who and what, in the middle of hell, is not hell and make it last and give it space to grow."

REFERENCES

Calvino, I. 1972. Le città invisibili. Giulio Einaudi Editore.
Horton, R. 2005. Violence as a health issue: Interview with Dr. Richard Horton, editor of *The Lancet. Bridges* 1 (1).

MacQueen, G., and J. Santa Barbara. 2001. Peace building through health initiatives. PGS Briefing Paper. Available online at the www.pgs.ca website.

Pascal, R. 1990..LIC 2010—Special operations and unconventional warfare in the next century. *Future warfare studies*. Published with the Institute of Land Warfare Association of the US Army. Washington, DC: Brassley's.

Santa Barbara, J., and G. MacQueen. 2004. Peace through health: Key concepts. *The Lancet* 364 (July 24):384–86.

NOTES

1. Low-intensity conflict is "armed conflict for political purposes short of combat between regularly organized forces" (Pascal 1990, 7).

2. On the occasion of *bridges*'s first anniversary, an evaluation survey was carried out externally, through interviews of key readers and members of the Advisory Board, as well as internally, in the form of a quantitative review.

3. Although all the *editorials* have naturally addressed and encouraged cooperation and have given enough room to the conflict in general and to the occupation, in the *main articles* Palestinian authors have talked openly about the violent conflict and the occupation, whereas Israelis have refrained from doing so. In the *special interviews*, eminent personalities from the international scientific community have been interviewed, all of whom spoke of the violent conflict or terrorism, and two-thirds of whom encouraged and proposed joint or cooperative activities between the two communities. In the *Day in the Life* section, all interviewees from both communities addressed aspects related to the violent conflict; few Palestinians spoke of cooperative efforts, whereas all Israelis did. The *Student Page* section presented articles from Palestinian and Israeli students (one was a joint contribution). The young authors from both sides nearly always mentioned at least one aspect related to the violent conflict, but only two articles urged cooperation.

4. The *Happening in Health* section informs and reports on many activities and initiatives that have the ambitious aim of overcoming the divide between the two populations, their health systems, the opportunities available to them, and their general living conditions. Among 27 items, 14 mentioned or were related to cooperative efforts, thus raising hope and setting good examples. Three items addressed the violent conflict, 9 addressed the occupation, and no news item dealt with or mentioned terrorism. This section links *bridges* to society at large and, one year from the beginning of the publication, reported on health initiatives of 58 organizations and institutions (universities, local and international NGOs, ministries, international organizations, various networks and programs), among which 27 were international, 15 Palestinian, and 16 Israeli.

Healing across the Divides: American Medical Peacebuilding in the Middle East ▪ Norbert Goldfield

IT MAY AT FIRST SEEM UNREALISTIC to speak about healing across the Israeli–Palestinian divide. But as executive director of an American charitable organization (www.healingdivides.org) that began operations in 2005, I refuse to accept the idea of unbridgeable divides. This idea is largely attributable to American engagement and complicity in the Israeli–Palestinian violent conflict. The United States is part of the problem and, more important, will be part of any resolution of the Israeli–Palestinian violent conflict. Yet at this point in the violent conflict, *no one* in the United States with power to move events in the Middle East is interested in listening to both sides of the violent conflict and in actively promoting a peaceful resolution that takes into account the cultural and historical barriers between the two parties.[1]

Healing Across the Divides (HATD) adapts the "peacebuilding through health" ideology by funding community-based health improvement projects for both Israelis and Palestinians. We aim to contribute to peacebuilding by encouraging groups of Americans to listen and learn from the conflict-related challenges faced in improving health.

Why bother trying to improve the health of Israelis and Palestinians? Why not just pursue an explicitly political strategy? By way of answering these questions, I would like to explain how improving diabetes care by collecting diabetes stories can fit into the three HATD objectives.

- For the patients themselves, as health professionals at the organizations that we fund repeat the diabetes stories to the patients: *improving the health of Israelis and Palestinians within a community framework. This can best be accomplished by empowering patients to decide that life is worth living and, working within their community, to improve the control of their chronic illness such as diabetes.*
- For the grantee organization from a planning and evaluation perspective: *measuring the results, both positive and negative (challenges), of efforts to improve health*
- From a political/policy point of view, to promote an understanding of the impact of societal forces (such as the ongoing violent conflict) on diabetes control: *bringing barriers to the attention of policymakers*

Consider the following anecdote involving a diabetic from the Palestinian village of Abboud.

> *Villager:* "Why can't I control my sugar? Well, it's obvious. It is the stress of Israeli occupation. You [addressing me] should go do something about it."

Me: "How can HATD work with you and the Palestine Medical Relief Society so that you will wish to live, feel better empowered to control your diabetes, and thus see the day that you will be in a country of your own?"

What has been accomplished thus far?

- *Improved outcomes:* Documented changes in HgbA1C (a measure of long-term control of blood sugar) for several hundred diabetics participating in the Palestine Medical Relief Society (PMRS) diabetes project (Ghosh et al. 2007).
- *Process improvement:* A detailed understanding of diabetics in a large Israeli Arab town (Khatib, Efrat, and Deeb 2007).
- *Structural improvement:* Formation of an advocacy group consisting of Israeli Jewish women living in Beersheva, Israel.

The community-based organizations that HATD funds, all of which already communicate across both sides of the Israeli–Palestinian divide, have accomplished significant health improvements. The PMRS, in particular, is ready to expand its diabetes project significantly, both in scope and in raising awareness among Americans (policymakers, Arab Americans, and Jewish Americans) of the challenges they face. It will take five years to evaluate the degree to which these two objectives have been achieved.

Now let's return to the question posed at the beginning of this case study: Why bother trying to improve the health of Israelis and Palestinians? *Answer:* Without health, one cannot be an empowered citizen taking charge of one's own life and trying to improve the lives of others—including efforts to influence the ongoing violent conflict. Why not just pursue an explicitly political strategy? *Answer:* Today, there is no political strategy that is worth pursuing—(unless you like talking to yourself), because some parties to the conflict refuse to participate in dialogue. In saying this, I don't mean to criticize those who advocate an explicitly political approach. However, I know that I am not one of the 25–50 individuals with the power to push the political process from the top down. I believe that without the clout of these 25–50 people, the United States simply will not move toward facilitating a resolution of this tragic conflict. In the meantime, HATD and I will attempt to impact the Israeli–Palestinian conflict from the bottom up—at a minimum, to improve the health of both Palestinians and Israelis. As part of this long-term strategy, we bring Palestinian and Israeli health professionals to speak before mainstream Jewish-American, Arab-American, and general/politically engaged audiences (such as the World Bank). In so doing, we hope to influence American communities and leaders within those communities to take the next step and strongly encourage both of these Semitic peoples to arrive at a historic compromise. This may not happen in my lifetime, but as a Jewish-American health-care professional, I have a moral and political obligation to help improve the health of these two peoples in a manner that can contribute to peacebuilding.

REFERENCES

Ghosh, H. A., A. Shaar, J. Mashal, K. Dheidil, N. Barghuti, N. Shalaldeh, S. Aqabneh, and N. Goldfield. 2007. Diabetes control in three villages in Palestine: A community-based quality improvement intervention. *J Ambul Care Manage* 30 (1): 74–78.

Khatib, M., S. Efrat, and D. Deeb. 2007. Knowledge, beliefs, and economic barriers to healthcare: A survey of diabetic patients in an Arab–Israeli town. *J Ambul Care Manage* 30 (1): 79–85.

Wittes, Tamara. 2005. *How Israelis and Palestinians negotiate: A cross cultural analysis of the Oslo peace process.* Washington, DC: USIP Press.

NOTE

1. For further details on a negotiating approach that the United States could adopt, see Wittes 2005.

A Model for Improving Mental Health in Palestine— An Alternative View on Peace and Health?

▪ Hana Saab and Viet Nguyen-Gillham

INTRODUCTION

PEACE THROUGH HEALTH (PTH) peacebuilding projects may involve bringing parties in conflict together, having both health goals and peace goals in mind. The extent to which both of these goals are realized depends on a broad range of factors that go beyond good intentions. The World Health Organization's Health as a Bridge for Peace (HBP) efforts, for example, have been seen to have varying degrees of success because of inconsistency in the aims, strategies, and processes underlying these efforts and because of a lack of consensus as to their overarching goals (Hess and Pfeiffer n.d.).

Our thesis is that during ongoing conflict characterized by overwhelming differences in power, such endeavors may not always represent the most successful promotion of peace. On the other hand, in the Palestinian context, the promotion of societal cohesiveness, together with the principles of dignity and justice, may help foster resilience. Even though such efforts may not lead directly to political peace, they might create the conditions that set the stage for peace.

ANALYZING PEACEBUILDING

Expanding on Santa Barbara's conflict analysis (Chapter 12), peacebuilding efforts need not only to account for the multiplicity of factors that influence how these efforts unfold but also to consider the following analytical questions:

- Who are the players in the peacebuilding discourse?
- What framework serves as the backdrop for these initiatives?
- Who is involved in these initiatives?
- How relevant are the players to the local context?
- Do the players' conceptualizations of peacebuilding resonate with those of the stakeholders?

The principles underlying the prevalent PtH or HBP initiatives sometimes assume a process whereby groups perceived to be on opposite sides of a conflict come together through outside intermediaries in what are known as *contact projects*. Although these well-intentioned efforts differ in their funding process, the nature and type of health problems they address and in the peace deficits identified as a priority for a particular context, the projects share a common belief. Underlying this belief is an implicit agreement to work toward peace by health professionals, schoolchildren, teachers, or interested parties representing both sides of a conflict. Moreover, it is thought that the ripple effect resulting from such initiatives may broaden sufficiently to benefit other sectors of the population on either side of the conflict.

In certain instances, however, some members of a community who constitute primary targets of these interventions, and are benefiting from the health gains, may be unaware of the ambitious peace goals and efforts underlying the programs. Under these circumstances, many who are crucial to the ultimate peacebuilding are excluded from the peace discourse.

Ricigliano (2003) urges organizations not to view peacebuilding "through the narrow lens of their own core competencies" (446) and proposes a more integrated and holistic approach where peacebuilding interventions operate at political, social, and structural levels:

- *Political peacebuilding* is directed at realizing agreements (over disputes or ceasefire, for example) between political factions.
- *Structural peacebuilding* is directed at restoring, rebuilding, or reforming the fundamental organizations that are crucial in supporting and sustaining a peacefully functioning society.
- *Social peacebuilding* is about relationship building, is directed at changing long-held perceptions and attitudes adopted by those on each side of the conflict, and will eventually result in a shift in relationships between these groups.

According to Ricigliano, *structural peacebuilding* encompasses the wide variety and forms of traditional humanitarian and development assistance. These traditional models might be only "band-aid" solutions that conceal differences rather than contribute to enhancing the foundation for a peaceful society in situations of prolonged and protracted conflict. Such is the case for the Occupied Palestinian Territories (OPT), where violence threatens the very existence and viability of society itself. However, when such assistance is combined with advocacy, as well as with the call for justice and dignity of all parties, the meaning and effect may be more positive.

CAPABILITY DEPRIVATION AND TRADITIONAL MODELS OF AID

Borrowing the concept of *capability deprivation* developed by Amartya Sen and Martha Nussbaum, we see the need to establish capability within the Palestinian society as a prerequisite for survival, justice, and then peacebuilding. Capabilities comprise what a person is able to do or be (Sen 1984) particularly in relation to basic needs, education, and participation in society. Capability deprivation is a lack of access to resources and the resulting limitation in functioning. The capability deprivation framework has been applied to issues in development, health, and economic and social themes, but not to peacebuilding efforts per se. In our minds, an alternative model for peace recognizes that for peace to be achieved, capabilities need to be strengthened in conjunction with targeting health improvements.

When humanitarian and health programs are predicated on the goal of peacebuilding, there is the risk of "allowing the tail to wag the dog," which could compromise the intention of these initiatives (Rushton and McInnes 2006). Moreover, traditional models for the distribution and provision of aid, operating through a top-down decision-making approach with little involvement of communities in the process, do not enhance local capability. They could also lead to the alienation and isolation of certain community members and have in fact, often proved ineffective (Demichelis 1996).

THE PACT PROJECTS

Palestinian Adolescents Coping with Trauma Project (PACT) is a joint initiative between the Institute of Community and Public Health at Birzeit University and the Social Program Evaluation Group (SPEG) at Queen's University.

Our underlying premise is that capability deprivation, as manifested in the Palestinian context by lack of voice, lack of access to social supports, and limited mobility—exacerbated by exposure to traumatic events—leads to a sense of powerlessness and despair. The interaction of these factors contributes to psychosocial and mental health problems in young Palestinians. Accordingly, the goal of the project is to establish a comprehensive initiative, one that not only empowers community members but also rebuilds the social fabric of the community through a participatory research-to-action model that responds to the psychosocial needs of youth. Because Palestinians themselves identified the problem and conceived the plan of action with minimal interference from the Canadian partners and funders, this model avoids the imbalance inherent in some partnership power structures.

One of the goals of the project is to highlight the distinction between psychosocial problems and mental illness. Although these concepts often overlap, mental illness entails psychiatric disorders and chronic conditions (such as psychosis and depressive and anxiety syndromes) and the utilization of specialized treatment. Psychosocial problems, on the other hand, comprise a broader range of emotional well-being and psychological problems, while taking into account a spectrum of social, political, and cultural determinants.

PACT I

The first phase of PACT was a research project that surveyed close to 3500 Palestinian youth aged 14 to 18 in the Ramallah district of the OPT.

This occurred during and after the second Intifada, during a period of reoccupation by the Israeli military of towns in the Ramallah district. In addition to the usual checkpoints, roadblocks, travel restrictions (permits), and curfews, there was evidence of collective punishment, mass detentions, house demolitions, and incidents of direct abuse, both individual and collective (Giacaman et al. 2004).

We identified a strong relationship between the individual and collective trauma that Palestinian youth experienced and psychological indicators such as depression, anxiety, and problematic coping styles (Giacaman et al. 2007).

Development of Appropriate Models of Mental Health Intervention. Psychological rehabilitation models are usually based on Western values and principles, even though "the notion of the self, and its relationships to others and to the outside world is different in many non-Western cultures" (Parker 1996). Cross-cultural differences exist in the manner by which emotional and behavioral disorders are expressed or exhibited in physical symptoms (Bracken, Giller, and Summerfield 1995; Rahman et al. 2000). Interventions based on inappropriate models of trauma interventions are unlikely to be productive (Giacaman, Arya, and Summerfield 2005). On the contrary, research suggests that when compared to counseling and clinical interventions delivered by humanitarian agencies, social support networks and a sense of community can be of greater value in providing needed help (Children and War 2004; Raphael, Meldrum, and McFarlane 1995; Save the Children Alliance Working Group on Children Affected by Armed Conflict and Displacement 1996; Summerfield 1999).

More important, a special focus on youth is warranted in view of their high proportion within the general Palestinian population and their constitution as a particularly vulnerable group. Nonetheless, because of their continuing experiences of severe emotional distress, a psychosocial intervention that is most effectively provided at the community level can contribute to the well-being of Palestinians.

Pact II

Rather than adopting approaches to mental health shaped by Western models and operating on a disease treatment paradigm, the second phase of PACT has adopted a social and community approach by utilizing existing communal structures, a local NGO, and in this case the community-based rehabilitation program (CBR). By involving youth in the different phases of the project, PACT II addresses the psychosocial problems among Palestinian youth. PACT II builds on the successes of CBR in the West Bank and its expansion into other aspects of community development—specifically, culturally sensitive psychosocial programs for youth.

PACT II utilizes an Action Research framework that fosters collective action and the involvement of various stakeholders at different points of the research process. At the same time, it systematically integrates practice and interventions with research development by

- Reinforcing the capacities of institutions and community agencies to work together
- Connecting community members directly with the research process and model building
- Using the knowledge, culture, traditions, and resources of the community to understand psychosocial health problems and to design interventions
- Providing immediate benefits from the results of the research to the communities that participate in the project
- Reconstructing a social web and a sense of community that helps bring people together to improve their lives
- Putting knowledge in the hands of those who need to make changes

The PACT II project reinforces the capabilities model in that the list of envisioned capabilities was developed and prioritized through general social discussion and public engagement, not through theoretical assumptions derived from a predetermined list (Sen 2004).

PACT AS A PEACEBUILDING PROJECT

The PACT project did not set off as a PtH or HBP project, although it did unfold in a manner that exhibits the structural and social elements of peacebuilding outlined above. Peacebuilding efforts do not necessarily have to start with two opposing groups with conflict as a backdrop; they can also focus on building communal strengths and helping communities deal positively with difficult circumstances. In the process, peace is created within local communities as a first step, rather than peaceful relations developing across communities. We see the potential of such an initiative within current-day Palestine, which has suffered recent conflicts between political factions, military repression, and years of material deprivation that have contributed to the dismantling of internal cohesion. Peacebuilding dialogue has to be directed at the rebuilding of trust and communication to bridge the hostilities and rivalries that have developed between members of the same community.

By empowering community members, youth, and health service providers to assess need and to collaborate in planning, designing, and mobilizing resources, local capacity is established and developed. At the same time, support networks are established and the social fabric of communities strengthened. Providing a safe space for youth to express their feelings of anxiety, anger, and frustration is seen as a means of improving their psychosocial health.

Measures of social capital[1] have been used as interim short-term indicators of progress toward desired long-term community health goals (Petersen 2002). It might be logical to suggest that enhancing social capital is a critical first step in "building a human infrastructure of people who are committed to engendering a new culture, a 'peace culture,' within the fabric of communal and intercommunal life" (Hess and Pfeiffer n.d.).

Santa Barbara (2005) asserts that "peace needs a little expansion. It will clearly include the value of nonviolence. It will also include the goal value of justice, in both the sense of righting wrongs and the sense of being treated equally. These goal values may be furthered by other human goods that are both means to health and peace as well as being goal values in their own right. These would include *education, democracy, and ecological sustainability.*" We propose expanding the list of human "goods" to include capabilities in the sense of Sen's use of the term: honor, dignity, and hope, which are essential for peace efforts to be realized. PACT, which might not have begun as a peacebuilding project, nonetheless has the potential to strengthen the capability for peace within Palestinian society.

ACKNOWLEDGMENT

We would like to thank our collaborator Rita Giacaman for inspiration and guidance in developing our understanding of peace and community and the IDRC, which has funded three cycles of PACT.

REFERENCES

Bracken, P. J., J. E. Giller, and D. Summerfield. 1995. Psychological responses to war and atrocity: The limitations of current concepts. *Social Science and Medicine* 40 (8): 1073–82.

Children and War. 2004. *Children and War: Impact, protection and rehabilitation.* Phase I: Impact Report. Available online at the www.arts.ualberta.ca website.

Demichelis, J. 1996. *NGOs and peacebuilding in Bosnia's ethnically divided cities: Special report.* Washington, DC: United States Institute of Peace.

Giacaman, R., A. Husseini, N. Halaby-Gordon, and F. Awartani. 2004. Imprints on the consciousness: The impact on Palestinian civilians of the Israeli Army invasion of the West Bank. *European Journal of Public Health* 13 (3): 286–90.

Giacaman, R., N. Arya, and D. Summerfield. 2005. Establishing a mental health system: The Occupied Palestinian Territories. *International Psychiatry,* 16–18. Available online at www.rcpsych.ac.uk/publications/ip/ip9.pdf

Giacaman, R., H. Shannon, H. Saab, N. Arya, and W. Boyce. Individual and collective exposure to political violence: Palestinian adolescents coping with trauma. *European Journal of Public Health* (accepted October 2006).

Hess, G., and M. Pfeiffer, n.d. Comparative analysis of WHO "Health as a Bridge for Peace" case studies. Available online at the www.who.int website.

Parker, M. 1996. The mental health of war-damaged populations. *Institute of Developmental Studies (IDS) Bulletin* 27 (3): 77–84.

Petersen, D. 2002. The potential of social capital measures in the evaluation of comprehensive community-based health initiatives. *American Journal of Evaluation* 23 (1): 55–64.

Rahman, A., M. Mubbashar, R. Harrington, and R. Gater. 2000. Annotation: Developing child mental health services in developing countries. *Journal of Child Psychology and Psychiatry* 41 (5): 539–46.

Raphael, B., L. Meldrum, and A. McFarlane. 1995. Does debriefing after psychological trauma work? *British Medical Journal* 310: 1479–80.

Ricigliano, R. 2003. Networks of effective action: Implementing an integrated approach to peacebuilding. *Security Dialogue* 34 (4): 445–62.

Rushton, S., and C. McInnes. 2006. The UK, health and peacebuilding: The mysterious disappearance of Health as a Bridge for Peace. *Medicine, Conflict and Survival* 22 (2): 94–109.

Santa Barbara, J. 2005. Working for peace through health—Ethical values and principles. *Croatian Medical Journal* 46 (6): 1007–9.

Save the Children Alliance Working Group on Children Affected by Armed Conflict and Displacement. 1996. *Promoting psychosocial well-being among children affected by armed conflict and displacement: Principles and approaches.* Working Paper No. 1, March.

Sen, A. K. 1984. Resources, values, and development. Cambridge, MA: Harvard University Press.

———. 2004. Capabilities, lists and public reason: Continuing the conversation. *Feminist Economics* 10 (3): 77–80.

Summerfield, D. 1999. A critique of seven assumptions behind psychological trauma programs in war-affected areas. *Social Science and Medicine* 48: 1449–62.

NOTE

1. The two core constructs of social capital identified by Coleman (1990) and Putnam (1993, 1995) are civic engagement and levels of mutual trust among community members. Civic engagement is the degree to which citizens are committed to their communities, as reflected in their involvement in community activities.

The Iraq Body Count Project:
A Citizen Initiative in Response to Government
Indifference and Inaction ■ John Sloboda and Hamit Dardagan

ASSESSING POPULATION MORTALITY, the ultimate health data, would seem to be of fundamental importance to political and humanitarian actors involved in armed conflict. Yet no statute under international law requires invading or occupying powers to record, count, or even estimate—let alone identify—the civilian casualties of their wars. When pressed by electors or civil society, governments typically deny their responsibility or capacity to account for civilians who have been harmed. In Iraq there is an official tally of coalition military deaths, but no comparable record of civilians killed.

In early 2003, during the run-up to the invasion of Iraq, a group of concerned British and US volunteers, determined to record and publicize the war's inevitable toll on innocent lives, founded the Iraq Body Count project (IBC). The project was also intended to demonstrate that even with minimal resources it is possible, via the latest information technology, to count many of the deaths our governments refused even to attempt to record.

The project's website (www.iraqbodycount.org) fully describes IBC's methodology and some of the controversy surrounding the work. Briefly, the project team extensively scans news media, including news wires, on a daily basis for reports of violent civilian deaths in Iraq. Whenever an incident is corroborated by two sources, it is added to an online database. The updated totals are then instantly transmitted to IBC web-counters that can be uploaded to and displayed on any website.

The project does not claim to have recorded every directly war-related civilian death in Iraq, but it offers an irrefutable baseline of deaths that are verified to a minimum standard of evidence (Dardagan et al. 2005, 2006; Sloboda et al. 2006). At the time of this writing (July 2007), the cumulative toll of violent civilian deaths so far reported is around 70,000.

A number of other research studies have also provided data on civilian casualties in Iraq. The most often cited of these are the two Johns Hopkins University studies, published in *The Lancet* in October 2004 (Roberts et al. 2004) and October 2006 (Burnham et al. 2006), which estimated, respectively, 100,000 and 650,000 war-related "excess deaths" among Iraqis up to that point. Like the less-cited but larger UNDP study of 2004, these estimates were derived by multiplying data from random-sample surveying by a factor. It is not straightforward to compare these studies, because of differences in time scale, types of death included, and other methodological details. Nonetheless, the most rigorous of these studies complement each other and provide converging evidence regarding the overall picture (Rai 2005).

In the years since 2003, IBC has remained the only ongoing public project that is methodically recording casualties in Iraq. Its figures are now widely used by governments, media, and NGOs, yet no government or official agency has so far come forward to offer any funds or material support for the work.

REFERENCES

Burnham, G., R. Lafta, S. Doocy, and L. Roberts. 2006. Mortality after the 2003 invasion of Iraq: A cross-sectional cluster sample survey. *The Lancet* 368 (9545): 1421–8.

Dardagan, H., J. A. Sloboda, K. Williams, and P. Bagnall. 2005. A dossier of civilian casualties in Iraq: 2003–2005. Iraq Body Count. Available online at the www.reports.iraq bodycount.org website.

Dardagan, H., J. Sloboda, and J. Dougherty. 2006. Speculation is no substitute: A defense of Iraq Body Count. Available online at the www.iraqbodycount.org website.

Rai, M. 2005. Iraq Mortality. Available online at the www.iraqmortality.org website.

Roberts, L., R. Lafta, R. Garfield, J. Khudhairi, and G. Burnham. 2004. Mortality before and after the 2003 invasion of Iraq: Cluster sample survey. *The Lancet* 364:1857–64.

Sloboda, J. A., and H. Dardagan. 2006. On Iraq Body Count. Presentation to working group meeting on methodologies used by researchers to estimate numbers of armed conflict deaths. Geneva, Small Arms Survey: February. Available online at the www .iraqbodycount.org website.

UNDP. 2005. Iraq living conditions survey 2004. Available online at the www.iq.undp .org website.

Doctor as Witness:
Opposing Economic Sanctions on Iraq (1990–2003) ■ Neil Arya

INTRODUCTION

Economic sanctions are increasingly being used in international affairs, supposedly as a more humane and less aggressive form of coercion than conventional warfare. Sanctions are seen as cheaper than war and more politically feasible. In Iraq, however, sanctions ultimately acted as a weapon of mass destruction, killing on the order of 1.5 million people in order to prevent nonexistent weapons of mass destruction from being employed. Nobel Peace Prize winner Mairead Corrigan Maguire holds the international community ultimately culpable. "In fifty years the next generation will ask, what were you doing when the children of Iraq were dying?" (Maguire 2000).

Epidemiologists conducted studies on the sanctions' impact. International Physicians for the Prevention of Nuclear War (IPPNW) doctors went to Iraq bringing medication, but they also bore witness to the use of sanctions as a weapon of violence. Each of them sought to publicize the consequences of sanctions. Although these initiatives prevented neither sanctions nor, ultimately, war, lessons were learned that may be applied to future initiatives. This chapter presents the effect of sanctions through the eyes of these doctors and illustrates some of the images employed to mobilize public and political opinion.

BACKGROUND

Prior to 1990 and even during the catastrophic Iran–Iraq war in 1988, investments in health, education, and physical infrastructure meant that 93 percent of the Iraqi population had access to health care in a clinic or hospital; 92 percent of the Iraqi people had access to safe drinking water; education was free at all levels, and Iraq's literacy rate of 95 percent earned it the United Nations Education, Social and Cultural Organization (UNESCO) Literacy Prize three years in a row; there was ample electricity. Its people were blessed with bountiful food resources. Between 1984 and 1989, Iraqis consumed 3372 calories per person per day, whereas the minimum caloric intake suggested by the World Health Organization is 2100 calories per person (van der Gaag 1999).

IMPACT OF FIRST GULF WAR AND SANCTIONS

On August 6, 1990, four days after the Iraqi invasion and annexation of Kuwait, the UN Security Council passed Resolution 661 imposing a full trade embargo on Iraq, freezing all its foreign assets except medical supplies, food, and other items of humanitarian necessity. To a country that was recovering from war with Iran and had imported roughly 70 percent of its food, medicine, and chemicals for agriculture, this was particularly damaging.

The United States led a coalition of thirty nations authorized by the United Nations on January 16, 1991. The war ended by the end of February of that year. The impact of the 1991 war included an estimated 40,000 direct casualties, both military and civilian. In postwar uprisings encouraged, then abandoned, by the United States, a further 20,000–35,000

Kurdish and Shiite civilians died, and 1.8 million refugees fled (Hoskins 2000). Massive bombing systematically destroyed nearly all of the country's civilian infrastructure: roads, railways, bridges, hospitals, water and sewage treatment facilities, and factories, reducing the country to a "pre-industrial state" (UN 1991). Financially, the damage was estimated at $170 billion (Global Policy Forum 2002). The country's GDP fell from $66 *billion* in 1989 to less than $245 *million* by 1992. Baghdad, a city of 5 million, was left virtually without electricity for three months, with no refrigeration, ventilators, or air conditioning, thereby critically damaging vaccines, blood supplies, and medicines.

After the Gulf War, Resolution 687 continued the sanctions, ostensibly to eliminate WMDs (weapons of mass destruction) and ensure inspections. These most stringent and comprehensive economic sanctions ever imposed on a country controlled virtually every aspect of Iraq's imports and exports and continued for another twelve years. The resultant de-development reduced the country, which had entered the period with a health and education system and per capita income close to those of southern Europe, to on par with Haiti. This was reflected in Iraq's unprecedented drop in UNDP ranking from 50th to 126th (UNDP 2000; van der Gaag 1999). By the time the sanctions regime was finally ended on May 22, 2003 (with certain arms-related exceptions) by paragraph 10 of UNSC, approximately 1.5 million people had died (Arya and Zurbrigg 2003).

OIL FOR FOOD

Four months after the end of the Gulf War, initially with what was considered to be a stop-gap proposal, UNSC Resolution 706 permitted Iraq oil sales of $1.87 billion a year (approximately 19 cents per person per day) for food, medicines, and all other basic needs. This was one-third the amount recommended as the bare minimum requirement by the secretary-general's humanitarian envoy (UN 1991). Iraq refused to comply, in part because of the inadequate amount, but also because UN administration of the plan would mean a UN takeover of nearly all economic activity in the country.

The Security Council agreed to the Oil-for-Food Program in April 1995, allowing the government of Iraq to administer the food distribution program. This was intended to mitigate the suffering of civilians without allowing Iraq to rebuild its military. By May 1996 the Iraqis signed on, and beginning in December 1996, thanks to UNSC Resolution 986, the UN Oil-for-Food Program allowed Iraq to export US$4.2 billion of oil every six months to purchase humanitarian items needed to sustain the civilian population. Because production was hampered by materials embargoes, this limit was never reached, and although it was removed in 1999, the effect of this move was meaningless. However, a rise in oil prices did mean somewhat more money for the program. After deduction of reparations to victims of the 1991 war (notably the government of Kuwait), the cost of UN administration and WMD search teams, and allowance for the Kurdish areas, the amount for south central Iraq was 29 cents per person per day (UNICEF 1998) for a population conservatively estimated at 18 million. Twenty-one of the 29 cents went for food contracts inadequate to meet even bare minimum caloric needs, and 8 cents was allotted for everything else—medicines, health care, sanitation and water supply, education, and agriculture supplies. The 29 cents per person was supposed to administer, to rebuild, and to provide work and livelihood to an entire country of 22 million (Boone, Gazdar, and Hussain 1997).

Although corruption is often cited as responsible for the dire situation that ensued for Iraqis, the US General Accounting Office estimated that the Iraqi regime generated only $10.1 billion in illegal revenues, including $5.7 billion from oil smuggling to neighboring countries and $4.4 billion in illicit surcharges on oil sales. Even here, the US was not only aware of the 'smuggled' oil exports, but had brokered such deals to secure the cooperation of neighbouring countries severely affected economically by the embargo (Zurbrigg 2007, pp. 53–54).

WERE SANCTIONS LEGAL OR MORAL?

Sanctions have been imposed on countries such as Rhodesia, South Africa, Haiti, and Yugoslavia to protect human rights and to promote peace. Article 16 of the United Nations Charter permits the UN Security Council to impose economic measures to address "threats of aggression" and "breaches of peace," and Article 39 asserts that "massive and systematic violations of human rights constitute a threat to peace."

Joy Gordon (Gordon, Crosscurrents weblink) argues that ethically, sanctions must be considered "a bureaucratized, internationally organized form of siege warfare, and should be seen, and judged, as such." Gordon argues that they should be subject to the same rules as warfare. *Jus ad bellum* (right to wage war) requires the belligerent party to have valid grounds—"a real and certain danger," such as protecting innocent life, preserving conditions necessary for decent human existence, and securing basic human rights. *Jus in bello* (justice in war) would require that sanctions be used with certain standards of conduct, proportionality, and probability of success.

Sanctions would also be illegal under current international law, violating not just the (nonbinding) **Universal Declaration of Human Rights, Article 25,** which states that "[e]veryone has the right to a standard of living adequate for the health and well-being of himself and of his family, including food, clothing, housing, medical care and necessary social services" but also many binding laws. These include the **International Covenant on Economic, Social and Cultural Rights, Articles 11 and 12,** which recognize "the fundamental right of everyone to be free from hunger," "the right of everyone to the enjoyment of the highest attainable standard of physical and mental health," and that necessary steps must be taken for "the creation of conditions which would assure to all medical service and medical attention in the event of sickness." These binding laws also include the **Convention on the Rights of the Child** as well. Sanctions also violate the Geneva Conventions that impose constraints on harm to civilians, including the **Geneva Convention relative to the Protection of Civilian Persons in Time of War (1949) (the "Geneva Convention IV"), Article 23,** which states that each party "shall allow the free passage of all consignments of medical supplies and hospital stores . . . intended only for civilians . . . [and] shall likewise permit the free passage of all consignments of essential foodstuffs, clothing and tonics intended for children under fifteen, expectant mothers and maternity cases." **Article 54(1) of Protocol I Additional to the Geneva Conventions (1949)** states that "[s]tarvation of civilians as a method of warfare is prohibited." **Article 70(2)** provides that parties to a conflict "shall allow and facilitate rapid and unimpeded passage of all relief consignments, equipment and personnel."

Peace Studies definitions would certainly include sanctions as a form of violence—"an unnecessary insult to basic needs," because they are intended to harm civilians, restrict the economy of the entire community, create shortages of food, potable water, and fuel, manifesting in malnutrition, sickness, and exhaustion, all resulting in a reduction in human potential, including shorter life expectancy. The intent of sanctions may be to prevent violence rather than to exacerbate it, but their methods damage the health of a population directly in the hope that the sanctions will influence the leadership indirectly by triggering political pressure or uprisings of the civilians.

HEALTH EFFECTS

In the first year after the war, more than 170,000 children under five died from contaminated water that caused diarrhea, including cholera, typhoid, amoebic dysentery, and giardiasis, as well as hepatitis and respiratory infections such as tuberculosis. These were exacerbated and rendered highly lethal through malnutrition, both acute and chronic. Consistent access to clean water was available to only 41 percent of the population—less than half the 1990 figure (UN 1999). Vaccine-preventable illness such as measles, mumps, pertussis, rubella, and poliomyelitis became more common after imposition of sanctions. It was not until 1999, however, that indisputable data on child mortality in Iraq under sanctions became available. A United Nations International Children's Fund (UNICEF) cross-country household survey documented a rate of 131 deaths per 1000 live births, meaning that nearly one child in seven died before reaching the age of five years, compared to a rate of 63 deaths per 1000 live births in the period 1986–90 (UNICEF 1999). Based on this, UNICEF estimated that 500,000 "excess" (above expected levels) deaths in the under-five population had occurred between 1991 and 1998.

Yet Madeleine Albright, then US ambassador to the United Nations and later secretary of state, felt the sanctions were justified. She was asked by *60 Minutes* correspondent Leslie Stahl, "We have heard that a half million children have died. I mean, that's more children than died in Hiroshima. And, you know, is the price worth it?" And she responded, "I think this is a very hard choice, but the price—we think the price is worth it" (CBS 60 *Minutes*).

Others disagreed. Denis Halliday, the first UN Humanitarian Coordinator until he resigned in protest in October 1998, called the program genocide. "We are in the process of destroying an entire society. It is as simple and terrifying as that. Hans Von Sponeck, Halliday's successor, who also resigned in protest, stated that "what is proposed at this point in fact amounts to a tightening of the rope around the neck of the average Iraqi citizen." Von Sponeck addressed the issue of dual use, under which items of military utility were arbitrarily denied the Iraqi people, asking rhetorically, "Air is dual use too; should we deny them air?" He considered it a dereliction of duty for the UN Security Council to impose sanctions but not to monitor their effects or to protect people (Von Sponeck 2006).

STUDIES

But consequences were known. As Rob Chase describes in Chapter 18, when the International Study Team went in barely two months after the end of the Gulf War, the subsequent tragedy from war and sanctions should have been anticipated. They described a situation where "the destruction of the country's power plants had brought its entire system of water purification and distribution to a halt, leading to epidemics of cholera, typhoid fever, and gastroenteritis, particularly among children. Mortality rates doubled or tripled among children admitted to hospitals in Baghdad and Basra. Cases of marasmus appeared for the first time in decades. The team observed "suffering of tragic proportions . . . [with children] dying of preventable diseases and starvation" (Harvard [International] Study Team 1991).

Five months later a UNICEF-supported group carried out a more comprehensive household survey. The age-adjusted relative mortality rate among children under five in the eight months after the war, as compared with the five years before the war, was 3.2, meaning that an excess of 47,000 deaths had occurred in just those eight months. The deaths resulted from infectious diseases, the decreased quality and availability of food and water, and an enfeebled medical care system hampered by the lack of drugs and supplies (Eisenberg 1997).

The Food and Agriculture Organization and the World Food Program reported in July 1993 that the sanctions had "generated persistent deprivation, chronic hunger, endemic undernutrition, massive unemployment and widespread human suffering" and that "a grave humanitarian tragedy is unfolding" (Food and Agriculture Organization 1993). A World Health Organization (WHO) study released in March 1996 stated that health conditions were deteriorating at an alarming rate and that malnutrition among young children was widespread (WHO 1996).

Demographers at the London School of Hygiene and Tropical Medicine confirmed the finding of the 1998 UNICEF household study in July 2003 of a rising trend in child mortality in 1998, in spite of the Oil-for-Food Program (Ali, Blacker, and Jones 2003). Child mortality in the Kurdish areas remained stable after war, even before implementation of the Oil-for-Food program in 1997 because of smuggling and that region's greater self-sufficiency in food.

MISSIONS

Many NGOs worked to try to end sanctions, but sanctions' effects remained largely hidden from Western eyes at least until 1997. The practice of sending medical investigating teams to war zones is quite old. Médecins Sans Frontières (MSF, "Doctors Without Borders") and the Red Cross have provided eyewitness reports for years. IPPNW doctors motivated by religious faith, conviction, family, and friends went to Iraq to get a first-hand understanding of the situation and to deliver aid. Direct flights to Baghdad were forbidden, and it was illegal for Americans to bring in supplies, which made such missions risky. These physicians returned to decry the plight of the health system.

Canadian family physician Larry Willms (LW) was part of a delegation with Jubilee Partners delivering US$45,000 worth of medicines in March 1998, and he met some of the women and children who crowded the halls of Iraq's children's hospitals. Vancouver general practitioner and psychotherapist Allan Connolly (AC) went for a second time in April 1999 as part of a multinational IPPNW delegation. Halifax physician and famine historian Sheila Zurbrigg (SZ) visited Iraq in November 1999. Calgary public health doctor David Swann (DS), who later became a member of the Alberta Provincial Legislature, accompanied former US Attorney General Ramsay Clark and 50 others in January 2000. Retired Frankfurt professor emeritus of internal medicine Ulrich Gottstein (UG), co-founder of the German affiliate of IPPNW, went to Iraq nine times during the sanctions period. The following represent observations that these physicians delivered, in written and verbal form, to media and public groups on their return.

Poor Facilities

DS: We saw the poorly functioning, unsafe water system and broken sanitation system which cannot be fixed because sanctions prevent needed materials from being imported; and under-used hospital wards because of lack of materials, supplies, electricity, medicines and staff.

LW: A nauseating stench from blocked and broken sewerage pipes pervaded many hospital wards. With adequate plumbing supplies and chlorine and other chemicals for water purification either blocked by the sanctions or unaffordable, it is very difficult to control fecal–oral spread of infections.

In the hospitals we visited, most of the basic drugs and medical and surgical supplies, including antibiotics and intravenous fluids, were in short supply or unavailable. At Saddam Pediatric Hospital, in Baghdad, clinicians to whom we spoke stated that cholera, gastroenteritis, tuberculosis, measles, pertussis, rubella, poliomyelitis and other infectious illnesses have become more common since the imposition of sanctions. Vaccination programs have suffered from a lack of refrigerated transport.

AC: In a hospital in Basra, the Iraqi physician takes me to a room off the ward. Two terminally ill children are lying on a bare, soiled mattress. "The children only come here to die. There is no medicine," he says. A mother emerges from the shadows and lays her child beside the two. It mirrors their emaciated state, the result of severe malnutrition. She looks at me with a fading glimmer of hope. The kindly, accomplished physician glances at me. "There is great sorrow . . . We can only practice hands-on medicine because our hands are all we have to work with."

Lack of Drugs

UG: I visited a ward with children with leukemia, who have very little chance of beating their illness, while for example in Germany about 90 percent are cured. Expensive and effective chemotherapy, laboratory diagnostics and radiation therapy are all lacking. Everything has to be ordered via the Sanctions Committee in New York, and they work very slowly and unreliably. The same is true for the adult cancer patients. The central radiation institute has only two 17-year-old radiation units, no gamma cameras [or] other modern ones. The Security Council does not allow "dual use" articles. There are 2200 articles on "dual use" lists and therefore on hold.

LW: In one pediatric hospital, I met Ali. He was eleven and had leukaemia. His father had sold his house to pay for the first year of a two-year course of chemotherapy. Now Ali was dying of his disease because his father could not afford further treatment. Before the 1991 Gulf War and the sanctions that followed, the treatments would have been provided free to Ali under Iraq's universal healthcare system. I saw a whole ward of children like Ali. His oncologist said what was most difficult for her was that she had the knowledge, but not the resources, to help the children. She did not have the heart to send them away, yet often could not provide even a simple aspirin in order to remove their pain.

SZ: I spoke with Maiada, whose malnourished four-month-old was admitted to Baghdad hospital for dehydration. Her husband earns 7000 dinars a month as a janitor. Unable to breastfeed her son after forty days, she fed him with infant formula provided under food rationing. The ration is insufficient, and she ends up buying additional cans on the open market for 500 dinars each. When I met her, for her diabetes she was receiving two vials of insulin free from the government but had to purchase two additional vials per month, each costing 2000 dinars.

Malnutrition

SZ: Food imports fell to less than a third of what they were prior to 1990 in a country that has been dependent on imports for two-thirds of its food. The Iraq government responded to sanctions even before the Oil-for-Food (OFF) program by shifting the entire civilian population onto a public dole of bare subsistence food rationing. The neurological effects of chronic malnourishment may never be completely reversed. Infant mortality and under-five mortality which correlated with levels of acute malnutrition figures were not reduced by OFF. The impact on people's health has been catastrophic. The International Red Cross estimated that by 1994, 24 percent of Iraqi babies weighed less than 5 pounds at birth, compared to 4 percent before sanctions (UNICEF 1998). This low-birthweight rate is among the highest in the world, signaling severe hunger throughout Iraq.

Economic Situation

SZ: The United Nations (UN) blockade of Iraq ("sanctions") began in August 1990. With the country dependent on imports for two-thirds of its food needs, sanctions instantly triggered rampant inflation. Within weeks most Iraqi families were shut out from the food market. The Iraq government responded by shifting the entire civilian population (22 million) onto a public dole of bare subsistence food rationing. Today, a liter of milk, which before sanctions cost one Iraqi dinar, costs 850 dinars; a kilogram of bananas, 3000 dinars; a handful of peanuts, 500. With average household income estimated at 7000 dinars a month, the "market" is largely meaningless for most Iraqi families.

Since the massive 1991 bombing most real jobs have disappeared. The sanctions prevent rebuilding factories, water, sewer and electrical systems destroyed by the bombs while unemployment is 70 percent. Parents and children are forced to take on two or three makeshift "jobs" for basic survival—and, yes, [they are] resorting to prostitution in increasing numbers.

UG: More than 60 percent of the people are very poor, mostly unemployed, because there were very few functioning industries and no trade with foreign countries, and because 40 percent of the population earned an average of 2000–4000 dinars per month, which is the equivalent of 1–2 dollars. Sixteeen eggs cost 2000 on the open market. Every person gets a free food package from the state every month, consisting of peas, flower, sugar, oil, tea but without eggs, meat, milk, so that they either have to buy them on the market or suffer protein deficiency.

Those who are close to the government or the Baath party, who are officers or legal smugglers or who practice legal-illegal trade across the borders, especially with Turkey and Jordan, or who have relatives in foreign countries who send hard currency, can buy what they need on the market and in the shops.

On their return each of the doctors lectured extensively to lay and medical audiences, organized petitions, gave media interviews, and wrote articles all detailing consequences. Thus they employed many of the mechanisms referred to by MacQueen and Santa Barbara in Chapter 4, such as broadening altruism, putting a human face on suffering, and extending solidarity.

CONCLUSIONS

In 1997 the *New England Journal of Medicine* stated, "Like John Snow, we have a responsibility to petition the authorities to remove the known causes of epidemics—in this case, by ending US restrictions on trade in nonmilitary supplies. Doing so will not make us popular in some circles. But neither the Hippocratic oath nor its contemporary versions contain clauses that make self-interest grounds for exempting physicians from acting for the benefit of the sick . . . and keeping them from harm and injustice" (Eisenberg 1997). The IPPNW physicians represented the best tradition of doctors acting as witnesses and trying to promote peace.

REFERENCES

Ali, M., J. Blacker, and G. Jones. 2003. Annual mortality rates and excess deaths of children under five in Iraq, 1991–98. *Population Studies* (July).

Arya, N., and S. Zurbrigg. 2003. Operation infinite injustice: The effect of sanctions and prospective war on the people of Iraq. *Can J Pub Health* 94 (1): 9–12.

Boone, Peter, Gazdar Haris, and Hussain Athar. 1997. *Sanctions against Iraq: Costs of failure.* New York: Center for Economic and Social Rights.

CBS *60 Minutes.* 1996. May 12. Available online at the www.democracynow.org website.

Eisenberg, Leon. 1997. The sleep of reason produces monsters: Human costs of economic sanctions. *New England Journal of Medicine* 336 (17): 1248–50.

Food and Agriculture Organization of the United Nations. 1993. *Crop and food supply assessment.* Special Alert No. 237- FAO/WFP. July.

Global Policy Forum. 2002. *Iraq sanctions: Humanitarian implications and options for the future,* August 6. Available online at the www.globalpolicy.org website.

Gordon, Joy. 1999. Economic sanctions, just war doctrine, and the fearful spectacle of the civilian dead. *Cross Currents* (Fall) 49(3). Available online at www.crosscurrents.org/gordon.htm

———. 2002. Cool war: Economic sanctions as a weapon of mass destruction. *Harper's Magazine* (November). Available online at www.crosscurrents.org/gordon.htm

Harvard (International) Study Team. 1991. The effect of the Gulf crisis on the children of Iraq. *New England Journal of Medicine* 325:977–80.

Hoskins, Eric. 2000. Public health and the Persian Gulf War. In *War and public health,* ed. Barry S. Levy and Victor W. Sidel, 254–78. Washington, DC: American Public Health Association.

International Herald Tribune. 2002. March 20, 7.

Lopez, George A., and David Cortright. 2004. Containing Iraq: Sanctions worked by foreign affairs, July/August 3(4). Available online at http://www.foreignaffairs.org/20040701faessay83409/george-a-lopez-david-cortright/containing-iraq-sanctions-worked.html (83)4.

Maguire, Mairead Corrigan. 2000. *Fellowship of Reconciliation Newsletter,* September–October.

Rieff, David. 2003. Were sanctions right? *New York Times* Magazine, July 27. Available online at www.nytimes.com/2003/07/27/magazine/27SANCTIONS.html

Sacks, Bert. 2003. *Seattle-Post Intelligencer,* August 7. Available online at www.commondreams.org/views03/0807-01.htm

UNDP. 2000. Available online at the www.hdr.undp.org website.

UNICEF. 1998. *Situation analysis of children and women in Iraq.* Baghdad.

———. 1999. *Child and maternal mortality report,* July.

United Nations. 1991. *Report to the secretary-general on humanitarian needs in Iraq.* Prepared by a mission led by the executive delegate of the secretary-general for humanitarian assistance in Iraq. [Sadruddin Aga Khan]. S/22799. July 17.

———. 1999. *Report of the second panel established pursuant to the note by the president of the Security Council concerning the current humanitarian situation in Iraq.* S/1999/100. paragraphs 43, 49, January 30, quoted in SCFAIT.

Van der Gaag, Nikki. 1999. Iraq: The pride and the pain. *New Internationalist* 316 (September): 10. Available online at the www.newint.org website.

Von Sponeck, Hans Christian. 2006. *A different kind of war: The UN sanctions regime in Iraq.* New York: Berghahn.

World Health Organization. 1996. Health conditions in Iraq "serious," WHO study finds. Press Release 23. March 25.

Zurbrigg. Sheila. 2007. Economic sanctions on Iraq: Tool for peace, or travesty. *Muslim World Journal of Human Rights* 4 (2): 1–63.

18

Tertiary Prevention

Psychosocial Healing ▪ Paula Gutlove

PSYCHOSOCIAL HEALING IN A POSTWAR CONTEXT

REBUILDING A SOCIETY in the aftermath of violent conflict requires reconstruction of social, physical, and political structures. Social reconstruction includes rebuilding the fabric of human interactions that allow a society to function, restoring or creating new opportunities for productive social functions, and preventing cycles of vengeance and violence. An important component of social reconstruction is psychosocial healing, the promotion of psychological and social health for individuals, families, and communities. Psychosocial healing encompasses trauma healing and related psychological and social support activities to empower survivors and reconnect them within a functional society. Ultimately, psychosocial-healing programs can provide opportunities for postconflict societies to recreate themselves, replacing destructive habits and belief systems with constructive interactions and laying the foundation for a peaceful, sustainable society.

Health professionals are particularly well suited to develop and conduct psychosocial-healing programs in postwar societies. Health professionals can integrate trauma healing and social support into a range of community-based health services. Furthermore, activities that feature cooperation between health professionals from different sides of a conflict can serve as a model for collaborative action and help to create broader intercommunal interactions that can contribute to sustainable peace (Gutlove 1998a, 1999, 2000a).

TRAUMA HEALING AND PEACEBUILDING

Trauma healing is a central pillar of psychosocial healing. It should be noted that trauma healing is closely related to peacebuilding; both are

225

ultimately about developing or restoring healthy human relationships. Trauma healing implies the reduction of loneliness; mood improvement; a sense of inner peace; a decrease in isolation, anger, and bitterness; and a decrease in feelings of animosity and hatred toward others. Such healing does not occur in isolation, because healing the psychological faculties that were damaged by the trauma can best occur in connection with other people (Herman 1997; Sider 2001; Volkan 1999).

Stages through which individuals move as they heal from a traumatic experience include safety—moving from a feeling of unpredictable danger to one of reliable safety and security; acknowledgement—moving from a sense of dissociated trauma to acknowledged memory; and reconnection—moving from feeling isolated and stigmatized to a state of restored meaningful social connections (Herman 1997).

The need for safety underlies all other aspects of the healing process. In an evaluation of psychosocial-assistance programs during and immediately after the Croatian and Bosnian wars in the former Yugoslavia, it was noted that the most important benefit these programs could provide was a safe space—psychologically and physically—in which people could rebuild their previous social contacts and make new contacts. The safe space was more important than any particular type of psychological intervention or therapy (Mimica and Agger 1997).

Storytelling is an important aspect of acknowledgment. When a survivor tells the story of her trauma, it can transform the traumatic memory so that the survivor can then integrate the memory into her life story (Herman 1997). Societies also need to discuss, acknowledge, and mourn traumatic societal events (Montville 2001).

Reconnection is crucial within a violence-ravaged community, where the ultimate goal is the restoration of healthy human relationships and the building of trust, hope, and mutuality. Empowerment is an important byproduct of reconnection. It is empowering for people to feel that their collective actions can promote positive societal change. Experience shows that people feel good when they are in productive relationships with colleagues (Gutlove 2000a). Engaging in cooperative actions that have the power to change the course of events feels even better. Thus empowerment and reconnection can operate in a healthy cycle, each building on the other (Gutlove and Thompson 2004, 2005).

PSYCHOSOCIAL HEALING AND COMMUNITY REGENERATION

Societies, just like individuals, are susceptible to stress and trauma. A traumatized society can undergo "psychosocial degeneration," in which a large fraction of the population loses its sense of trust, or faith, in their society or the wider world. Feelings of rage and revenge often alternate with feelings of helplessness, humiliation, and victimization (Volkan 1999). Psychosocial healing of the individual and society requires embedding trauma healing within a program of community support. Psychosocial-healing programs can be synergistic with related programs and, through a process of ever-expanding cycles, can promote psychosocial assistance to wider and wider segments of the community (Gutlove and Thompson 2003a, 2003b, 2005).

The experience of the Institute for Resource and Security Studies (IRSS) in psychosocial healing derives from our work with health professionals in violence and postwar situations through our Health Bridges for Peace (HBP) project. IRSS founded HBP in 1996 to create sustainable programs for community reconstruction through the integration of health-care delivery with peacebuilding. In the first HBP field program, IRSS helped to launch the Medical Network for Social Reconstruction (MNSR) in the former Yugoslavia.

Founded in 1997, MNSR is a region-wide peacebuilding NGO with a diverse, representative governing council. A training program for psychosocial support to promote trauma recovery was one of the first cooperative projects of MNSR (Barsalou 2001). Psychosocial healing has evolved as one of the network's most important program activities. MNSR has also reached out to healers in other regions of violent conflict, including Chechnya, Ingushetia, Iraq, Israel, and Palestine, to exchange experience and offer assistance (Gutlove 1998b, 2000b). Through MNSR's efforts, health professionals in these areas of violent conflict formed the International Partnership for Psychosocial Healing in 2004.

SELECTED MNSR PSYCHOSOCIAL-HEALING PROGRAMS

Distinct aspects of MNSR's psychosocial-healing process were developed by different member organizations. Three important contributions are described below.

Volunteer Action

The Slovene Philanthropy (later the Together Regional Center) in Ljubljana, Slovenia, pioneered the development of volunteer action, promoting training for local community leaders, teachers, health-care providers, and social workers. Volunteer action is a strategy to train and empower individuals to volunteer to support postwar reconstruction. Individuals in difficult or traumatic situations frequently derive satisfaction from volunteering to help fellow sufferers. However, this sort of spontaneous volunteer activity often extends only to one's own family and closest friends, because people instinctively provide first for their own safety and welfare. Therefore, a more systematic means of providing consistent and organized volunteer aid is required. Volunteer action aims to harness the full capacity of humankind's instinct to help fellow citizens, while directing this help where it is most needed (Kos, Gutlove, and Russell 2003).

In programs of psychosocial healing, volunteers collaborate with professionals to reassure victims of trauma that their plight is not unrecognized, to provide practical assistance to refugees adapting to new environments, and to help reconcile communities during a postwar transition. In postwar situations, volunteers can help combat the effects of poverty, unemployment, social inequities, disintegration of families, and the corruption and associated challenges that may characterize public institutions. If volunteers are chosen from diverse backgrounds, their joint activities may create a sense of "togetherness" between two otherwise-opposing sides, building trust and dispelling notions of segregation or antagonism. Moreover, volunteers can help to rebuild and reconcile communities during a postwar transition. Through a variety of functions—such as providing psychosocial assistance, practical aid, or education—volunteers can exert a positive influence on society and public attitudes, thereby expediting the process of social reconstruction.

Training

The Society for Psychological Assistance (SPA), in Zagreb, Croatia, offered training in trauma healing, together with training of trainers and provision of support services to healers. Postwar social reconstruction requires the identification, empowerment, and activation of large cadres of health professionals and volunteers, trained to meet the unique psychosocial needs of the postwar community. SPA demonstrated in former Yugoslavia that such a training program can lay the foundation for a psychosocial-healing program for a postwar society, providing countless rewards for the trainees, their clients, and the society as a whole (Ajdukovic 1997).

SPA learned many lessons as training programs evolved to meet the needs of the caregivers and the communities with whom they were working. One crucial, early lesson was the necessity of integrating healing of the individual (psychological healing) with healing of the community (social healing). This contrasted with the traditional medical model that focused on treating trauma as an individual disorder. Another lesson was that building networks of mutual support among trainees was an important component of successful training efforts. SPA found that support networks improved the mental health of the population and significantly increased the potential for peace in the region. Also, SPA found that the self-esteem of most health providers grew as they tested their new skills and knowledge in practice and, later, became trainers themselves (Ajdukovic 1999).

SPA found that gains from training in the psychosocial model extended far beyond the initial focus on trauma healing and that they involved positive changes within the professional community and at the societal level. SPA noted that building a community-based psychosocial-assistance program often led to the growth of the nongovernmental sector. This is an important spin-off effect of trauma relief efforts, whose long-term impact on democratization and the development of civil society will be fully appreciated only in the future. Thus, ongoing support to the professionals and paraprofessionals who are engaged in psychosocial healing should be viewed as an important long-term social investment (Ajdukovic and Ajdukovic 2000).

Community Integration

The OMEGA Health Care Center, in Graz, Austria, a MNSR founder and member, conducted community integration and refugee support programs. Community integration is a process whereby vulnerable or marginalized groups, such as refugees, are integrated into a community in a manner that strengthens the overall social fabric of that community. Community integration programs aim to establish strong social networks made up of empowered individuals who can function productively in their new environment. Integration is achieved through local psychosocial projects that empower members of the target groups and help them adapt to new environments. OMEGA pioneered community integration projects in Austria whose beneficiaries were refugees from the former Yugoslavia. Psychosocial projects were found to be especially useful in helping refugees adapt to a new culture. The challenges of adapting to a host country are typically a source of stress to refugees that is exceeded only by the trauma that was experienced in their region of origin. In order to ease the process of adaptation, community integration promotes safe and supported contact with the new environment, which might otherwise be perceived as strange or hostile (OMEGA 2000; Wagner, Gutlove, and Russell 2003).

CONCLUSIONS

IRSS's experience demonstrates that psychosocial-healing programs, implemented through local health professionals, can contribute significantly to social reconstruction. In the former Yugoslavia, for example, the Medical Network's psychosocial-support programs have involved more than 10,000 volunteers over a five-year period, bringing together Serb, Muslim, Bosnian, Kosovar, and Croat participants for a wide range of social-reconstruction projects. Experiences in the former Yugoslavia provide valuable lessons for the development of psychosocial-healing programs in other violence-afflicted communities. Key among these lessons is that program development should be guided by a broadly representative group of indigenous personnel. Only local people can identify the crucial health needs of their communities. Moreover, important resources for understanding and transforming conflict can be found within the culture from which a conflict has emerged.

After violent conflict, trauma healing and related psychological and social support activities are essential to the development of a stable, peaceful, and functional society. The psychosocial-healing process can provide postwar communities with hope and a basis for believing that the promise of a shared future can shine brightly enough to begin to heal the painful memories of a violent past.

REFERENCES

Ajdukovic, D. 1997. Challenges of training for trauma recovery. In *Trauma recovery training*, ed. D. Ajdukovic. Zagreb, Croatia: Society for Psychosocial Assistance.

———. 1999. Psychosocial assistance to children. In *Empowering children: Psychosocial assistance under difficult circumstances*, ed. D. Ajdukovic. Zagreb, Croatia: Society for Psychological Assistance.

Ajdukovic, D., and M. Ajdukovic. 2000. *Why is the mental health of helpers at risk?* In *Mental health care of helpers*, ed. D. Ajdukovic, and M. Ajdukovic. Zagreb, Croatia: Society for Psychosocial Assistance.

Barsalou, J. 2001. *Training to help traumatized populations.* Washington, DC: United States Institute of Peace.

Gutlove, P. 1998a. Health bridges for peace. *Medicine, Conflict and Survival* 14:6–23.

———. 1998b. *Health as a Bridge for Peace in the North Caucasus.* Final Report on a Workshop for Health Professionals, Pyatigorsk, Russia, October 29 to November 2. Cambridge, MA: Institute for Resource and Security Studies; and Copenhagen, Denmark: World Health Organization, Regional Office for Europe.

———. 1999. Health bridges for peace: Integrating healthcare with conflict prevention and community reconciliation. In *Training to promote conflict management: USIP-assisted training projects,* ed. D. Smock. Washington, DC: United States Institute of Peace.

———. 2000a. Health as a bridge to peace: The role of health professionals in conflict management and community reconciliation. In *Violence and health: Proceedings of a WHO global symposium, October, 12–15.* Kobe, Japan: World Health Organization.

———. 2000b. *Application of the Peace through Health approach in the North Caucasus.* Report of an Interagency Consultation, Moscow, April 4–5. Cambridge, MA: Institute for Resource and Security Studies; and Copenhagen, Denmark: World Health Organization, Regional Office for Europe.

Gutlove, P., and G. Thompson. 2003a. Human security: Expanding the scope of public health. *Medicine, Conflict and Survival* 19 (1): 17–34.

———. 2003b. *Psychosocial healing: A guide for practitioners.* Cambridge, MA: Institute for Resource and Security Studies.

———. 2004. Psychosocial healing and post-conflict social reconstruction in the former Yugoslavia. *Medicine, Conflict and Survival* 2–2, 136–50.

———. 2005. Psychosocial healing in postconflict reconstruction. In *The psychology of resolving global conflicts: From war to peace,* ed. M. Fitzduff, and C. Stout. *Vol. 3: Interventions,* New York: Praeger.

Herman, J. 1997. *Trauma and recovery.* New York: Basic Books.

Kos, A. M., P. Gutlove, and J. H. Russell. 2003. The theory and practice of volunteer action. In *Psychosocial healing: A guide for practitioners,* ed. P. Gutlove and G. Thompson, 99–105. Cambridge, MA: Institute for Resource and Security Studies.

Mimica, J., and I. Agger. 1997. NGO perspectives: An evaluation of psychosocial projects and a retrospective. In *Trauma recovery training,* ed. D. Ajdukovic, 251–59. Zagreb, Croatia: Society for Psychological Assistance.

Montville, J. 2001. Peace, justice, and the burdens of history. In *Reconciliation, justice, and coexistence: Theory and practice,* ed. M. Abu-Nimer. Lanham, MD: Lexington Books.

OMEGA Health Care Center and Society for Victims of Organized Violence and Human Rights Violation. 2000. *European guidelines on empowerment and integration programs for refugee children and adolescents.* Graz, Austria: OMEGA Health Care Center.

Sider, N. G. 2001. At the fork in the road. *Conciliation Quarterly* 20 (2): 7–11.

Volkan, V. 1999. Post-traumatic states: Beyond individual PTSD in societies ravaged by ethnic conflict. Presented to the Eighth International Conference on Health and Environment, April. New York: United Nations.

Wagner, A. M. M., P. Gutlove, and J. H. Russell. 2003. Community integration for psychosocial assistance. In *Psychosocial healing: A guide for practitioners,* ed. P. Gutlove, and G. Thompson, 91–9. Cambridge, MA: Institute for Resource and Security Studies.

Community-Based Rehabilitation ■ Will Boyce

INTRODUCTION

War, by its very nature, is intended to produce death and disability—the latter directly from injuries in violent conflict or indirectly through disruption to health services, vaccination delivery, nutrition, and water supplies (Rehabilitation International/UNICEF 1991; UNHCR 1992; UNRWA 1992). But can appropriate rehabilitation for persons with disabilities actually lead to peace?

Community-based rehabilitation (CBR) programs aim to rehabilitate and train individuals with disabilities, as well as to find ways to integrate them into their communities. In effective CBR programs, persons with disabilities collaborate with their families, the community, and health professionals to provide supports in a noninstitutional environment. Thus the essential feature of CBR is its focus on the mechanisms supporting community participation and the partnership of diverse groups (Helander et al. 1989). In situations of armed conflict, where services for persons with disabilities are seriously limited or totally absent, a CBR program typically works with other agencies that are active in emergency aid and reconstruction (Boyce and Ballantyne 1997). However, a clear understanding of this context of violent conflict, and adaptation of CBR programs so that they contribute to the process of peacebuilding without unintended negative consequences, is crucial (Ballantyne 1999; Boyce 2000).

For example, the focus of many Peace through Health strategies has been on prevention of childhood disability caused by polio. Negotiated cessation of armed conflict allows mass vaccinations to protect children against unnecessary infection and lifelong disability, permitting a temporary reduction of violence. In these situations, childhood disability is used as a powerful emotive lever that can mobilize cooperation between warring factions. Consequently, a Queen's University research team has been investigating other rehabilitation initiatives, to examine their peacebuilding properties, in a number of countries (Boyce, Koros, and Hodgson 2002). The following section describes some apparent mechanisms of peacebuilding that may explain how and why CBR can lead to peace.

MECHANISMS OF PEACEBUILDING IN CBR ACTIVITIES

There are at least four mechanisms for achieving peacebuilding impacts in CBR: psychological, social, organizational, and political.

Psychological

The immediate impact of CBR interventions with a critical vulnerable group, whose immediate human security is in jeopardy, is significant from a psychological perspective. Humanitarian response toward those with disabilities demonstrates compassion for individuals and may provide important symbolic and tangible catharses to warring factions, thus gaining their interest and support. Those who have been engaged in, or affected by, violent conflict as combatants or as civilians can then come to grips with the need to integrate persons with disabilities as part of the psychological healing of the population at large.

As an example, over the past twenty years of war in Sri Lanka, CBR approaches to improve community attitudes to disability have facilitated the integration of disabled refugee children into schools and have supported alternatives to institutionalization for disabled, displaced, and orphaned children. Inclusion, rather than exclusion, has become the model. Similarly, in Palestine, legislative and bureaucratic measures that include access to public services for all persons with disabilities, whether injured in the Intifada or not, have become symbols of equality. This strategy has helped to reduce inequities between disabled combatants and civilians and has led to gains for all persons with disabilities that previously had been difficult to achieve in an Arab context (Ballantyne 1999).

In other areas of violent conflict, national development programs (for example, primary health care, food and agriculture, and rural and urban reconstruction) have been integrated with CBR programs so that the needs of persons with disabilities, including ex-combatants, are considered and there is less chance of their exclusion from mainstream humanitarian assistance. Before 2001 in Afghanistan, disabled persons' organizations were linked to such national reconstruction planning and were consequently seen as legitimate and among the neediest (Coleridge 2000).

Social

The social context of persons with disabilities is a broad one: they live in families and neighborhoods, work in occupational and professional settings, and belong to religious or spiritual groups. The process of de-emphasizing the differences of impairment, by integrating persons with disabilities in these contexts, is a strategy that transcends gender, cultural, social class, religious, and political divisions. This process can illustrate how to lower perceived barriers between other social groups, thereby reducing the legitimacy of exclusionist political rhetoric.

A core practice in CBR involves building peer support networks. In areas of violent conflict, this has been extended to include groups that were previously at war. For example, in southern Africa, intercountry disability programs sponsored by Disabled People South Africa (http://www.dpsa.org.za) have brought together former political and military adversaries for policymaking, sports, and cultural exchanges and have demonstrated to other parties the possibilities for reconciliation.

CBR training modules for areas of violent conflict have necessarily focused on major traumatic musculoskeletal impairments arising from head injuries, multiple fractures, peripheral nerve injuries caused by projectiles, traumatic amputations from landmines, and torture injuries. In Sri Lanka, training in these CBR skills was jointly held for both Sinhalese military and Tamil community groups. This exposed these different factions to commonalities of the disability experience and also promoted unexpected mutual assistance between the groups after the training. However, such cooperative training can be achieved only during specific windows of opportunity before separate rehabilitation services are established for different groups, which then become difficult to amalgamate.

Organizational

CBR promotes a multisectoral organizational approach to complex problems, such as the interacting causes of poverty—war and disability—which require negotiations and priority setting. The community-based delivery of rehabilitation services in war zones can also have a major influence on reconstruction of the health-care sector, often conferring significant economic benefits through increased local employment. These interactions can alter the disposition of key managers who control the health and social service infrastructure, by increasing their propensity to view local cooperative action as beneficial to the wider community and worthwhile to support.

CBR programs in areas of violent conflict need to prioritize quick action over lengthy planning if they are to reach persons in urgent need and also have a peacebuilding impact. Community-based assessment and evaluation methods for physical disability and psychosocial trauma have been developed to assess these needs, as well as local response capacities (Boyce and Weera 1999). Rapid assessment teams have been used for responding quickly to disability in emerging war zones in Central Africa, as well as in large-scale disasters such as earthquakes in El Salvador

(Rose 2004). More recently, CBR efforts in disseminating information, networking, and strategic planning in Afghanistan have demonstrated the benefits of a multisectoral approach to other national planners as they gain insight into the complex interaction among disability, education, and employment (Coleridge 2000).

At the local level, CBR programs have sought out tradespeople (such as carpenters and welders) to assist with rehabilitation devices during low-intensity warfare, instead of training new technicians or developing new orthopedic workshops that might fail to draw on existing local capacities. This approach has been used to reinforce local support for economic development by disability organizations in Angola and El Salvador. Moreover, refugees from countries embroiled in violent conflict, who sometimes raise funds in their new homes to support warring parties, have been mobilized to donate rehabilitation equipment, prosthetics, and orthotic supplies.

Political

Through its focus both on personal change in people with disabilities and on social adaptation of communities, CBR demonstrates opportunities for health, social, economic, and political reforms in a noncontentious arena. This can also heighten the expectation in local communities that they will be consulted in the design of longer-term social reconstruction and development projects. CBR enters postwar situations with an implicit assumption of the value and abilities of all persons and a fundamental respect for cultural integrity. It can lend confidence to groups whose self-assurance and identity have been critically compromised during periods of violent conflict. Thus CBR offers the model of establishing open and trusting dialogue that can aid in resolving political conflicts and discourage future violence.

In Sri Lanka, for example, reconstruction efforts in war areas have tried to address disability access problems, such as the need for ramp access to buses. However, this reconstruction occasionally required moving valued public services, such as transportation and recreation facilities, from one area to another. Such relocation had to be done with particular sensitivity and openness, or there was a risk of increasing tensions within communities that were still suspicious of each other (Chase et al. 1999).

In other politically dynamic situations, such as Cambodia, Afghanistan, Mozambique, and Lebanon, members of Disabled Peoples' International have assisted national disability organizations in improving their abilities to develop self-help programs and to advocate, before their governments, the improvement of local rehabilitation efforts (Driedger 1989). Different political factions in Afghanistan and El Salvador have been pressured by national disability organizations to support a common understanding of the consequences of violence, as expressed in International Disability Day on December 3. This strategy, then, utilizes injured persons' status and visibility as victims of war to promote peace.

CONCLUSION

The focus on disability offered by CBR addresses an extreme form of vulnerability that affects all sides during violent conflict, and thus it represents a learning opportunity for peacebuilding. This is particularly so when jointly held education and training in disability issues can bring together opposing factions. If public services and support can reach the most vulnerable in society, especially in difficult circumstances such as war and escalated conflict, then processes, systems, and relationships are established whereby other forms of vulnerability and their social impacts may also be addressed. Crucially, the impact of CBR as a peacebuilding activity will be enhanced only if it works in a complementary manner with other community-based initiatives.

REFERENCES

Ballantyne, S. 1999. Community-based rehabilitation under conditions of political violence: A Palestinian case study. Master's Thesis. Kingston, Ontario: Queen's University.

Boyce, W. 2000. Adaptation of community-based rehabilitation in areas of armed conflict. *Asia Pacific Disability Rehabilitation Journal* 11 (1): 17–20. Available online at www.aifo.it

Boyce, W., M. Koros, and J. Hodgson. 2002. Community-based rehabilitation: A strategy for peacebuilding. *International Health & Human Rights* 2:6. Available online at www.biomedcentral.com/1472-698X/2/6

Boyce, W., and S. Ballantyne. 1997. Community-based rehabilitation in areas of armed conflict. *8th World Congress of the International Rehabilitation Medicine Association.* Bologna: Litosei-Rastignano: 65–9.

Boyce, W., and S. Weera. 1999. Issues of disability assessment in war zones. In *Disability in different cultures—reflections on local concepts,* ed. B. Holzer, A. Vreede, and G. Weigt, 332–42. Bielefeld, Germany: Transcript-Verlag.

Chase, R., A. Doney, S. Sivayogan, V. Ariyaratne, P. Satkunanayagam, and A. Swaminathan. 1999. Mental health initiatives as peace initiatives in Sri Lankan school children affected by armed conflict. *Medicine, Conflict and Survival* 15:379–90. Available online at the www.humanities.mcmasteru.ca website.

Coleridge, P. 2000. Disability and culture. In *CBR in transition,* ed. M. Thomas and M. J. Thomas, 2–38. Newcastle Upon Tyne: Action for Disability.

Driedger, D. 1989. *The last civil rights movement*. New York: St. Martin's Press.

Helander, E., P. Mendis, G. Nelson, and A. Goerdt. 1989. *Training in the community for people with disabilities*. Geneva: World Health Organization.

Rehabilitation International/UNICEF. 1991. Effects of armed conflict on women and children: Relief and rehabilitation in war situations. *One in Ten* 10:2–3.

Rose, W. I. 2004. *Natural Hazards in El Salvador*. Boulder, CO: Geological Society of America.

UNHCR (United Nations High Commissioner for Refugees). 1992. *UNHCR guidelines on assistance to disabled refugees*. Geneva: United Nations.

UNRWA (United Nations Relief and Works Agency for Palestinian Refugees). 1992. *Community rehabilitation programs for disabled Palestine refugees—report and recommendations of UNRWA/NGO Conference*. Amman: United Nations.

Butterfly Peace Garden:
Healing War-Affected Children in Sri Lanka ▪ Rob Chase

MCMASTER UNIVERSITY'S 1994–1996 "HEALTH REACH" PROJECT undertook field work in three of the world's zones of armed conflict (Santa Barbara 1999). In Sri Lanka the research consisted of a survey of 308 school children within three different ethnic communities in eight conflict-affected locations; it focused on psychological distress in children (Chase et al. 1999). A primary research site was Batticaloa district on the eastern coast, where the civil war had incited communal tensions between minority Muslim villages and ethnic Tamils since 1983, including a wave of village massacres in 1989, as well as civilian displacements, abductions, and "disappearances" perpetrated by militant factions, the government army, police, and special forces. In the sample of 170 children (ages nine to eleven) in four affected villages, 95 percent had experienced threatened death or serious injury, 19 percent had lost a close family member through violent death or "disappearance," and 20 percent of the children suffered severe or very severe levels of posttraumatic stress disorder (PTSD), with similar levels of severe depression and unresolved grief reaction. Results and recommendations of the 1994–1996 project were published and disseminated to key government and nongovernmental organizations (Health Reach 1996).

The team was committed to a parallel, responsive "intervention" because it was felt that study alone would be unethical and insufficient. Recognizing the stigmatizing effects of labeling psychological distress as mental illness, the limits of resource-intensive counseling, and the impact of ongoing conflict, explorations shifted to using creative arts in a community-based response to children's psychological needs, to foster resiliency and reconciliation. Canadian artist Paul Hogan from the Spiral Garden, Toronto,[1] was engaged to explore the idea of a children's peace garden as a refuge for an expressive arts and cultural program. In 1996 the Butterfly Peace Garden (*Vannathupoochi Poonga,* in Tamil) opened. The first 150 children to attend the program for nine months came from the survey cohort.

Children from the divided communities are brought together and encouraged to share their imaginations freely (Hogan 2003). The Health Reach report facilitated dialogue with local school principals and village leaders about the children's psychosocial needs; twenty more schools were invited to select troubled children to participate over the first several years.

Once a week the Butterfly Garden Bus collects fifty boys and girls, from both Tamil and Muslim schools, to deliver them to a day program with creative activities in mixed groups of ten or twelve. The Butterfly Garden is the only place in the Sri Lankan conflict zone where Tamil and Muslim children are brought together to learn from each other. The fourteen full-time staff (they are called animators) are local, artistically inclined individuals trained by visiting teachers and other professionals, who are guided by their practical experience with children in the garden and the transformative potential of creative expression. Over the six-to-nine-month cycle, the process interweaves art, narrative, and theater into one collective operatic performance that concludes the program. The program's intent is to have a sustained presence; children, parents, and teachers often seek this. An evaluation of the impact on children and communities, which included a follow-up case series of twenty participants with interviews among caregivers and teachers, demonstrated impressive improvements and satisfaction levels (Chase 2000).

Learning a path of reconciliation and healing, the children also become a means for healing the wider society. As Hogan says, "most adults who come to the garden carry more inimical psychological and cultural baggage with them than do the children. It is the children who lead the way out." Witnessing the children learning to deal with adversity, fear, and conflict brings hope to others and reinvigorates family, teachers, religious leaders, community, and staff at the garden. Some village voices may oppose children attending, but whereas in the past they simply refused to discuss the matter or made veiled threats, they are now willing to talk about their concerns.

Ten years after the Butterfly Garden opened, more than 1200 children have attended the nine-month program, 3000 in single school visits and thousands more unscheduled visitors from throughout the district. The dynamics of armed conflict continue to grind on the morale of the community, and the area was hard hit by the December 2004 Asian tsunami, after which conflict tensions paralyzed relief assistance. The Butterfly Garden now provides mobile programs that travel to several resettlement camps. Alumni from earlier years—now young adults—offer a resource pool for staff and volunteer support. More broadly, the Butterfly Peace Garden is a demonstrably successful approach to mental and social rehabilitation for children, peacebuilding and community reconciliation (Chase 2002; Chase and Bush 2002), which has inspired initiatives elsewhere in Sri Lanka, Canada, and Cambodia.

REFERENCES

Chase, R., 2000. The Butterfly Garden, Batticaloa, Sri Lanka: Final report of a program development and research project (1998–2000). ISBN 955-599-197-9 Sri Lanka. Available by request or as downloadable zip file from www.robertchase.ca

Chase, R., A. Doney, S. Sivayogin, V. Ariyaratne, P. Satkunanayagam, and A. Swaminathan. 1999. Mental health initiatives as peace initiatives in Sri Lankan school children affected by armed conflict. *Medicine, Conflict and Survival* 15:379–90. Available online at the www.humanities.mcmaster.ca website.

Chase, Robert. 2002. Healing and reconciliation for war-affected children and communities: Learning from the Butterfly Garden of Sri Lanka's eastern province. In *Helping children outgrow war*. Technical Paper No. 116, Human Resources and Democracy Division, Office of Sustainable Development, Bureau for Africa, US Agency for International Development, 39–52. Available online at the http://pdf.usaid.gov website.

Chase, Robert, and Ken Bush. 2002. The mental health of war-affected children: A community-based rehabilitation and reconciliation program in Sri Lanka's eastern province. *Asia Pacific Journal on Disability and Rehabilitation* (February). Available online at the www.aifo.it website.

Health Reach. 1996. The health of children in war zones in Sri Lanka: A study by Health Reach of McMaster University, Canada. Published in Sri Lanka. Available online at the www.humanities.mcmaster.ca/peace-health/Resources/ref.htm website.

Hogan, Paul. 2003. Ashoka Fellowship award profile. Available online at the www.ashoka.org website.

Santa Barbara, J. 1999. Helping children affected by war. *Medicine, Conflict and Survival* 15 (4): 352–4. Available online at the www.humanities.mcmaster.ca website.

NOTE

The Butterfly Peace Garden is a project of the Jesuits of Batticaloa http://www.aid srilanka.info/wst_page6.html and supported by the Dutch nongovernmental organization Hivos (www.hivos.nl) and by War Child Canada (www.warchild.ca).

1. The Spiral Garden at the Bloorview MacMillan Children's Center, Toronto, is a outdoor creative arts program that since 1984 has integrated children with disabilities attending the physical rehabilitation center with neighborhood children. More information is available online at www.bloorview.ca/programsandservices/communityprograms/centreforthearts/spiralgarden.php

The World Health Organization:
Health as a Bridge for Peace   ■   Neil Arya

IN THE 1980S THE PAN-AMERICAN HEALTH ORGANIZATION (PAHO) initiated the concept of Health as a Bridge for Peace (HBP) based on the principle that "shared health concerns can transcend political, economic, social and ethnic divisions among people and between nations" (WHO 1997). This concept developed into a multicountry, multiagency process with cross-border surveillance of populations, joint procurement, and the exchange of medicines and vaccines among Central American countries. PAHO's leadership was essential to bringing health to the forefront of the peacebuilding agenda, while the actions of UNICEF, the International Committee of the Red Cross (ICRC), and nongovernmental organizations (NGOs) were important in coordinating efforts at the field level. The international community [the Organization of American States (OAS), Spain, the United States, other European countries, and UN agencies] invested between $50 and $100 million in this project in the late 1980s and was also integral to the conceptualization and implementation of HBP efforts.

Although the WHO has embraced the concept of Health as a Bridge to Peace since 1997 (WHO Health Action in Crises www.who.int/hac/about/mission/en/index.html), HBP remains minimally operationalized and funded within WHO. However, WHO has facilitated training workshops on HBP in the Caucasus/Russia (1998), Sri Lanka (1999–2004), and Indonesia (2001) and considers many of its field activities to be carried out in the name of HBP. Even prior to this, WHO attempted to embrace its peacebuilding potential, however imperfectly. Let us examine some of the relevant fieldwork of WHO.

When a military junta overthrew the democratically elected Haitian government of Jean-Bertrand Aristide and ruled from 1991 until 1994, WHO and international NGOs were torn as to whether or not they should cooperate with the junta in order to deliver needed aid. Some in the international community (supported by many in Haitian civil society) felt that the best response was strict noncooperation, enforcement of sanctions, and evacuation of foreign personnel. In the end, a decentralized, strictly apolitical Health/Humanitarian Assistance Program involving Haitian professionals of different backgrounds, and targeted to the most vulnerable segments of the population, contributed to the development and stabilization of the health sector. Opponents of such an approach argued that maintaining relations with the de facto government may have legitimated it and weakened civil society. In the name of maintaining peace and well-being, the program has been criticized as perpetuating violence.

During the 1992–1995 war in Bosnia-Herzegovina, government buildings, civilian homes, hospitals, and other public institutions on all sides were targeted and destroyed. A severe refugee crisis ensued with hundreds of thousands fleeing to Croatia and the rest of Europe and many others being internally displaced. As the war ended, the health sector remained divided, and WHO again worked to unify staffing, service provision, training, and health-care delivery. With European partners, it facilitated "decentralized cooperation," a community empowerment bottom-up initiative to link local communities (institutions, health and social services, professionals, and lay people) in Europe, primarily in Italy, with twenty-two diverse towns in Bosnia-Herzegovina (particularly Croat and Muslim) to create and/or consolidate long-term cultural, technical, and economic partnerships. WHO assisted in the coordination of preliminary meetings, needs assessments, planning exercises, and training sessions and provided technical assistance meant to strengthen the trend toward reconciliation. The importance of WHO and the health sector and the ultimate success of this venture is still not clear.

In 1996–1997 WHO led an effort to reintegrate health services in Eastern Slavonia, the largely ethnic Serb part of Croatia, according to principles of the Dayton, Paris, and Erdut agreements. Chairing the Joint Implementation Committee, it called upon governments, civil society leadership, and health NGOs to bring together Croat and Serb health workers in confidence-building activities. These included joint health situation analysis, planning, and implementation. In the public health domain, ethnic Croatians and Serbs worked together on the organization of a subnational immunization day against polio and provision of essential drugs, along with epidemiology and other health research. The administrative reintegration of the health sector included physical rehabilitation, mental health, and health information systems.

By providing a safe space for dialogue on technical issues, WHO hoped to create a basis for mutual understanding and cooperation within the health sector. This included emphasizing the respect for both sides' roles as health professionals and for their traditional neutrality and impartiality in situations of armed conflict. Although this seemed to increase the number of Serb and Croat health employees working together and to provide for more equal opportunities for local Serb health workers, few Serbs were employed by the Croatian administration, none were selected for key positions in the health system, and only half of the Serb population were covered by the Croatian National Insurance System.

WHO also tried to help integrate health systems in Mozambique and Angola. From 1992 to 1996, cooperation of the government and RENAMO (Resistencia Nacional Mozambicana) rebels in Mozambique led to a comprehensive effort to re-train RENAMO health workers, to reintegrate them within the National Health Systems government health workers, and to increase the accessibility of basic health care to demobilized soldiers and their families in order to defuse political tensions.

After the signing of the Lusaka protocol with UNITA (União Nacional pela Independência Total de Angola) rebels, the Angolan government worked with UNICEF and WHO to disarm and demobilize soldiers from armies on both sides of the conflict. The latter brokered arrangements for the development and implementation of a health program. This included joint data collection activities, designing common protocols between groups, the adoption of national guidelines on priority health issues (sleeping sickness, malaria, TB), and a common simplified health information system (early warning system). Integrated activities, meant to promote dialogue, trust, and common goals, included in-service training, working with communities to develop public health programs, and setting up a joint medical team to assess and classify disabilities, thus supporting a legal basis for institutionalizing benefits to disabled war victims and demobilized soldiers. When fighting broke out again in 1998, "days of tranquility" once again allowed for immunization.

WHO has identified the following characteristics as important for success: working with health authorities and professionals on all sides openly and transparently according to geographic (not political) boundaries to create a safe space for health (neutral environments), addressing human rights and ethics through health, fostering and empowering responsibility for health and environment with action based on best available information, and flexibility to correct when necessary.

However, the WHO has not been able to properly evaluate the success of the above measures or to develop a framework for assessment.

REFERENCES

Arya, N. 2007. "Peace through Health" Chapter 24 in *Handbook of peace studies*, ed. Charles Webel and Johan Galtung. London: Routledge.

Hess, Gregory, and Michaela Pfeiffer. Comparative analysis of WHO "Health as a Bridge for Peace" case studies. Available online at the www.who.int website.

Large, J. 1997. Considering conflict: Concept paper for first Health as a Bridge for Peace consultative meeting, Les Pensières, Annecy, October 30–31.World Health Organization. Available online at the www.who.int website.

Manenti, A. 2001. *Health as a potential contribution to peace: Realities from the field: What has WHO learned in the 1990s?* World Health Organization, Health and Conflict, Department of Emergency and Humanitarian Action.

Peters, M. A. 1996. A health-to-peace handbook. *The Journal of Humanitarian Assistance.* Hamilton, Ontario: McMaster University. Available online at the www.humanities .mcmaster.ca website.

Rodriguez-Garcia, R., J. Macinko, F. X. Solórzano, and M. Schlesser. 2001. *How can health serve as a bridge for peace?* Washington, DC: School of Public Health and Health Services, The George Washington University.

World Health Organization. 1997. *Report on the first WHO consultative meeting on Health as a Bridge for Peace.* Les Pensières, Annecy, October 30–31.

NOTE

Further reading and source material for this chapter include Hess and Pfeiffer, Large 1997, Manenti 2001, Peters 1996, and Rodriguez-Garcia 2001. Each of these articles refers to the above project's attempt to evaluate their success. This material has previously been used by the author in Arya 2007.

PART VI

Evaluation

19

Evaluation of Peace through Health Initiatives

Joanna Santa Barbara

WHY EVALUATE?

Evaluation is not a special activity; we do it all the time. We look at the consequences of actions and base our future behavior on what we learned. Most of our everyday evaluations are simple linkages of cause and effect: "If I hold the nail that way, I bang my thumb with the hammer; if I hold it this way, I don't." If our action involves time elapsing between cause and effect, we are more deliberate about evaluation. "The seedlings of this variety of tomatoes have given me better fruit than the other varieties." Now if our intervention involves many people, over a period of time, and with outcomes that aren't easily observable, we have to be *much* more deliberate in our evaluation. If we want the learnings from it to be reliable for the use of others, and not subject to our bias and other errors, we have to observe certain rules of science to make them so. This brings us to the kind of evaluation we have in mind in appraising the outcomes of Peace through Health interventions.

Formal definitions of evaluation encompass these ideas. Scriven (1991) defines evaluation as "the process of determining the merit, worth or value of something." More specifically, program evaluation is defined as a systematic inquiry that describes and explains policy and program operations, effects, justifications, and social implications for the purpose of social betterment (Mark, Henry, and Julnes 2000).

We evaluate in order to learn from our actions and therefore to pursue our goals more effectively. If we set out to try to improve people's lives in areas of health and peace, we need to know whether we have accomplished our goals—whether we have made things better in unexpected ways, made things worse, or made no difference at all. If the latter is the case, the outcome is not neutral, because the resources expended on our activities might have been used on a more beneficial action. A good argument could be made for a duty to evaluate.

In Peace through Health work we will have dual sets of goals, aiming at both health and peace. For some, peace goals may be intermediate to the ultimate goal of health; for others, peace and health are held jointly as interdependent goals. For example, the health professionals throughout the world who work on the abolition of nuclear weapons do so in order to prevent the catastrophic impact on health that would result from the use of such weapons. They employ dissemination of knowledge of health effects in order to accomplish that goal. Their success will be measured by indicators related to that goal. A health professionals' organization for work on landmines may hold goals of adherence to the Mine Ban Treaty (peace), the clearing of landmines (peace and health) and the rehabilitation of landmines victims (health). Evaluation of their work would involve all three areas.

Evaluation of health interventions is a well-developed area and the subject of much literature, but the evaluation of peacework is a new area with a paucity of literature. Although the principles of evaluation are very similar for both areas, this chapter will focus on evaluation of peacework. Using an evaluation perspective sharpens thinking in an area in which it may be vague and fuzzy.

We should begin with a theory of change. What is the route between proposed action and hoped-for outcome? For example, in the Afghanistan schools program discussed in Chapter 16, we might suggest that the following goals exist:

Health Goal
Identifying with and discussing stories with themes of mental health problems → reconstructions in a child's mind that are more conducive to mental health → improved mental health

Peace Goal
Identifying with and learning ideas from stories with themes of peace processes → expanded understanding and valuing of peace processes → more use of peace processes in child's life and more support of peace processes in child's environment → more experience of peaceful relationships (with the latter goal seen as maturing over many years)

Each of these linkages is testable. Evaluation methods can be applied at any point in the process of accomplishing these health or peace goals. Some of the best tools evaluation has to offer are methods of building program models that show how a goal is to be accomplished and what it takes to accomplish that goal. Such a "logic model" helps people clarify and understand program interventions.

Programs of intervention often have more than one goal and involve multiple activities. They can be evaluated at various stages of their development. The logic model for a Peace through Health program or project will have the following elements:

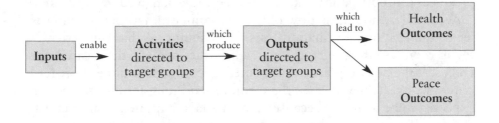

Inputs are those elements that go into a program: money, time, knowledge, creativity, and the like.

Activities are what the program does with the inputs to achieve the goal. They include tasks, actions, campaigns, and interventions undertaken to accomplish the program goals. For example, if you were running a campaign to outlaw cluster bombs, the activities might consist of a series of conferences on the health effects of these devices. There may be different audiences for different activities. In this case the audience would be the general public, journalists, and other peace organizations.

Outputs are the direct products of the activities and are usually measured in terms of work accomplished—for example, number of media appearances on the topic and number of articles written for medical journals and the popular press.

Outcomes may be short-term, medium-term, or long-term. A *short-term outcome* might be that journalists picked up the issue, and activist organizations adopted the campaign. A *medium-term outcome* might be a shift in public awareness and public opinion favoring the banning of cluster bombs. The *long-term outcome* would be an international treaty, possibly an additional protocol to the Mine Ban Treaty, outlawing cluster bombs. The outcomes will be affected, not only by the outputs of the program, but also by many factors in the environment of the work being done. Sometimes such effects can be large and unpredictable. In the campaign by health professionals and many others to ban landmines, Princess Diana's adoption of this cause had a large positive effect. This effect was further enhanced by sympathy for her cause after her unfortunate death.

The essential understanding to be gained from this model is the "cause and effect" linkages among what goes into a program (inputs), what the program does (activities) and who the audience is, what the program produces (outputs), and what is expected to be achieved (outcomes).

With clarity about the flow of the program, evaluation becomes easier to think about. Evaluation tests the assumption that the activities, focused on specific target groups, will in fact achieve the desired outcomes. If the activities are implemented as planned, and the short-term outcomes are achieved, then the medium- and long-term outcomes are expected to be achieved because planners have built in a "cause-effect" relationship between what you do and the health or peace goals you want to achieve. As we have noted, long-term outcomes are often a result of multiple interventions and various other contextual factors. Therefore, although we need to prove the connection to them, we are rarely able to claim that we are the only, the direct, or the main contributor to that level of change.

One way to think about this is in terms of what we **control** (the activities we undertake), what we **directly influence** (the short-term outcomes most closely linked to the activities), and what we **indirectly** influence (the longer-term outcomes).

Process (or formative) evaluation focuses on a variety of questions: (Are we delivering the program we planned? Who are the recipients of our activities? Are we reaching those we wanted to influence?) We must monitor these issues to remain faithful to the plans and to identify barriers to delivery of the program. Such evaluation may also lead to refinements of the theory of change.

Then we turn to **outcome (or summative)** evaluation and ask other questions: Is this program making a difference? Are the hoped-for changes occurring? Are there any unintended effects, good or bad? What aspects of the outputs are working and which are not?

METHODS OF EVALUATING PEACE THROUGH HEALTH WORK

Suppose you were involved in rebuilding health-care systems in a society that has come to the end of a period of interethnic violence over land and resource use. There is a peace plan. One of your team's goals in rebuilding the health system is to reduce interethnic antipathy and thus decrease the probability of further outbreaks of violence. How will you know whether you have accomplished this? You will need to know the state of interethnic hatred and interethnic peace before you begin your intervention and then compare the state of affairs afterward. How will you measure this?

You may look at episodes of violence that erupt between groups or at accounts of friction that appear in the press. You may do a survey to find out about people's attitudes. Then you will look at the same things at a later point in your program and see whether they have changed. You might already have noticed a difficulty here: You are not the only game in town. Others may be working toward the same goals (and indeed this is to be hoped for). Maybe religious leaders are preaching sermons on social unity and ending prejudice. Maybe the schools system has a program directed to the same end. If there is a change after a year, will you know what brought it about? No. You have to put up with this uncertainty. Pure scientific experimentation demands that all other conditions that might affect the outcome be held constant, so that if there is a change, we know what caused it. But it is very hard to reproduce those circumstances in interventions we do in a society, with all its complex and ever-changing dynamics. We simply do the best we can and acknowledge the uncertainty. (See Chapter 15 on epidemiology.)

In the schools project in Croatia (see "Peace Education as Primary Prevention" in Chapter 16), the children showed a positive change in acceptance of other ethnicities after a year of the program. Meanwhile, radio and TV programs focused heavily on the superiority of being Croatian (and the inferiority of others). In these circumstances, we felt more confident that it was the program that brought about the positive change.

How did we know that it wasn't just the passage of time after the end of the war that produced the change? We did the same measurements on another, similar group of children at the beginning and end of the same time period. These children had no peace education input from us, and they did not show the changes seen in the group that received the program. This is known as using a control group to compare with an intervention group.

It is possible that the measurements were done by people who were so enthusiastic about the program that they accidentally biased the results to look positive? This is one form of bias in evaluation work. To eliminate it, we had another team, different from the one who delivered the program, do the evaluation. The people on this team did not know which children had received the program and which had not. Such "blinding" is a device to eliminate bias.

The hoped-for outcome may be an event, such as a change in government policy, which either does or does not occur. More often it is a change in people's awareness, attitudes, understanding, knowledge, skills, and behaviors.

Suppose we introduced peer mediation to a school and our long-term outcome was decrease in physical fights in the playground and improvement in "school climate" (a cluster of qualities that include individuals feeling respected and liked, and people working cooperatively). The phenomena we select to represent our intended changes are called indicators. We might decide that the number of children sent to the principal's office each day was a suitable indicator of the number of physical fights. Or we might decide to do a systematic playground observation and actually count the number of physical fights. How will we measure the positive qualities we hope have developed from the program? Once we know what we are looking for, we might find an instrument already developed to measure it. In the case of "school climate," there are several. The Mental Measurement Yearbook, available in university libraries, is a compendium of such instruments, although it is always necessary to consider whether an instrument developed for one culture will be applicable in another. Sometimes there is no ready-made instrument to measure what we are looking for, so we need to develop our own instrument. Then we need to go through the process of ensuring that it is a valid and reliable way of measuring the dimension of interest. Methods of doing this can be found in texts relevant to the area of study.

Our evaluation design should also have a way of discerning unintended good and bad effects of the program. Because we do not know what to ask for, much less measure, a good way to arrive at this knowledge is through a focus group. This is a group of recipients of the program who are invited to a free-flowing, but structured, discussion of what the program meant to them. Researchers sometimes learn surprising things. In the Croatia schools program, teachers changed their general teaching methods to become less authoritarian as a result of the training to deliver the program.

There are other ways of gaining knowledge in the realm of evaluation that are quite different from the approach described above. Suppose you wanted an answer to the question "Did the Western antinuclear movement influence former Soviet President Mikhail Gorbachev to introduce his stunningly comprehensive plan to eliminate nuclear weapons in 1986?" One way of finding out would be to interview Gorbachev and ask him. Happily, he has spontaneously told us that the International Physicians for the Prevention of Nuclear War influenced him in this direction (Gorbachev 1987). But there are other instances when it would require a reading of diaries, autobiography, or interview transcripts to establish a causal relation of interest. This is one of many methods of **qualitative evaluation.**

WORKING WITH PARTNERS IN EVALUATION

Many projects described in this text involve partnership with other organizations and may involve delivery of programs to participants. The goals, methods, and theory of change will have been worked out with the partners. The evaluation too must involve partners and (in some cases) recipients. Involving everyone shows respect and reflects the equal status of all members of the partnership. It is possible that a partner organization has had little experience in evaluation. In this case, hosting a preliminary workshop would be useful. Involving partners in the questions for evaluation, in identifying the indicators, and in choosing the instruments is important.

FOR WHOM IS THIS EVALUATION?

So far we have treated the evaluation as though its sole purpose were to yield information that will benefit the recipients or participants. This should surely have first priority. But there are others who have an interest in evaluations, particularly funders. This is laudable, in that funders have a responsibility to ensure that their funds are used to benefit recipients. Sometimes, however, funders want workers to use instruments that are uniform across a wide range of projects. This may conflict with both the specifics of a particular project and the creative elements that might be generated by a participatory project. Workers may also gain academic credentials from work on evaluation projects. This is a worthy purpose, but it must always be subordinate to the interests of the intended beneficiaries of the program Conflicts over goals in evaluation need to be dealt with through respectful dialogue.

EVALUATIONS IN OTHER CULTURES AND LANGUAGES

Working in other cultures and languages complicates the task of evaluation considerably. Great care must be taken to ensure that the form of the evaluation is culturally appropriate and that any translation of instruments or of exchanges in focus groups is of high quality. Working with a partner may overcome these problems, because these functions will be carried out by native speakers and culture bearers.

BARRIERS TO EVALUATION

Evaluation of peacework is a new field, and little has yet been accomplished, except in the area of conflict resolution. Heather Farrell (2005) interviewed Peace through Health workers in an effort to understand barriers to undertaking a meaningful evaluation of their work. Some of the problems were the evaluators' inadequate knowledge of evaluation; peace workers' reluctance to make the peace goals of the project explicit; program recipients' negative prior experience of coercive interrogation, such that a structured interview might recall those memories; and the fact that participants might have a cultural aversion to criticism and therefore be unwilling to offer any negative feedback. There is also an assumption that anything done with good intentions must produce good effects. We certainly have enough evidence to debunk this myth; indeed, many development projects do unintentional harm to recipients (Anderson and Olson 2003). There may also be an insistence that urgent humanitarian work is more important than evaluation (even though evaluation may subsequently make the humanitarian work more efficient).

CONCLUSION

- If you intend to intervene, you have a duty to evaluate what you do.
- Consider the evaluation from the earliest stage of planning the project (and build it into the budget).
- Include partners in developing the evaluation plan, and when possible, include recipients as well.
- Consider a broad range of effects—intended and unintended, good and bad.

ACKNOWLEDGMENT

I am grateful to Sharon Campbell for many helpful comments on this chapter.

FOR FURTHER INFORMATION

A recommended text on program evaluation is Bamberger, Rugh, and Mabry 2006. The World Bank (2004) has some very good evaluation tools available online, as does the United Way.

REFERENCES

Anderson, Mary B., and Lara Olson. 2003. *Confronting war: Critical lessons for peace practitioners*. Cambridge, MA: Collaborative for Development Action, 20.

Bamberger, M., J. Rugh, and L. Mabry. 2006. *Real world evaluation: Working under budget, time, data and political constraints*. Newbury Park, CA: Sage Publications.

Farrell, Heather. 2005. Towards a framework for Peace-through-Health evaluation: Current thinking in the field. Master's Thesis.

Gorbachev, Mikhail. 1987. *Perestroika: New thinking for our country and the world*. London: Collins, 154.

Mark, Melvin M., Gary T. Henry, and George Julnes. 2000. *Evaluation: An integrated framework for understanding, guiding and improving policies and programs*. San Francisco: Jossey-Boss.

Scriven, M. 1991. *Evaluation Thesaurus*, 9th ed. Newbury Park, CA: Sage.

World Bank. 2004. *Monitoring and evaluation: Some tools, methods and approaches*. Washington, DC. The World Bank. Available at the lnweb18.worldbank.org website.

PART VII

Expanding the Bounds of
Peace through Health

20

Expanding the Bounds
of Medical Peace Practice

Klaus Melf, Neil Arya, and *Caecilie Buhmann*

For many years medical peace activists and academics have sought to bring peace issues into the research and education of medical and public health schools around the world. They have developed several frameworks to understand and analyze the health sector's contribution to peace. Depending on the local, institutional, national, political, and cultural context, the frameworks for research, teaching, and action may be called Health and Human Rights, Violence Prevention, Peace Medicine, Global Health, or Ecosystem Health. These theoretical constructs vary in the types and levels of violence they address, the phase of conflict in which they act, and whether they use a preventive or a curative approach.

Recently, academics on both sides of the Atlantic have chosen to expand the scope of their inquiry to develop a holistic framework to embrace all the different kinds of peacework performed by health professionals. This approach coincides with the broadening of concepts and activities in the medical peace movement and mirrors the integrative efforts within peace research and peace studies in general. To understand this development, we need to go beyond traditional definitions of peace and health. This chapter offers an overview of the theoretical considerations behind Peace through Health by briefly describing relevant concepts and disciplines and elaborating on holistic understandings of peace and health.

WORKING FOR DISARMAMENT

The international medical peace movement gained momentum during the coldest period of the Cold War when physicians from both sides of the Iron Curtain formed IPPNW (International Physicians for the Prevention of Nuclear War). Bolstered by the Nobel Peace Prize in 1985, the membership grew rapidly to more than 200,000 individuals, united in the medical struggle for nuclear disarmament. Aiming to inject awareness of the nuclear threat into medical education, IPPNW produced and disseminated a model curriculum titled *Medicine and Nuclear War* (IPPNW 1988). Over the years, IPPNW has broadened its focus from nuclear abolition to the disarmament of all weapons of mass destruction and of vast public health impact. This includes the fight against small arms and landmines.

Disarmament is insufficient, however, if the goal is the prevention of (nuclear) war. Peace educators have stressed the need for addressing militarism at its roots: "Thus, disarmament education will have to delve into the roots of arms build-ups and arms races, not simply the arms per se which are no more than a symptom of more fundamental problems" (Haavelsrud 2004, 47).

FROM DISARMAMENT TO WAR PREVENTION

Besides arms proliferation and militarism, there are other risk factors for violence and armed conflicts, which are addressed in various concepts and frameworks. Frances Stewart, for instance, divides risk factors for war into the following categories:

- Group motivation (inter- or intrastate resentments, divisions along cultural or religious lines, by geography, or by class)
- Private motivation (Young, uneducated men with no alternatives and those with little income and no hope for gainful employment may seek the opportunity to profiteer.)
- Poor governance
- Failure of the social contract (With economic stagnation, the state fails to deliver services and to provide reasonable economic conditions, including a robust employment rate and livable incomes.)
- Environmental degradation (Rising population pressure and falling agricultural productivity may lead to land disputes and a growing scarcity of water.) (Stewart, Holdstock, and Jarquin 2002).

In other words, violations of human rights, poverty, disparity, and ecological disruption are also risk factors for war and armed violence.

Using a public health model, disarmament and addressing the root causes of violent conflicts may be referred to as **primary preventive intervention**

(Levy and Sidel 1997). Some scholars even distinguish risk factors for violent escalation of a conflict (primary prevention) from root causes for conflicts in the first place (primordial prevention) (Yusuf, Anand, and MacQueen 1998).

Health-related frameworks that deal with different root causes of violent conflicts include the Global Health, Health and Human Rights, and Ecosystem Health frameworks. Also, the discipline of Social Medicine may cover peace-relevant issues such as the reduction of poverty and social inequality.

FROM PRIMARY PREVENTION
TO CONFLICT INTERVENTION AND PEACEBUILDING

In addition to the struggle for war prevention, health professionals have engaged in harm prevention during armed conflicts—secondary prevention. The International Committee of the Red Cross established the tradition of health professionals entering battlefields in the service of humanity. Since its formation in 1863, it has brought medical and other humanitarian aid to the sick and wounded. Through initiating the Geneva Conventions and monitoring adherence to them, it has contributed to reducing impunity for war crimes and to protecting noncombatants.

Other forms of **secondary preventive interventions** have been developed and tested largely in the last two decades. They present a curative approach to the conflict itself and focus on health diplomacy, relationship building, and conflict resolution. This is reflected in another model curriculum supported by IPPNW; *Medicine and Peace* deals not only with disarmament issues and the root causes of warfare, but also with the possibility of secondary prevention (UN Commission on Disarmament Education, IPPNW, and PSR 1993). The most influential actor in this field is the World Health Organization, which has developed the framework of Health as a Bridge for Peace. It has organized various on-the-ground training for health workers in violence-prone regions, using the "Active Learning Package" (International Training Programme for Conflict Management of the Scuola Superiore S. Anna 1999).

Tertiary prevention of violent conflicts consists often of peacebuilding activities in the postwar period and embraces the terms *reconstruction,* *resolution,* and *reconciliation.* However, most such interventions, like McMaster University's Peace through Health field projects, start while war and violent events are still going on. Clear allocation to one prevention phase is therefore difficult, and many initiatives during and after violent events also have primary prevention purposes.

FROM MACRO LEVEL TO MICRO LEVEL

Even in areas where war prevention, conflict mediation, and reconciliation are successful, for many people there is still no peace. Despite the absence of violent conflicts on a macro level (societal, regional, and global levels), they are suffering under violence on a micro level (individual and community levels), such as abuse of power, high crime rates, or domestic violence.

Cases of torture and ill-treatment by security forces, police, and other state authorities are not limited to theaters of war and have been documented in more than 100 countries (Amnesty International Report 2007; The State of the World's Human Rights 2007). The framework of Medicine and Human Rights demonstrates that health professionals may be at risk of complicity in human rights violations merely by fulfilling official functions as prison doctors, psychiatrists, or public health specialists. This framework has been promoted by Physicians for Human Rights and by Amnesty International, and it has been supported in particular by the British Medical Association (BMA 2001). Even the discipline of Medical Ethics covers many aspects of medical practice, teaching, and research, where the rights and dignity of individuals either have been violated in history or are currently in danger. Therefore, Medical Ethics can also be understood as a peace-related framework.

Millions of women worldwide suffer from physical and/or sexual abuse in their homes or communities. Feminist critiques brought the attention of peace research to the "war against women" as a form of violence on a grand scale (Brock-Utne 1997, 151). Prevention of interpersonal violence not only entered into the scope of peace science but also became a subject in medical training and public health. By 1994 most medical schools in the United States reported curricular components on adult domestic violence, and the issue of child abuse has been more systematically addressed in medical education around the world (Alpert, Sege, and Bradshaw 1997).

Most recently, suicide prevention is no longer limited to the sphere of psychiatry but has been identified as a major public health challenge (Krug et al. 2002). Within peace research there is a growing interest in intrapersonal violence and the relationship between inner and outer peace.

FROM DIRECT VIOLENCE
TO STRUCTURAL AND CULTURAL VIOLENCE

We elaborate here on definitions of violence given in Chapter 1. Noted peace theorist Johan Galtung begins with "violence" as the antithesis of "peace." War is merely considered to be the extreme form of collective violence, impacting a huge number of people and analogous to epidemics in public health. Violence may be defined as unnecessary insults of basic human needs, including violations of survival needs (death), well-being needs (misery), freedom needs (repression), and identity needs (alienation) (Galtung 1996, 197).

Just as there are many types of diseases, acute and chronic, there are many types of violence or violations: direct, structural, or cultural. **Direct violence** consists of violent acts or events, usually referred to in public and in the media as simply violence. In health literature, this is defined as "the intentional use of physical force or power, threatened or actual, against oneself, another person, or against a group or community, that either results in or has a high likelihood of resulting in injury, death, psychological harm, maldevelopment or deprivation" (Krug et al. 2002, 5).

Structural violence is considered to be processes built into the socioeconomic or political structure. These processes express themselves in exploitation, repression, or unequal opportunities for individuals or groups. **Cultural violence** consists of those elements in our cosmologies, such as religion, ideology, language, art, and science, that justify and legitimize the use of direct and structural violence (Galtung 1996, 31).

Understanding violence and peace in this way makes it clear that peacework is not limited to disarmament efforts and the prevention or ending of war and direct violence. Peacework also challenges violent socioeconomic and political structures, as well as violent aspects in our cultures, whether or not they are root causes of war. Violent structures might include the inaccessibility of health care and life-saving drugs or the spending of scarce resources for military purposes. Examples of cultural violence include paternalism, racism, and sexism. Health professionals and organizations are challenging violent structures and cultures by fighting for equal access to health services for all and everywhere, by giving research priorities to the major health obstacles of the poor, and by promoting tolerance and intercultural understanding in the clinical setting and the society at large.

FROM CONTEMPORARY CONFLICTS
TO VIOLENCE AGAINST FUTURE GENERATIONS

Violence in its different forms can be targeted at people, cultural heritage, infrastructure, or biological species. It can include ecological violence that, in anthropocentric terms, sets the current generation in conflict with the needs of succeeding human generations. Sustainable development and environmental protection are therefore interrelated with peace.

We might even look at both peace and health in their biophysical and socioeconomic contexts, with each representing balance or resiliency. Noted public health pioneer John Last defines health as a "sustainable state of equilibrium or harmony between humans and their physical, biological and social environments that enables them to coexist indefinitely. Implied in this is the capacity to adapt or adjust harmoniously to changes in aspects of the environment" (Last 2006, 154)

A HOLISTIC PEACE CONCEPT

Peace has many different meanings, depending on culture and context. *Shalom* in Hebrew, for instance, is related to well-being and spiritual wholeness, whereas the Greek word *eirene* stands for ethical social relationships. The predominantly Western concept of peace derives from the Latin term *pax,* connoting law, order, and mutual duty.

Analogous to the World Health Organization's definition of health as much more than the absence of disease, a holistic definition of peace entails much more than the absence of war and all types of violence (this might be termed negative peace). Peace also means the presence of loving, harmonious acts (direct peace), of equitable, horizontal relations (structural peace), and of life-enriching cultures that promote peace and nonviolence (cultural peace). This is what Galtung calls positive peace (Galtung 1996, 33).

Contrary to the mainstream use of the term *conflict* as synonymous with violence and war, peace scientists consider conflict merely as the clash of incompatible goals in a goal-seeking system. Conflict is neutral, but it challenges the status quo and can even catalyze improvement. The problem is not the conflict in itself, but its "resolution" by violent means (Barash and Webel 2002). Peace is therefore also described as creative and nonviolent conflict transformation (Galtung 1996, 9).

The teaching of human values, empathy, communication skills, and social harmony can be construed as peace capacity building. These terms, therefore, can complement the aforementioned peace-related frameworks within medical and health science education.

Defined holistically, peace and health have many conditions in common, such as well-being, harmony, security, fulfillment of needs, and human dignity. Peace and health are interdependent and at the very least fraternal, if not identical twins.

UNIFYING THE DISCIPLINE

The frameworks of Peace through Health and Medical Peace Work, and for some the concepts of Health and Human Rights or Health and Human Security, are able to unify medical peace engagement on all levels and to link theory and understanding to action and advocacy, research and field projects. These frameworks, although they still often focus on war zones, could deal with the prevention or reduction of all kinds of violence and with the promotion of all kinds of peaceful behaviors, structures, and cultures. They could encompass the aforementioned concepts, such as Global Health, Ecosystem Health, Medicine and Human Rights, Medical Ethics, and Violence Prevention.

Even though the different concepts complement each other, each emphasizing particular aspects of violence prevention and peace promotion, some argue that such frameworks should not be united into one overall framework. This perspective may be grounded in a more conservative understanding of the term *peace* as the absence of war or in concern that the new field might lose focus and strength. Some peace researchers have also stated that a holistic concept of peace, which encompasses everything, blurs distinctions and makes research unfeasible (Müller 2005, 55).

Advocates for this inclusive and holistic approach, on the other side of this debate, do not wish to prioritize the expertise of one particular set of peacework experience or practice. They take equitably into account different knowledge traditions and celebrate the richness of health professionals' potential for building peace.

REFERENCES

Alpert, E. J., R. D. Sege, and Y. S. Bradshaw. 1997. Interpersonal violence and the education of physicians. *Academic Medicine* 72 (1 Suppl): S41–50.

Amnesty International Report 2007: The State of the World's Human Rights. 2007. London: Amnesty International.

Barash, David P., and Charles P. Webel. 2002. *Peace and conflict studies*. Thousand Oaks, CA: Sage Publications.

BMA. 2001. *The medical profession and human rights: Handbook for a changing agenda.* London: Zed Books.

Brock-Utne, Birgit. 1997. Linking the micro and macro in peace and development studies. In *The web of violence: From interpersonal to global,* ed. Jennifer Turpin and Lester R. Kurtz. Chicago: University of Illinois Press.

Galtung, Johan. 1996. *Peace by peaceful means: Peace and conflict, development and civilization.* London: Prio/Sage.

Haavelsrud, Magnus. 2004. Target: Disarmament education. *Journal of Peace Education* 1 (1):37-57.

International Training Programme for Conflict Management of the Scuola Superiore S. Anna. *Health as a Bridge for Peace: Active learning package.* WHO 1999 [cited 2007-06-28. Available from http://www.who.int/hac/techguidance/hbp/99CAFEA3_full.pdf.

IPPNW. 1988. *Medicine and nuclear war: A medical curriculum.* Cambridge, MA: IPPNW.

Krug, Etienne G., Linda L. Dahlberg, James A. Mercy, Anthony B. Zwi, and Rafael Lozano. 2002. *World report on violence and health.* Geneva: WHO.

Last, John M. 2006. *Dictionary of public health.* New York: Oxford University Press.

Levy, Barry S., and Victor W. Sidel. 1997. Preventing war and its health consequences: Roles of public health professionals. In *War and public health,* ed. B. S. Levy and V. W. Sidel. New York: Oxford University Press.

Müller, Harald. 2005. Theories of peace. In *Peace studies: Critical concepts in political science,* ed. M. Evangelista. Oxon and New York: Routledge. Original edition, Lettres de Byblos 1, Byblos, Lebanon: Centre International des Sciences de l'Homme, 2003.

Stewart, Frances, D. Holdstock, and A. Jarquin. 2002. Root causes of violent conflict in developing countries. Commentary: Conflict—from causes to prevention? *BMJ* 324 (7333):342–345.

UN Commission on Disarmament Education, IPPNW, and PSR. 1993. Medicine and peace: A model curriculum for medical students (draft).

Yusuf, S., S. Anand, and G. MacQueen. 1998. Can medicine prevent war? Imaginative thinking shows that it might. *BMJ* 317 (7174):1669–70.

21

Social Injustice and the Responsibility of Health-Care Workers: Observation, Assessment, Action

Evan Lyon, Jim Yong Kim, and Paul Farmer

THE CHALLENGES

"When I give food to the poor, they call me a saint. When I ask why the poor have no food, they call me a communist."
—Dom Helder Camara, Brazilian Archbishop

We are sometimes prevented from recognizing the root causes of illness by the modern sciences of medicine and public health. Medical interventions—from the miracles of antibiotics and anti-hypertensives to the benefits of aseptic surgery—cannot keep up with the flood of sick and poor patients if people remain poor and sick. Furthermore, well-designed disease prevention efforts based on education, hygiene, infrastructure improvements, environmental stabilization, and adequate nutrition are doomed to fail if they are not supported with adequate resources. Analyses based purely on quantitative epidemiology and cost-effectiveness parameters may not take into account the specific vulnerabilities of individuals and communities in need.

Health-care workers committed to health and social justice are responsible for understanding—and directly addressing—the root causes of poor health. Like Dom Helder Camara, an early thinker in what became Catholic Liberation Theology, we must ask such questions as "Why don't the poor have enough food?"

Social injustice cannot be addressed without first considering poverty and inequality (Fort, Mercer, and Gish 2004; Kim et al. 2000).[1] The health of poor populations is measurably worse than the health of those with wealth, whether comparisons are made between or within nations.[2] And inequality is a powerful engine that creates poverty worldwide. It

267

also exerts a powerful effect on health independently (Banks et al. 2006; Lynch et al. 1998).

Consider a single disease to help illustrate this point. HIV was first recognized in marginalized groups that suffered the consequences of social exclusion in the rich world: gay men, injection drug users, commercial sex workers. Twenty-five years later, the vast majority of people living with HIV live in poor countries, and nearly all HIV-related deaths are among the poor.[3] In the United States, where general HIV infection rates are relatively low, the virus continues to concentrate down the steep gradient of inequality that persists into the twenty-first century. Black women (who tend to be economically, politically, and socially excluded in the United States) carry the highest burden of HIV of any single demographic group and account for the greatest increase in new HIV infections.[4] If we consider economic status—or even political access—Black women in the United States may not be as poor or as excluded as their sisters in poorer countries, but the risks imposed by inequality and poverty have proved just as deadly. Furthermore, on a global scale, gender inequality has made HIV a disease of women.[5]

OBSERVATION

Looking for new ways to address a complex disease like HIV requires first asking the right questions. To begin this process, Liberation Theology—a social and religious movement rooted in the small communities of Latin America where we have spent a large part of our careers—recommends a simple prescription for people of any spiritual faith, or simply the faith in human capacity for social change. When beginning any work of service, we are urged to observe, judge, and act.[6]

Perhaps the most radical concept embedded in this simple formula is where it begins, with observation. In this context, observation is an inherently local practice. Whereas analysis may integrate information and experience from other sources, endeavoring to understand a health problem using this prescription begins with a place in addition to a problem. Careful observation must consider all the varied forces—historical, colonial, economic, social, cultural, gendered, disease-related, and so on—that contribute to the creation and persistence of health problems, and it must include listening deeply to local people. Community input, from the beginning of engagement to ongoing priority setting, helps ensure that the right problems are being addressed and in useful ways.

For example, Partners In Health—a not-for-profit, nongovernmental organization that two of the authors (J. Y. K. and P. F.) founded more than twenty years ago—settled in the village of Cange in Haiti's Central Plateau for a variety of reasons. Haiti is the poorest nation in the Western Hemisphere.[7] Largely as a consequence of this deep poverty, Haiti also remains at the bottom of world's health and development indices. But the village of Cange has been a place of particularly intense poverty, even in a setting of universal need. The village and its citizens were displaced, from the fertile Artibonite valley below the current village to the rocky hillsides where Cange now sits, by an internationally financed hydroelectric dam project completed in the 1950s (Farmer 1992). The first Partners In Health (PIH) clinic in Cange, of course, focused on providing direct service to a population in need. We trust that it has also helped shed light on the historical, political, social, and economic forces that create poor health in Haiti generally, and more specifically, in a place like Cange. The health inequities and innumerable injustices suffered by one poor village are not unique. But the village of Cange, both for the people of the Central Plateau and for foreign volunteers and visitors, has become a focal point for continued engagement with the suffering of the poor and for analyses aimed at understanding why poor health and suffering persist.[8]

ASSESSMENT

Once a problem is understood, judgment and analysis can often follow naturally and productively. A limited set of principles—such as considering health care as a human right, or judging all forms of structural violence as risks to human health—can guide this process. Judgment should also mean standing in solidarity with communities in need, and against the powers that create and maintain their oppression. This stance can be the beginning of action.[9]

By comparison, the majority of health and human rights dialogues begin with analysis, not observation. Public health experts and politicians usually identify health problems from a distance—in a conference room or ministerial office, extracting data from a report or spreadsheet—and invariably prescribe standard solutions. Many successful global health campaigns have focused, for example, on "vertical" or disease-specific programs. It is impossible to argue with the success of vaccine initiatives and disease eradication efforts, especially because much of the world still lacks vaccines and simple disease prevention infrastructure. Furthermore, vaccines and specialized treatments are judged to be most effective, both from a narrow medical perspective and in terms of cost, so these are doled out to the masses first. But beyond curing or preventing a single disease, do these initiatives and technological fixes begin to address social and economic injustice? Do these interventions, in any way, address how a population was left vulnerable to illness?

Economic globalization in the latter half of the twentieth century, the creation and propagation of massive international debt, and the constraints imposed on debtor nations in the form of structural adjustment programs have much to do with the persistence of preventable diseases (Kim et al. 2000). For example, polio persists only in a few nations suffering from economic and/or political turmoil: Iraq, Congo, Afghanistan, Somalia, Nigeria, northern India, Ethiopia, and Bangladesh (WHO 2005). Massive and sincere international efforts have eradicated it elsewhere. Likewise, tuberculosis—still a leading infectious killer of adults worldwide—began to decline in the developed world decades before the first antibiotic treatments were discovered. Improved nutrition, housing, and public hygiene are largely responsible for this change (Herbert 1983; Daniel 1997). In fact, many diseases that fall under the modern rubric of "tropical diseases" (malaria, tuberculosis, endemic typhoid, and so on) were problems in the temperate north prior to economic development. Although they persist in poor nations, wealthier places in the tropics, such as Australia and some regions of southeast Asia, do not suffer unduly from these "tropical" afflictions.[10]

Rather than replicating the approaches of others or propagating an incomplete paradigm such as "tropical diseases," health-care workers who begin with observation—not predetermined analyses or the simple desire to act—have the potential to make original, innovative, and successful interventions. Through this threefold process of observation, judgment, and action, health-care workers have the capacity to support social justice. A first step is to set priorities differently. Our job should be to ensure that the needs of the sick and poor, instead of the priorities of international funders, politicians, or health economists doing cost–benefit analyses, are placed at the center.

Another principle of Liberation Theology, making a preferential option for the poor, has been adopted as a long-standing motto for Partners In Health. Consequently, all PIH projects *preferentially* begin with the poor. Choosing to address a most difficult or most neglected problem is an act of solidarity from the first step. In rural Haiti, this kind of engagement has led PIH to a broad array of health and social justice programs beyond the traditional realm of the clinic. The board of *Zanmi Lasante* ("Partners In Health" in Haitian Kreyol) and many of its leaders are community members, so programmatic priorities are set locally. *Zanmi Lasante* (ZL) received a million patient visits in 2006.[11] In addition to offering free comprehensive primary care to the population, ZL cared for more than 5000 individuals living with HIV, and provided home-based [directly observed] therapy for everyone in our region who had been diagnosed with tuberculosis or needed highly active antiretroviral therapy (Walton et al. 2004). ZL also maintains four functioning operating rooms and a staff of general surgeons and obstetricians, even though surgical services are not usually part of the public health "standard package" deemed important for the health of the poor. Because the people we serve in Haiti have demanded surgery as part of their care, it has been on ZL's agenda since the beginning. ZL has also worked to improve health through primary school education, popular education, clean water initiatives, providing housing, and food security and sustainable agriculture projects.[12] Recognizing that shamefully inadequate housing can lead to poor health, the Program on Social and Economic Rights, which was founded by an activist from the village of Cange, has built over 200 homes in the past year and has plans to build hundreds more.

DIFFERENT ANALYSIS, LOCAL PRIORITIES, SIMILAR SOLIDARITY

PIH also supports several autonomous indigenous communities in Chiapas, Mexico. These communities, where living conditions are very similar to those in rural Haiti, have never requested direct clinical services. Instead, our colleagues in Chiapas have focused on promoting community health and disease prevention, popular education, and retention of local, indigenous medical traditions (Farmer 2003, 91–114). The PIH projects in Chiapas therefore have developed very differently.

In 1994, PIH founded a community-based health project in the densely packed, politically chaotic slums of Carabayllo in northern Lima, Peru. The project initially intended to provide general health care in a setting of intense poverty. After surveys uncovered the extent of active tuberculosis in the community, and the death of one of our co-workers from multidrug-resistant TB (MDRTB) tragically revealed that a standard approach to TB treatment was likely to be ineffective, the need for a more focused intervention was quickly recognized. The first patients were enrolled for community-based MDRTB treatment in 1995.

What began as a primary care project quickly evolved into a ground-breaking community-based program to treat a single complex disease. Many of our nurses and doctors took on multiple roles, doing home visits in the steep, dusty streets of Carabayllo, participating in exhaustive meetings with the Peruvian Ministry of Health, and representing their patients in the halls of the World Health Organization and the boardrooms of pharmaceutical manufacturers and universities around the world. Direct care for a small number of patients in northern Lima and advocacy on their behalf led to changes in global policy on MDRTB treatment, the manufacture and distribution of medicines to treat MDRTB, and improved access to MDRTB treatment worldwide (Mitnick et al. 2003; Partners In Health 2002).

A commitment to social justice has led our nurses and doctors to advocacy work beyond the "traditional" scope of health care. Staff from PIH have advocated locally and internationally for the basic right to health care, against military and structural violence, against trade and aid embargos, for the social and health rights of prisoners, and against the international political and financial structures that maintain poverty and inequality. The privileged position of health-care workers, witnessing in intimate detail the physical and psychological suffering of victims of injustice, demands that we speak out about these injustices.

Rudolf Virchow—an early-nineteenth-century proponent of what has become the discipline of social medicine, connecting health to society and encompassing many of the ideas addressed here—famously remarked that "the physician is the natural attorney of the poor."[13] In the role of attorney or advocate, and sometimes the only advocate available to poor and vulnerable people, health-care workers should confront social injustice as seriously and carefully as they confront clinical disease. The two are inextricably linked. Like Virchow endeavoring to uncover the "artificial" causes of a typhus outbreak in the 1840s, health-care workers are continuously close to physical suffering and its social dimensions.[14] This gives us great opportunities and a great responsibility to investigate the cases in front of us like a dogged attorney preparing for trial. If we observe carefully and tirelessly ask why a problem is concentrated in a particular place and time, then we have a chance to understand the problem to its foundations. From this understanding, common cause and action can follow, with the hope of transforming the unjust social and economic structures at the root of most sickness and suffering.

REFERENCES

Anderson, Matthew R., Lanny Smith, and Victor W. Sidel. 2005. What is social medicine? *Monthly Review* 56 (8). Available online at www.monthlyreview.org/0105anderson.htm

Banks, James, Michael Marmot, Zoe Oldfield, and James P. Smith. 2006. Disease and disadvantage in the United States and in England. *JAMA* 295 (May): 2037–45.

Black AIDS Institute. 2006. *AIDS in blackface: 25 years of an epidemic,* ed. Kai Wright. Available online at the www.blackaids.org website.

CDC (Centers for Disease Control). 2006. *Fact sheet: HIV/AIDS among African Americans.* Available online at the www.cdc.gov website.

Daniel, Thomas M. 1997. *Captain of death: The story of tuberculosis.* Rochester, NY: University of Rochester Press.

Dubois, Laurent. 2004. *Avengers of the new world: The story of the haitian revolution.* Cambridge, MA: Belknap Press.

Farmer, Paul. 1992. *AIDS and accusation: Haiti and the geography of blame.* Berkeley: University of California Press.

———. 2003. *Pathologies of power: Health, human rights, and the new war on the poor.* Berkeley: University of California Press.

Farmer, Paul, Margaret Connors, and Janie Simmons, eds. 2005. *Women, poverty, and AIDS: Sex, drugs, and structural violence.* Monroe, ME: Common Courage Press.

Fort, Meridith, Mary Ann Mercer, and Oscar Gish, eds. 2004. *Sickness and wealth: The corporate assault on global health.* Cambridge, MA: South End Press.

Herbert, Frank. 1983. *The white plague.* London: Gollancz.

James, C. L. R. 1989. *The black Jacobins: Toussaint L'Ouverture and the San Domingo Revolution* (Originally published in 1938). New York: Vintage Books.

Kim, Jim, Joyce Millen, John Gershman, and Alec Irwin, eds. 2000. *Dying for growth: Global inequality and the health of the poor.* Monroe, ME: Common Courage Press.

Lynch, John W., George A. Kaplan, Elsie R. Pamuk, Richard D. Cohen, Katherine E. Heck, Jennifer L. Balfour, and Irene H. Yen. 1998. Income inequality and mortality in metropolitan areas of the United States. *American Journal of Public Heath* 88 (July): 1074–80.

Lyon, Evan, and Paul Farmer. 2005. Inequality, infections, and community-based health care. *Yale Journal of Health Policy, Law, and Ethics* V (1): 465–73.

Mitnick, C., J. Bayona, E. Palacios, et al. 2003. Community-based therapy for multidrug-resistant tuberculosis in Lima, Peru. *New England Journal of Medicine* 348 (2): 119–28.

Partners In Health. 2002. *A DOTS-plus handbook guide to the community-based treatment of MDR TB.* Available online at the www.pih.org website.

UNAIDS (Joint United Nations Program on HIV/AIDS). 2006. *Report on the global AIDS epidemic.* Available online at the www.unaids.org website.

UNDP (United Nations Development Program). 2006. *Human development report 2006: Beyond scarcity: Power, poverty and the global water crisis.* Available online at the www.undp.org website.

Walton, David A., Paul E. Farmer, Wesler Lambert, F. Léandre, Serena P. Koenig, and Joia S. Mukherjee. 2004. Integrated HIV prevention and care strengthens primary health care: Lessons from rural Haiti. *Journal of Public Health Policy* 25 (2): 137–58.

WHO (World Health Organization). 2005. *Global polio eradication initiative annual report 2005.* Available online at the www.polioeradication.org website.

Zanmi Lasante. 2001. *Deklarasyon Kanj La/The Cange Declaration.* Available online at the www.pih.org website.

NOTES

1. These two forces are arguably responsible for more suffering, sickness, and early death than any other causes.

2. There are many examples of the connections between inequality and poor health. The United States, Canada, and most of Western Europe have similar levels of economic and social development. But the United States lags behind the rest of the developed world on most important health indicators. Much of this difference can be attributed to high levels of inequality in the United States. Some United States health measures are even surpassed by poor countries. **For example, life expectancy at birth in virtually the same in Cuba (77.6 years) as in the United States (77.5 years), even though per capita GDP is approximately 10 times higher in the United States (UNDP 2006).**

3. According to the most recent statistics from the Joint United Nations Program on HIV/AIDS (UNAIDS 2006), there were 38.6 million people living with HIV/AIDS (PLWHA) worldwide. Nearly two-thirds of all PLWHA (64 percent, or 24.5 million) live in sub-Saharan Africa alone. Ninety-nine percent of deaths from AIDS occurred outside North America and Western and Central Europe (UNAIDS 2006).

4. HIV is the leading cause of death among Black women between 25 and 34 years of age; HIV is among the four leading causes of death for Black women aged 25–54. Another dramatic sign of inequality is that 73 percent of all infants perinatally infected with HIV infections in the United States during 2005 were African-American. African-Americans in general make up 12.3 percent of the United States population but accounted for 50 percent of all new HIV/AIDS diagnoses and 43 percent of PLWHA in the United States (CDC 2006). See also Black AIDS Institute 2006.

5. For example, young women aged 15–24 in sub-Saharan Africa are infected at a ratio of 3:1 when compared to young men (UNAIDS 2006). Biology explains some of this difference; women carry a greater risk for infection than men with any single sexual exposure. But the concentration of HIV disease among women is also tightly linked to gender inequality and to cultural and sexual power dynamics (Farmer, Connors, and Simmons 2005).

6. The prescription to observe, judge, and act applies to a manner of engagement. PIH is not a faith-based organization; health-care workers and community members represent a variety of faith traditions, including no faith at all.

7. By any measure, Haiti is one of the poorest nations in the world. In 2006 Haiti ranked number 154 of 177 countries on the Human Development Index (UNDP 2006). Many of the roots of Haiti's current poverty lie in its unique colonial/anticolonial history. See James 1989 and Dubois 2004 for detailed discussions of the Haitian revolution and its consequences.

8. For the past twelve years, an annual forum on health and human rights has been held at Clinique Bon Sauveur in Cange. Many of the principles that guide Partners In Health's work are expressed in the "Cange Declaration," which was written and delivered by a group of HIV patients in August 2001 (*Zanmi Lasante* 2001).

9. There is a long history of physicians becoming directly involved in political struggle. Rudolf Virchow—considered the founder of social medicine—became a political

activist after connecting epidemic infectious disease to poverty and exclusion from democratic decision making. Salvador Allende was a public health physician before becoming the short-lived president of Chile in 1970. Che Guevara was also a physician by training and advocated widely for health care as a pillar of an equitable society. More recent movements, such as International Physicians for the Prevention of Nuclear War, Physicians for Social Responsibility, Physicians for Human Rights, and the International Campaign to Ban Landmines, have pushed health-care workers to the forefront of political debates.

10. This same dynamic is at work in the concept of "emerging infectious diseases." From the perspective of the poor, a disease like TB or HIV or even the ebola virus is not an emerging problem. These diseases have been constant, deadly companions for a long time.

11. *Zanmi Lasante* administers and maintains a series of hospitals and clinics throughout the Central Department of Haiti. ZL's services are staffed almost entirely by Haitian-trained workers: 3000 national staff supported by 5–6 foreign volunteers. Money and logistical support come from outside because the local economy is too poor—due almost entirely to the influence of outside forces—to sustain the cost of supplies, staff, building, and so on. What has been "sustainable" for ZL/PIH is the commitment to keep these projects going, even in times of political instability. This is in contrast to fee-for-service clinics and most charity hospitals in Haiti, which have been shut down by political violence and are less well used in general (Lyon and Farmer 2005).

12. Partners In Health has published widely on the range of programs and services in Haiti and in the other places where we work. Links to most publications can be found at the http://www.pih.org website.

13. Virchow had this to say in the mid-1800s: "Artificial epidemics . . . are attributes of society, products of a false culture or of a culture that is not available to all classes. These are indicators of defects produced by political and social organization, and therefore affect predominantly those classes that do not participate in the advantages of the culture" (in Anderson, Smith, and Sidel 2005).

14. He is also quoted as saying "[P]olitics is nothing more than medicine on a grand scale," suggesting that the two fields of human endeavor are completely inseparable.

22

Living in Harmony
with the Earth and with Each Other

John Last

Two challenges tower above all others confronting us. Putting an end to violent armed conflicts that kill and maim millions is the lesser; the accelerating crisis of global climate change is the greater of the two. Unless we control both, the future for humanity is bleak.

Health professionals have the same self-interest and obligation as other people to safeguard the life-supporting ecosystems that sustain us. Moreover, stressed ecosystems lead to conflict over shrinking resources (Homer-Dixon and Percival 1996). If humans are to survive, we must learn how to live in harmony with our ecosystem and with each other, and we must stop trying to conquer or subdue one another and the world around us. Health professionals also have special skills to help others learn how to do this.

Many changes in my lifetime of 80 years have improved the human condition: reduced infant mortality; increased life expectancy; control of many previously fatal diseases; breathtaking progress in medical and other technologies; reduction of financial barriers between sick people and the care they need; a more gender-balanced, culturally diversified medical profession, rather than one dominated by white men in suits. But other changes are ominous portents. Profligate misuse of nonrenewable resources; worldwide chemical pollution; widening gaps between rich and poor; escalating species extinction; savage, costly, and unnecessary wars; and climate change do great harm (Last 1997). In the twentieth century, wars killed over 100 million and maimed many times that number (70–80 percent of whom were noncombatants) drained wealth and talent, and did terrible environmental damage (Chapter 5). Climate change, however, is the gravest danger facing us and other living things. Signs of planetary stress and climate-related risks to health are obvious everywhere (McMichael, Woodruff, and Hales 2006). These are humanmade, and everyone must help to undo the harm we have done to the Earth, to each other, and to future generations.

Multiple interconnected forces are responsible, and we may have only a few decades to stop the headlong rush toward what may be an irreversible tipping point that will change our world forever (Lovelock 2006). The worrying changes are physical, biological, demographic, social, cultural, behavioral, economic, and political. All interact and reinforce each other in many complex ways.

Physical changes in the atmosphere include the increasing burden of carbon dioxide that causes climate change (global warming), acid rain that kills our lakes, smog that rots our lungs, and contamination with chlorofluorocarbons (CFCs) that destroys the stratospheric ozone layer shielding the biosphere from lethal ultraviolet radiation. Of these the rising burden of atmospheric carbon dioxide is the gravest danger. It comes from combusted carbon-based fossil fuels that we use to generate electricity; in airplanes and cars; for cooking, heating, and cooling; to power televisions and computers; and to make and drive our war machines. We are fouling and destroying our habitat with our addiction to fossil fuels (Gore 2006). Our economy, our political systems, and our entire way of life are so dependent on fossil fuels that *addiction* is the only apt word. Our civilization risks perishing just like others that relied on unsustainable customs and policies (Wright 2004).

Biological changes include species extinctions, reduced biodiversity, and the emergence, since 1970, of dangerous new pathogens: HIV (the virus that causes AIDS) and about thirty other new infectious agents, such as those responsible for Ebola-Marburg disease, viral hemorrhagic fevers, Legionnaires' disease, hantavirus pulmonary syndrome, severe acute respiratory syndrome (SARS), transmissible spongiform encephalopathy (TSE), Lyme disease, and West Nile virus. Nearly all are potentially lethal and some are highly contagious. By mid-2006, HIV/AIDS had infected 42 million people and killed over 12 million since it was identified in the early 1980s (UNAIDS 2006). New and emergent infections have various origins. The HIV/AIDS pandemic is probably the result of a recent mutation of the causal retrovirus and its "species jump" from forest monkeys to humans in equatorial Africa. Several other diseases have arisen because humans have disrupted previously balanced ecosystems or because pathogens or vectors have invaded a new ecological niche.

The pressure of people and their consumption habits on fragile ecosystems is exceeding sustainable limits. Population numbers and distribution, social structure, and culture have been transformed. The population almost quadrupled—from 1.7 billion in 1901 to 6.5 billion in 2001. There has been unprecedented migration from rural to urban areas and from one country to another far from the migrants' birthplace and family traditions, as people are pushed by oppression and conflict and pulled by powerful economic forces. Wars can be both cause and consequence of these massive population shifts. The proportion of people living in cities rose from less than one in twenty in 1901 to about one in two by 2001. Tens of millions of new city dwellers live in abject squalor in slums and shanty towns in low- and middle-income countries. Over 20 million are refugees or internally displaced persons, who have been forced out of homes and habitat by conflict, ethnic cleansing, and even genocide. The age structure of populations in industrial countries has changed from predominantly "young" (high proportions of infants and children) to "old" (high proportions of middle-aged and elderly people, low proportions of children). Large extended multigeneration families that made their own entertainment have been replaced by small nuclear families that rely on mass entertainment—mass "culture" that undermines individual thought. We are bombarded by a confusing jangle of signals from TV and the Internet that ought to bring us all together in a global village but more often divide generations and nations. Cohesive family ties have fragmented; traditional faiths and loyalties have eroded. We rapidly tire of our political leaders, disillusioned by their failure to correct the discontents of our daily lives. The consequences include political volatility and unstable, frequently changing governments with different national and international policies, plans, and priorities, when we urgently need visionary leadership and long-range planning with a time horizon of at least several decades. Instead we seek scapegoats and are easily seduced by demagogues with empty promises, who distract the people by declaring "wars"—war on crime, war on drugs, war on poverty, war on terror, war on nations or ethnic groups with fabricated, fomented hostility and imaginary aggressive designs against us. Rarely our leaders get the priorities right and declare war on diseases, though seldom on conditions that kill and disable the largest numbers; cystic fibrosis and muscular dystrophy generate greater enthusiasm and more charitable donations from well-meaning but ill-informed benefactors than infant diarrhea. Until the Bill and Melinda Gates Foundation got involved, malaria, tuberculosis, and HIV/AIDS largely failed to attract the needed attention, expertise, and funding.

THE PUBLIC HEALTH RESPONSE

All these scourges confront humankind, in what may be the most complex and difficult cluster of social and public health problems of any time in human history. Reflecting on the social history of public health, I identified five essential elements that must be present for the successful control of every public health problem (Last 1991). We must

- Recognize that the problem exists
- Understand what causes it
- Be able to control the cause
- Believe it is important to control the cause
- Have the political will to do what is required

In the late nineteenth century, this combination of essential requirements produced the sanitary revolution. By the 1970s they were being deployed with some success to control the public health problems of tobacco smoking, impaired driving, child abuse, domestic violence, and occupational cancers such as those caused by exposure to asbestos.

Well-informed people agree that the problems associated with climate change and stressed ecosystems are real and dangerous, and many have some insight into what is causing them. Some can identify at least some aspects of the necessary corrective action. Many believe that climate change matters, perhaps more than any other problem we face. A few are willing to act, but often only in puny, almost irrelevant ways. What is lacking is the political will to tackle these problems at the societal level. At best, ruling parties—even in the most supportive nations—pay lip service but do little or nothing. The ruling parties in nearly all democracies and in all totalitarian states deny reality and take no meaningful action.

How and where can health workers intervene to break the vicious circles in which we seem to be trapped? We have the advantage that most people care about their health and want to preserve and protect it, so there is some goodwill toward health professionals, and we are trusted. When we mobilize, organize, and proselytize, we attract a following. And the efforts of organized health professionals are occasionally rewarded with the Nobel Peace Prize or similar honors.

We can start interventions with ourselves, our families, and our friends and neighbors. Because so many people care about their health, they ask health professionals for advice about other matters besides disease. Leading by example, we have a responsibility to educate everyone with whom we have professional and social contact. Actions we can encourage everyone to take to minimize climate change include basic dos and don'ts. Do walk or cycle, don't drive gas-guzzling cars; do invest in insulation to enhance efficient energy use for heating and cooling homes and workplaces; do eat locally grown food, don't eat processed junk food; do hang the washing out of doors in the breeze, don't use a clothes dryer; do turn off appliances when not in use, don't overheat homes and offices in winter, don't keep the air conditioning on all summer long. Always dispose of hazardous medical waste safely and responsibly. We must advocate with our political leaders for use of renewable energy sources, for energy saving and conservation, and for peaceful resolution of conflicts with adversaries, and we must collaborate in international activities aimed at these goals. Wars and preparation for war consume enormous quantities of nonrenewable fossil fuel and of financial and human resources that are desperately needed to educate children and prevent and treat disease, notably in Africa and South Asia (Lewis 2005). We must reject politicians whose policies are not oriented to sustainability and those who distract us with unnecessary wars and bribe us with short-sighted and irresponsible tax cuts.

These actions, multiplied throughout society, can help to reduce the impact of climate change, but they won't stop it. It is too late for that. Our immediate task is to prepare for inevitable changes and take all necessary actions to adapt to them. Much of what we can expect is predictable. Appropriate action by health professionals follows logically and is among the most crucial aspects of adaptation to the climate change that is happening now and will increase over the next few decades.

We know there will be more frequent, more severe extreme weather events such as heat waves, hurricanes, floods, and droughts. Heat waves—especially those associated with smog—kill isolated, frail, debilitated, and old people; premature and low-birth-weight infants; and poor and homeless people. The European heat wave of July 2003 caused the premature deaths of an estimated 35,000 people (International Federation of Red Cross–Red Crescent Societies 2005). Humid, wet weather increases the risk of vector-borne and water-borne diseases, causes an upsurge of malaria in vulnerable regions, and increases the risk of fecal–oral transmission of diarrheal diseases. Malaria kills 2 million annually, half of them children. Diarrhea kills another 2 million, mostly infants and children. Floods and hurricanes incapacitate and often destroy infrastructure and obliterate habitat, even entire human settlements. Floods disable sewage treatment plants and pollute water supplies. Both floods and droughts destroy food crops and endanger food supplies for large numbers of people. Rising sea levels and desertification devastate grain-growing regions and cause habitat loss and displacement of people, who become environmental refugees. The United Nations High Commissioner for

Refugees estimated in 2006 that there will be a tenfold increase in environmental refugees from 5 million in 2005 to 50 million by 2010 (UNHCR 2006). Movement on that scale and at that speed is a huge public health problem as well as a major logistic, security, and social problem. The cost of climate-related disasters is staggering. In the autumn of 2005, the US Congressional Research Services made a preliminary estimate that hurricanes Katrina and Rita would cost at least $65 billion in restoration and repair. The insurance industry's estimate was about double this, but it will be many years before all the claims are settled. The long-term human costs include regional depopulation: as several hundred thousand former citizens may never return because their homes and sources of livelihood are gone (Congressional Research Services 2005). They have become internally displaced persons—perhaps the first of many in the United States, because further massive storms are certain to occur.

The attenuated stratospheric ozone layer allows more harmful biologically active ultraviolet radiation to penetrate into the biosphere, where it increases the incidence of malignant melanoma, other skin cancer, and cataracts. Advisory messages about sun avoidance and warnings about high ultraviolet radiation have become routine in spring and summer weather forecasts. More ominously, increased UV solar radiation kills delicate small and single-cell organisms at the base of aquatic food chains—including the phytoplankton that are a vital component of the carbon cycle because they absorb large quantities of atmospheric carbon dioxide. Moreover, rising carbon dioxide levels lead to higher concentration of carbonic acid in seawater, and this kills oceanic phytoplankton, further impairing the carbon sink.

Actions to preserve and protect the environment can be lifesaving for people in vulnerable human settlements. The loss of life and homes in New Orleans from hurricane Katrina in 2005 would have been lower if wetlands that once acted as a sponge to soak up the impact of tidal surges had not been drained for housing and industrial development. Preserving, protecting, and (where possible) restoring wetlands and marshes is intelligent environmental planning and sound public policy. This sort of environmental protection may aggravate other health risks—for instance, by increasing mosquito breeding sites and thus requiring more pesticides for control—but natural predators such as fish, and other human protective measures such as the use of bednets and screened windows, can offset this. To achieve a balanced ecosystem where humans, other living species, and natural environments coexist in harmony is sound public policy and holistic public health practice.

Essential adaptive and reactive strategies by public health agencies and by primary health-care workers can be briefly stated. The public health services must perform systematic monitoring, surveillance, and analysis of all aspects of the health situation. Public health nurses can identify, register, and (when necessary) evacuate the most vulnerable to safer places when weather-related emergencies occur. After the Chicago heat wave in 1995, which killed over 700 mostly isolated, frail elderly people in low-lying rental housing, the city public health authorities created a register of similarly vulnerable people. In subsequent Chicago heat waves there have been no deaths, because vulnerable people were evacuated to air-conditioned shopping malls and similar places of refuge. Family physicians can advise patients and parents about sun exposure, especially about protecting infants and small children from excessive exposure to ultraviolet radiation. Environmental monitoring includes air quality assessment; routine surveys of the distribution and abundance of insect vectors; epidemiologic surveillance of communicable and exotic disease outbreaks and identification of pathogens; and monitoring of the occurrence of actinic cancer, cataract, and heat-related illness. Compiling a registry of vulnerable individuals (the frail elderly, infants, and so on) and the preparation and dissemination of advisory messages about UV radiation levels, sun avoidance, and routine precautions such as immunizations are other important functions. Disaster planning and preparation for adverse health impacts of extreme weather events are high priorities. Other essentials include food and nutrition policies, delineating health research policies and priorities, and standard setting—for example, standards for protective clothing.

The roles and responsibilities of primary health-care workers include vigilance and notification of exotic disease outbreaks (sentinel surveillance); advising on adaptation and helping to soften the impacts of social and cultural change; anticipating, preventing, and treating the adverse effects of extreme weather (such as heat waves, floods, and hurricanes); advising patients about sun avoidance and smog alerts; and participating in planning for emergency preparedness.

Most political leaders are in denial and avoid discussing the complex cluster of problems that accompany and cause global changes. Health professionals should use every opportunity to advocate and to remind political leaders that they must consider health problems in the context of everything else happening in the world. When opportunities arise, health professionals who occupy prominent positions in society can engage in advocacy in other forums. Such advocacy should include reminding everyone of the complexity and interconnectedness of political, economic, social, and cultural determinants with health problems, including those associated with armed conflicts and those due to climate change.

Aboriginal peoples possessed rich empirical wisdom about ways to live in harmony with their ecosystem, but since European colonization, much of this has been lost. Before it is too late, the colonizers must learn from those they subjugated what remains of this rich heritage. It is a tragic irony that many aboriginal people have been pushed to the margins of the most fragile environments in what were once their broad domains, their ancient wisdom suppressed by their conquerors and lost by the decimation of their people via imported diseases, smallpox, measles, and tuberculosis. Reparations for this injustice are long overdue.

REFERENCES

Congressional Research Services. 2005. *The costs of Hurricanes Katrina and Rita*. Reports to Congress. Available online at the www.cbo.gov website.

Gore, A. 2006. *An inconvenient truth*. New York: Rodale Press.

Homer-Dixon, T. F., and V. Percival. 1996. *Environmental scarcity and violent conflict: Briefing book*. Washington, DC: American Association for the Advancement of Science; Toronto: University of Toronto.

International Federation of Red Cross–Red Crescent Societies. 2005. *World disasters report*. Available online at the www.ifrc.org website.

Last, J. M. 1991. The future of public health. *Japanese Journal of Public Health* 38 (10): 58–93. Also published in Last 1997.

———. 1997. Human health in a changing world. In *Public health and human ecology*, 2nd ed., 395–425. New York: McGraw-Hill.

Lewis, S. 2005. *Race against time* (2005 Massey Lectures). Toronto: House of Anansi Press.

Lovelock, J. 2006. *The revenge of Gaia*. London: Allen Lane, Penguin.

McMichael, A. J., R. E. Woodruff, S. Hales. 2006. Climate change and human health: Present and future risks. *The Lancet* 367: 859–69.

UNAIDS. 2006. HIV/AIDS statistics. In *10th Annual Report of the United Nations Joint Program on HIV/AIDS*. Available online at the www.unaids.org website.

UNHCR (United Nations High Commissioner for Refugees). 2005. Asylum levels and trends in industrialized countries. Available online at the www.unhcr.org website.

Wright, R. 2004. *A short history of progress*. Toronto: House of Anansi Press.

PART VIII

Special Topics

23

A Role for Emergency Humanitarian Aid Organizations in Peace?

Ann Duggan

In violent conflict situations, the role of emergency humanitarian relief organizations is the provision of aid to save lives, alleviate suffering, and maintain human dignity. Engaging in peacemaking or peacebuilding activities is *not* considered to be the responsibility of those providing humanitarian assistance.

The concept of humanitarian aid was first articulated in 1859 by Henri Dunant, who organized emergency services for the victims he witnessed in the Battle of Solferino in northern Italy. Dunant later went on to found the Red Cross movement and to develop the Geneva Conventions that create the foundation of international humanitarian law. Within the midst of conflict, the Geneva Conventions and their additional protocols establish the "rules of war" and the responsibilities of persons involved in it, including humanitarian relief workers. This includes the right of impartial and humanitarian relief organizations to undertake humanitarian initiatives, while further protocols address neutrality and independence. Impartiality means the provision of aid to those who are in the most need, regardless of affiliation; neutrality means taking no side in the conflict either directly or indirectly; and independence means the ability to intervene on the basis only of humanitarian needs without any other consideration, including political influence.

In transforming these operational principles into action, emergency relief nongovernmental organizations (NGOs) provide assistance to war-affected persons based on a rapid assessment of critical life-saving needs and priorities. These needs and priorities include water (safe drinking water plus water for cooking and bathing), food (general rations and therapeutic feeding of the malnourished), sanitation (latrines, waste disposal, and vector control), shelter, curative medical care (hospitals and clinics), and preventive health care (such as vaccinations, prenatal care, family planning, and health education). They focus on those who are suffering, or are likely to suffer, the greatest morbidity and mortality from a lack of these essentials (such as children or the elderly). It is hoped that providing these basics will keep people alive until the violent conflict is over and peace has returned. NGOs are funded both privately and by public institutions, most commonly governments. It is critical that in accepting funding, NGOs ensure that receiving it does not carry conditions that would affect their neutrality, impartiality, or independence. Likewise, it is important that all relief actors respect these operational principles in order to maintain their protection under the Geneva Conventions.

SO WHAT ABOUT PEACE?

None of the well-known emergency aid organizations (such as the International Committee of the Red Cross (ICRC), Médecins San Frontières (MSF), the International Rescue Committee (IRC), Oxfam, Save the Children, and CARE) lists peace as an aim of its organization on its website. This is understandable, because it is aid agencies' goal to keep people alive until the war has ended, not to end the war itself. Although the vast majority of aid workers would acknowledge that the only true solution to the crises they face would be an end to the conflict, most would consider peace activities as distinct from the direct provision of aid with which they are entrusted. In the midst of a humanitarian emergency, peacemaking or peacebuilding activities move action into a political arena and could bring a relief agency's neutrality and impartiality into question, risking its protection under the Geneva Conventions and its ability to carry out relief efforts. Unfortunately, violence against aid workers is no longer uncommon, as has been demonstrated tragically by killings in the last few years in Chechnya, Afghanistan, and Iraq. Aid agencies being seen to be taking sides or assigning blame can compromise their security, and hence their ability to carry out their programs to help the most vulnerable.

Yet despite these reservations, relief organizations can, and do, impact peace in both positive and detrimental ways.

PERPETUATING AND WORSENING CONFLICT

Although emergency relief organizations working in violent conflict do not have peace in itself as a goal, they should all at least strive not to exacerbate or prolong the conflict in which they are working. It is the aim of most relief NGOs to be nonpolitical, but all action or inaction has political nuances that can affect the conflict directly and indirectly. Whether acknowledged or not, real or perceived, and no matter what is provided to whom, by whom, where, and how, all can have unintended political implications. Here are some ways in which aid organizations can inadvertently exacerbate conflict:

Diversion of Aid

In their desire to help as many people as possible as quickly as possible, many relief NGOs and individual aid workers may be blinded to the fact that their aid can be abused and hence may perpetuate the conflict. This may happen directly, through warring parties demanding a percentage of aid brought to an area, or indirectly, by belligerents looting warehouses, shipments, or trucks carrying supplies.

Manipulation of the Vulnerable

In Sudan, Ethiopia, and a number of other countries, conflicting parties have in the past purposefully created situations of hardship in order to attract aid into the area. Activities such as planned starvation, brought about by enclaving people and burning fields, create famine that the perpetrators know will draw a response from aid agencies, which can then be diverted. MSF was expelled from Ethiopia in 1985 for speaking out against the government's involvement in forced displacement of civilians and diversion of food aid that resulted in the starvation of tens of thousands of people.

Provision of aid can also create a potential opportunity to attack the civilian population. In Sudan in the 1990s, aid distribution sites, as well as locations of hospitals and clinics, drew large collections of civilians that too often attracted overhead bombings.

Distribution of Aid

Utilizing local community grassroots infrastructure to determine the most vulnerable in need of aid is a wonderful concept. However, in war situations, this system applied alone can unfortunately be abused and manipulated. Not all communities are equitable, and persons in power may divert aid to their friends, family, or political group. This became a dilemma in Zaire [now Democratic Republic of Congo (DRC)] in 1994, because the aid that was provided helped reestablish insurgents in the camps, reinforcing the old power hierarchy and enabling persons to continue to carry out acts of violence both within and outside the camps.

Just as in grassroots systems, staff put in charge of distributions, especially the distribution of food, have considerable power and are sometimes put under great pressure. Pressure exerted by family, community, security forces, and others may put the staff at great risk. Alternatively, staff members can potentially exploit their power in an unfair or abusive way, such as the sexual abuse documented in West Africa (UNHCR/Save the Children-UK 2001).

The struggle to empower and not disempower is highly complex. Because distributed relief items are of high value, they can make the recipients vulnerable to attack. In the Rwandan refugee camps in Zaire in 1995, food distributions were given to the woman of the house based on the theory that the food would thereby be more equitably distributed in the family. What was not foreseen was that this approach placed the women in a very precarious position. It made them vulnerable to abuse by husbands who felt emasculated, made them targets of thugs as they brought home their rations, and exposed them to late-night looters because it was general knowledge when provisions were distributed.

Mary Anderson (2006) and her colleagues in the "Do No Harm Project" have highlighted a multitude of other ways in which aid agencies can impact the conflict in which they work. From the staff they hire, to where they geographically establish services, from being influenced by the politics of their donors, to disrupting local economies, and allowing governments to avoid their responsibilities, provision of aid has complex repercussions that must be evaluated.

CONTRIBUTING TO PEACE

Even though peace is not their primary objective, emergency relief NGOs can have a significant effect on it, both directly and indirectly, whether or not they openly acknowledge their impact.

First, their mere presence as an international witness can provide protection to civilians. Warring parties, knowing that aid organizations are in the area, often will not attack for fear of their activities becoming known to the outside world and the possible repercussions. When relief NGOs are present during violent conflicts, they are able to bear witness to what has happened, recording and documenting, while at the same time doing their best to mitigate the impact of the violence. It is likely that the worst massacres in history are those we have no knowledge of because there were no surviving witnesses.

In the case where relief NGOs believe they may reduce or stop the violent conflict by advocating for the population, they can do this by speaking out publicly with hard facts about what they have witnessed. In an attempt to effect change, Médecins San Frontières has published numerous articles and books documenting what its members have witnessed around the globe. Recent examples include publishing the stories of violence-affected persons in Colombia; disseminating nutritional and mortality data for Katanga, DRC; and documenting the sexual abuse occurring in Darfur, Sudan (MSF 2006). Alternatively, when aid organizations feel their security or activities might be compromised by their directly speaking out, they can provide information to other organizations, such as the UN, which can then use this information on behalf of the populations affected.

Relief NGOs also help affect peace by serving as values models for the people they come in contact with. Humanitarian NGOs model peaceful existence throughout their activities, such as not allowing arms in hospitals, negotiating respect for hospitals and their workers, not using armed guards, not paying for protection, and not paying bribes. Ideally, aid organizations can demonstrate an alternative sort of existence by treating everyone with dignity and respect, regardless of affiliation, rather than showing biased, preferential treatment.

Medical aid NGOs are occasionally able to use health reasons to achieve temporary ceasefires; this can include vaccination programs (such as implementation of the World Health Organization's polio eradication campaign) or arrangements for the transport of wounded to receive hospital care. It is hoped that during these windows of calm, major actors in the violent conflict will experience the advantages of peace and advocate for it to continue.

In my experience, aid workers contribute to peace the most in providing people with hope. To be involved in a violent conflict situation is physically and emotional damaging for everyone. If left alone in suffering, it would be normal for people to give up hope of improvement and spiral into depression and inaction. Even if you cannot stop the war, to be present with the victims during the violence and to bear witness to their suffering can provide them with hope. This hope, built upon the knowledge that people outside of their situation know what is happening and are working in their best interest, empowers people to continue their efforts for a better future.

THE DILEMMA OF AID AT ALL

The humanitarian impulse to come to the assistance of people affected by war is one of the noblest human traits. Translating this impulse into action can lead to wonderful things, but if not done with knowledge and care, it can have the opposite effect of worsening violence at many levels. There are those who argue that any aid worsens a conflict. They maintain that aid postpones the end of the confrontation by allowing people to survive to continue the battle and enables governments to divert all of their resources into fighting. However, if it is done well with eyes wide open, aid can be a tool for peaceful transformation, empowering people to work toward a peaceful future.

Although the Geneva Conventions and their associated protocols do not allow for relief organizations to have peace as a goal, for war-affected people the mere existence of relief agencies attests to an existence other than war. The ideal of humanitarian aid being an agent for peace has been honored by the Nobel Peace Prize, which was awarded to Henri Dunant (founder of the Red Cross) in 1901, to the Red Cross in 1917, 1944, and 1963, and to Médecins San Frontières in 1999.

ACKNOWLEGMENT

Thank you to Eleanor Fitzpatrick, Luc Zandvliet, and Jane Little for their editorial input.

REFERENCES

Anderson, Mary. 2006. *Do No Harm Project*. Collaborative Learning Projects and the Collaborative for Development Action.

Bouchet-Saulnier, Francoise. 2002. *The practical guide to humanitarian law*. Lanham, MD: Rowman & Littlefield Publishers.

Human Rights Watch. 1999. *Famine in Sudan 1998, the human rights causes*. Available online at the www.hrw.org website.

Médecins San Frontières. All are available online at the www.msf.org website.
  a. *Living in fear: Colombia's cycle of violence*. 2006.
  b. *Food, nutrition and mortality situation of IDPs in Katanga, DRC*. 2006.
  c. *Crushing burden of rape: Sexual violence in Darfur, Sudan*. 2005.

Office of the United Nations High Commissioner for Refugees. 2006. *Humanitarian law*. Available online at the www.ohchr.org website.

UNHCR (United Nations High Commissioner for Refugees) and Save the Children-UK. 2001. *Note for implementing and operational partners on sexual violence and exploitation: The experience of refugee children in Guinea, Liberia and Sierra Leone*. Available online at the www.unhcr.org website.

24

Students and Peace through Health: Education, Projects, and Theory

Caecilie Buhmann and *Andrew D. Pinto*

A s Peace through Health (PtH) has developed as a field, students have played an important role in developing theories, interpreting them in the classroom and field, and contributing to research, education, and projects. This chapter offers an overview of student involvement in PtH, the challenges that may be encountered, and the rationale for increased engagement of students based on their special characteristics.

WHAT DRAWS STUDENTS TO PTH?

Students in both the humanities and the health sciences have found PtH to be applicable to their studies, and many call for more teaching in this area. Students are often attracted to the activist nature of PtH and to its unique way of addressing real-world problems from a medical perspective. Fundamentally, PtH goes beyond the traditional Western biomedical model of health (Arya 2006; MacQueen and Santa Barbara 2000). It challenges students to contemplate broader societal structures and determinants of health, such as political empowerment, structural violence, and human rights. These are often given scant attention in the traditional health science curriculum. Hence PtH appeals to a certain subgroup of students who are aware of politically motivated violence locally and globally, feel connected to such issues, and hope to take action on them.

STUDENTS AND PTH EDUCATION

Universities have been important in introducing students to the theory and practice of PtH. In addition to attending courses, students have been active participants by creating content, delivering lectures, acting as teaching assistants, and implementing elective programs. McMaster University in

Canada has played an especially important role through organizing two key conferences on PtH, in 2001 and 2005 (Neufeld and Yusuf 2004), and a number of faculty have mentored students locally and internationally.

Two undergraduate courses in PtH have been implemented in Canada, at McMaster University and the University of Waterloo. Their focus has been on addressing actions that health professionals can take to minimize the impact of war and actively promote peace (Arya 2004, 259; McMaster University 2006). In addition, an online PtH course has been designed by eleven European medical organizations and teaching institutions (Medical Peace Work 2006). Also the World Health Organization has organized a number of courses on Health as a Bridge for Peace and conflict resolution. However, these have mostly been aimed at field workers and few students have joined them over the years.

Education related to PtH also touches on bioethics, an area of study considered mandatory at most medical schools. However, students may find it challenging to consider the right thing to do when faced with state-sponsored violence and the political goals of war. Drawing on the existing literature of health and human rights and public health ethics, students in PtH may find it helpful to prioritize values of solidarity, social justice, and neutrality, alongside health promotion, disease prevention, and doing no harm (Santa Barbara 2005).

A discipline that is intimately linked to PtH education is the field of global health, where students have been actively calling for enhanced teaching for more than a decade (Bateman et al. 2001; Buhmann 2005). Students have been the crucial drivers behind the implementation of global health courses in Denmark, the United Kingdom, Ireland, Finland, and the Netherlands, as well as in the United States and Canada. These efforts have been fueled by medical students' desire to ensure that they are taught about issues relevant to the health of people in a globalized world.

Several challenges complicate bringing PtH into the "traditional" medical curriculum, whether in the form of electives or lectures. PtH exposes students to new concepts, such as peace, violence, and conflict resolution, and to new roles, such as being an advocate for peace. Because PtH is seen by many as being "political," students may question their ability to be "neutral" or "nonpartisan" while practicing PtH.

THE ROLE OF STUDENTS IN PROJECTS

Experiences in the classroom have inspired several students to get directly involved with PtH and even alter their career path. Broadly, student efforts can be divided into research projects and advocacy efforts, though the two areas often overlap. Students frequently use course research projects, elective opportunities, and travel grants to pursue such experiences overseas.

Within *research,* students have built on coursework to provide new insight into the theoretical basis of the discipline, such as devising strategies for evaluating PtH work. Students have also carried out studies, presented at conferences, and authored papers on PtH theory and practice (Buhmann 2005, Pinto 2003). Students have combined research and advocacy on the topic of small arms/light weapons (SALW). In Uganda, a collaborative initiative examined the impact of SALW on the health of the population (Pinto, Olupot-Olupot, and Neufeld 2006). In El Salvador, students have been involved in similar research, including prospective data collection, and in direct advocacy to the government (Paniagua et al. 2005).

Advocacy work has included educational initiatives, organizing public protests, and lobbying governments directly. Many projects discussed below were initiated and organized solely by students, and others have had the support of academic institutions and civil society organizations. Students have also helped plan large events, such as international conferences, and they constitute a large proportion of peace and health networks.

Students have helped organize workshops on PtH in organizations such as IPPNW, the International Federation of Medical Student Associations (IFMSA), and Physicians for Human Rights (PHR) (Buhmann 2007). "Peer education" has been an important component of advocacy efforts, where students are empowered by sharing knowledge and can create a space for honest dialogue on contentious issues. For example, the Nuclear Weapons Inheritance Project (NWIP) uses interactive training and dialogues with university students to increase awareness and the sense of relevance of disarmament among students (NWIP 2004). Human rights training by Physicians for Human Rights (PHR) and workshops on refugee health in Pakistan and Palestine (NWIP 2004; Buhmann 2007; IPPNW 2006) are two other examples of this form of advocacy.

The Refugee Camp Project (ReCap) combines work in a refugee camp in Palestine with training on refugee health (WMA 2003). It introduces students to these issues on a practical level, while building solidarity networks. "Peace Test" is an international project undertaken since 2000. It represents a partnership between numerous IPPNW and IFMSA student sections and the University of Texas, where students distribute questionnaires addressing intolerance and conflict resolution skills of high school students and discuss the results with the participants in nonconfrontational dialogues (Peace Test 2005).

In Canada, students have brought the concepts of PtH to high schools by organizing interactive presentations in several cities. The goal was to inspire youth to get involved and be aware, and the project was developed in collaboration with organizations such as War Child Canada and Médecins Sans Frontières (MSF). Health science students have also been involved with several advocacy campaigns, such as protesting the 2003 attack on Iraq (Brunham, Lee, and Pinto 2003; Lee 2003; Sibbald 2003) and speaking out against North American missile defense plans (Sibbald 2001) and in support of banning landmines.

Challenges include limited resources, time, and experience; the fluctuating schedules of students; and the rapid turnover of student leadership. However, small-scale projects that are handed over to new students, and that are tied to existing institutions and structures, can have a meaningful impact on PtH issues.

INCREASING STUDENT INVOLVEMENT

Several characteristics unique to students make them an important part of the PtH movement. They are often the most enthusiastic members of an organization, bringing energy and optimism to discussions and meetings. Students often belong to international networks, such as IFMSA and the student wings of organizations like PHR and IPPNW. They bring new perspectives to translating theory into practice, acting as a source for innovation, and may bring academia's questioning attitude to such work. Students are often able to tie their activism to their studies, particularly in settings with more flexible schedules and with bursaries and scholarships available for overseas work. For all of these reasons, students should be integrated into any PtH project, treated as full partners, and mentored in their efforts.

CONCLUSION

Students will continue to play an important role in the development of PtH and the application of its theories in the field. This discipline appeals to students as a dynamic and unique field that offers a way to combine academic work with activism. Students bring enthusiasm, international networks, and new perspectives to such work, and PtH should be open to student input and involvement with each new initiative.

REFERENCES

Arya, N. 2004. Peace through Health II: A framework for medical student education. *Medicine Conflict and Survival* 20 (3): 258–62.

———. 2006. The end of biomilitary realism? Rethinking biomedicine and international security. *Medicine, Conflict and Survival* 22 (3): 220–9.

Bateman, C., T. Baker, E. Hoornenborg, and U. Ericsson. 2001. Bringing global issues to medical teaching. *The Lancet* 358 (9292): 1539–42.

Brunham, L., P. Lee, and A. Pinto. 2003. Medical students not mum on Iraq. *Canadian Medical Association Journal* 169:541.

Buhmann, C. B. 2005. The role of health professionals in preventing and mediating conflict. *Medicine, Conflict and Survival* 21 (4): 299–311.

———. 2007. The Nuclear Weapons Inheritance Project: Student-to-student dialogues and interactive peer education in disarmament activism. *Medicine, Conflict and Survival* 23 (2): 92–102.

Gutlove, Paula, and Gordon Thompson, eds. 2003. *Psychosocial healing: A guide for practitioners.* IRSS. Available online at the www.irss-usa.org website.

IMCC Denmark, Final Report ITCMS, IMCC Denmark, 2002.

IPPNW, ReCap—The Refugee Camp Project, IPPNW 2006. Available online at www .ippnw-students.org/ReCap/ReCap.html accessed 11/2-2008.

Lee, P. P. S. 2003. An open letter from concerned medical students on Iraq. *Canadian Medical Association Journal* 168: 1115.

MacQueen, G., and J. Santa Barbara. 2000. *British Medical Journal* 321 (7256): 293–6.

McMaster University. 2006. Peace through Health Course. Available online at the www .humanities.mcmaster.ca website.

Medical Peace Work. 2006. Available online at the www.medicalpeacework.org website.

Neufeld, V., and S. Yusuf. 2004. The McMaster-*Lancet* health and peace conferences. *The Lancet* 364 (9431): 311–2.

NWIP. 2004. Activity report: The Nuclear Weapons Inheritance Project 2001–2004. Available online at the www.ippnw-students.org website.

Paniagua, I., E. Crespin, A. Guardado, and A. Mauricio. 2005. Wounds caused by firearms in El Salvador, 2003–2004: Epidemiological issues. *Medicine, Conflict and Survival* 21 (3): 191–8.

Peace Test. 2005. Available online at the www.peacetest.lsv.fi website.

Pinto, A. D., P. Olupot-Olupot, and V. Neufeld. 2006. Health implications of small arms and light weapons in eastern Uganda. *Medicine, Conflict and Survival* 22 (3): 207–19.

Pinto, A. D. 2003. Peace through Health. *University of Toronto Medical Journal* 80: 158–60.

Rodriguez-Garcia, R., J. Xavier Macinko, F. Solorzano, and M. Schlesser. 2001. How can health serve as a bridge for peace? CERTI. Available online at http://www.certi.org/publications/policy/2001-executive.pdf accessed 11/2-2008.

Santa Barbara, J. 2005. Working for peace through health—ethical values and principles. *Croatian Medical Journal* 46 (6): 1007–9.

Sibbald, B. 2003. MD group criticizes possible US attack on Iraq. *Canadian Medical Association Journal* 168:470.

Sibbald, B. 2001. Canadian MDs oppose US missile shield plan. *Canadian Medical Association Journal* 164: 1477.

WHO. 2006. Health as a Bridge for Peace—Training. Available online at the www.who
.int website.

WMA. 2003. Press release IFMSA http://www.wma.net/e/press/newsbriefs_2003_1.htm.
IFMSA (International Federation of Medical Students Association), International
training on refugees' health. Available online at the www.wma.net website.

25

Technology and Activism

Alex Rosen and *Tarek Loubani*

Peace through Health work involves dissemination of information, working with geographically dispersed groups, and work in dangerous areas. Modern technology offers activists and organizations new ways of coordinating projects, mobilizing members, and communicating with the public. Free and open-source software, a movement to share software and information, has also helped equalize use between rich and poor computer users. The movement has succeeded in giving the poorest users tools and voices equal to those of the largest companies. The advantages of free software for the less privileged should encourage socially aware groups and individuals to use it and participate in its development. Additionally, using modern means of communication such as Internet telephone calls and video conferencing can greatly reduce the need for face-to-face meetings when planning projects and can help cut down on carbon emissions from flights. In the following general comments on various tools, free software is suggested where possible.

Blogs (short for Weblogs—that is, Internet-based diaries) can be used to reach a larger public while maintaining intimacy with the reader. However, blogs require a great deal of work, because regular updates are vital to this medium.

Internal communication within a working group or organization can be facilitated by using mailing lists (Googlegroups, Yahoogroups), instant messaging (Jabber), chat forums (IRC), or even conference calls with programs such as OpenWengo or Skype, which require only an Internet connection, a microphone, and some headphones and allow for computer-to-computer conference calls free of charge and for calling to regular telephones at very low cost.

Using cell phones to send text messages is another effective, inexpensive, and fast way of reaching people, even internationally. Thus, when someone is abroad in a project site and wants to relay information back home very quickly (perhaps to someone uploading this information to a website or blog), he or she can do so either by logging in at an Internet café or simply by sending brief text messages by cell phone.

There's a saying that "if it's not on the Web, it didn't happen." Creating a Web presence has emerged as an important element in external communication. Websites can be used for general information about a project or organization, but they can also act as a valuable resource base, containing important documents, downloads, pictures, and other things that can be made available to activists around the globe around the clock. Furthermore, websites can inform the outside world of proper contact addresses, creating links between otherwise isolated communities around the world. The administration of websites can be done with relatively little technical knowledge using content management systems such as Drupal, or with HTML editors such as NVu or Bluefish.

In order to start a website, one needs a host server, which can provide server space for the website as well as administrative tools. The initial capital expense is modest and is recovered rather quickly if the website is properly kept and used. Most important for a good website are transparency, a clear structure, and regular updates. Unmaintained websites appear unprofessional and may even signal to outsiders the "death" of an organization or project. This can be avoided by regularly making minor changes, which update users on what is currently happening. In today's world, every small product, every political party, every politician, and every event has its own unique website, interlinked with many other connected sites in order to boost its Google rating. A Peace through Health initiative should have its own website—or at least a prominent place on some existing site with frequent links to related sites.

Wikipedia, a free, open, online encyclopedia, should also be considered for outward communication. A project can be added to the encyclopedia quite easily. After a project or organization is listed, the article on it can be edited by anyone. Wikipedia receives millions of hits each day, so having your project or organization adequately represented in this body of information is well worth the effort.

26

Educating Health Professionals in Peace

Neil Arya, Klaus Melf, and *Caecilie Buhmann*

Education of health professionals in prevention and public health, including the prevention of war and its public health consequences, has until recently been minimal. Now, however, there is a growing movement to educate health professionals in mitigating the adverse consequences of war (and other forms of violence) and in promoting peace, human rights, and social justice.

Health professionals and students in the health professions have expressed the need for more knowledge and skills in promoting peace and human rights—and in related subjects, such as global health and medical ethics (Leaning 1997; Mann 1997; Rowson 2002). Many medical students believe that war—and issues such as poverty, infectious disease, environmental pollution, and forced migration—have a tremendous impact on global health, and they seek education on these topics (Bateman et al. 2001; McMahon and Arya 2004; Melf 2004). The United Nations General Assembly supports the teaching of peace in all types and at all levels of education (UNGA 1978). The World Medical Association supports mandatory training for physicians in medical ethics and human rights (WMA 1999). Nevertheless, teaching of these subjects has not been a high priority at medical, nursing, or public health schools.

A good argument can be made for the teaching of peace knowledge and skills at all levels of health professional education. Health professionals care for the life, health, and well-being of their patients. Because war and other forms of violence endanger these goals, health professionals have a responsibility to work toward the prevention and reduction of violence and the promotion of peace. In addition, health professionals encounter the same level of workplace conflict as occurs in most settings and are among those whose professional practice may take them to arenas of large-scale violent conflict. In such arenas they need, at a minimum, to know how the context and their work interact and how to avoid worsening the violent conflict. However, with sufficient knowledge and skill, they may be able to work in ways that prevent or mitigate violence and that nurture peace.

ADDRESSING DEFICITS

In order to enable health professionals to work for peace, deficits in knowledge, skills, and values need to be addressed. For example, medical students and physicians, with their orientation to a pathophysiological basis for disease, often cannot see linkages between the health of their immigrant, refugee, or impoverished patients and such macrodeterminants of health as privatization of health care, criminalization of drug abuse, and promotion of the arms trade.

Knowledge deficits include concepts of peace, conflict, nonviolence, and reconciliation; international human rights norms; and humanitarian law. Deficits in skills include the ability to analyze conflicts, to use nonviolent communication, to act in a culturally sensitive manner, and to engage in conflict resolution, negotiation, and mediation. Deficits in values are obvious when health professionals become accomplices in inhuman acts ranging from human experimentation to torture of prisoners. Values that underlie medical ethics can help health professionals understand their responsibility to avoid participation in such violence—and, indeed, to condemn it (Miles 2004).

Learning from other disciplines, such as anthropology, sociology, and psychology, may help health professionals design conflict-sensitive and culturally appropriate interventions to prevent violence and to foster individual and societal empowerment and resilience (the capacity to do well in difficult circumstances). These interventions can address various forms of violence, such as exploitive and repressive social structures, as well as domestic violence, child abuse, youth violence, and suicide (Alpert, Sege, and Bradshaw 1997; Krug et al. 2002).

RECOGNIZING ASSETS

Health professionals have special assets that may help them prevent violence and promote peace. But in order to do so, they need to become aware of and nurture such specific knowledge, skills, and values (Arya 2004a).

There is much useful knowledge in the traditional curricula of health professional schools that can be adapted for this purpose. This knowledge includes concepts of public health, especially principles of epidemiology, which can be applied to documenting the health consequences of war and economic sanctions—and, if we act on what we discover, to minimize future adverse health effects of weapons on civilians. Such knowledge may be used to promote social change. Psychology and mental health concepts can provide an understanding of cycles of violence and can illuminate the roles of dehumanization and psychic numbing in group violence and even genocide (Lifton and Markusen 1990).

The skills education of health professionals can enhance their capacity to help communities heal through health-care and reconciliation activities that strengthen the social fabric. Health professionals can communicate knowledge and factual information to help counter oppressive governments, can help to humanize "the enemy," and can engage in diplomacy.

And the values education of health professionals can also be strengthened to promote their altruism, empathy, and integrity—each of which increases their credibility and effectiveness.

Health professionals can also be taught to develop and utilize superordinate goals and activities that warring parties may share and that may transcend opposing sides in conflict. Health also very naturally presents itself as a superordinate goal, to which opposing sides in conflict may subscribe.

EXISTING APPROACHES TO EDUCATION

Several approaches are currently being used for teaching health professionals and students in the health professions about peace-relevant issues.

One approach is to teach these subjects in the context of international health. But many schools do not teach international health. In 1993, for example, even though 61 percent of seventy medical schools in developed countries reported teaching international health, only 26 percent listed it as a separate curriculum entity (Bandaranayake 1993). Another approach is to utilize a Medicine and Human Rights framework, in which subjects such as torture and other violations of civil and political rights are addressed. A broader framework of Health and Human Rights—not limited to individual patients—is used to teach about human rights violations from a public, or population-based, health perspective (Mann, Gostin, and Gruskin 1994). Subjects that can be studied in this framework include access to AIDS medications and the Health for All initiative of the World Health Organization (WHO). Medical ethics courses represent another approach to addressing these issues at both the macro and the micro level.

A Global Health framework focuses on socioeconomic and political factors that influence health (Medact 2002). A Social Medicine framework (known in some areas of Europe as a Medical Sociology framework) focuses on social determinants of health. An Ecosystem Health framework focuses on the relationship between human health and the biophysical, socioeconomic, and political environments. These three approaches are similar and complementary, but in a given context, one of them may be more feasible or popular than the others.

CURRENT COURSES OF STUDY

A broad range of courses of study based on these principles cover many of these topics. For example, the Netherlands affiliate (NVMP) of International Physicians for the Prevention of Nuclear War (IPPNW) has organized a course at the Universities of Amsterdam and the Free University since 1992 titled "Health and Issues of Peace and Conflict." Recently partnering with the International Federation of Medical Students Associations (IFMSA), an umbrella group of more than 100 national medical students organizations with a deep interest in addressing medical education and global and public health issues, it plans to offer this course at all medical schools in the Netherlands. The course adapts curricular materials such as those of "Medicine and Nuclear War," developed by IPPNW in the 1980s, and "Medicine and Peace," developed by the United Nations Commission on Disarmament Education, in cooperation with IPPNW and its US affiliate, Physicians for Social Responsibility. At the University for the Basque region in Spain, which itself has a long history of a violent conflict, a similar course is taught at a preclinical level.

University College London offers an Intercalated Bachelor of Science in International Health. Students who are enrolled in an educational institution, such as a medical school, can earn a bachelor of science degree within one year. Many students in this program are enrolled in medical schools outside the United Kingdom. The program has been inspired by modules from the text *Global Health Studies* (now available free on the Internet) and addresses the health effects of globalization, national debt, poverty, environmental degradation, armed conflict, and forced migration, as well as the concepts of human rights and humanitarian assistance. The Karolinska Institute in Sweden offers a course in International Health with components in both theory and practice, the latter of which must be taken in a low- or middle-income country.

Numerous US institutions of higher education, including Harvard, Johns Hopkins, the University of California at Berkeley (UCB), and Emory, utilize the Health and Human Rights framework, often as part of their master of public health programs or certificate courses.

The first such course in the United States was developed in 1992 at Harvard. Both Harvard and Johns Hopkins offer week-long certificate courses in Health and Human Rights, and Harvard's has a public policy orientation. The UCB course focuses on all types of human rights—political and civil rights as well as economic, social, and cultural rights.

The Emory University School of Medicine offers second-year medical students a course titled "Human Rights, Social Medicine, and the Physician." This course, like other Social Medicine courses in the United States, focuses on individual responsibility and professional ethics. The Emory University Institute of Human Rights also offers students a transdiciplinary graduate certificate program in human rights that may focus on health.

As part of its Health as a Bridge for Peace program, WHO organizes training sessions for health professionals and field workers addressing peacebuilding, conflict resolution, and human rights. This training is designed to increase knowledge and to change attitudes and practice in zones of violent conflict. It is intended to encourage field workers to promote peacebuilding (WHO 1997).

The International Committee of the Red Cross has trained field workers, since 1986, in international humanitarian law and human rights with its Health Emergencies in Large Populations program. Over time, these courses have been decentralized to several countries.

Medécins sans Frontières (MSF) has begun to brief its delegates in the prevention of gender-based violence before sending them to work in refugee camps. The World Medical Association disseminates an international online course "Doctors Working in Prison: Human Rights and Ethical Dilemmas," which was produced by the Norwegian Medical Association (Hoftvedt and Reyes 2004).

A course on Global Health and Human Security at the University of British Columbia includes lectures on Peace through Health, and the Global Health course at the University of Waterloo for the master's in public health focuses on what public health personnel can do to reduce direct and structural violence. A four-week summer school in global health at Copenhagen University covers several aspects of violent conflict, including the role of health professionals and primary prevention of the health consequences of war. Many universities in Central and South America have expressed interest in developing Peace through Health courses. At the time of this writing, it is uncertain what the prospects for these courses will be.

COURSES IN PEACE THROUGH HEALTH
AND MEDICAL PEACE WORK

The frameworks of Peace through Health and Medical Peace Work attempt to unify this training at the micro and macro levels, linking theory and understanding to action, advocacy, research, and field work. At McMaster University, a Peace through Health course was first offered in 2004 to third-year undergraduate students (Arya 2004b). It aims to teach peacebuilding and reconciliation skills. Students bring experience from various disciplines, such as Peace Studies and Health Studies, Drama, Language and Literature, and Engineering. The course involves group work and a group presentation of Peace through Health materials, some didactic teaching, and frequent guest lectures. Medical students and Occupational Therapy students at McMaster have each developed their own problem-based elective course. McMaster students and faculty have also created an interactive online introduction to Peace through Health (http://65.39.131.180/ContentPage.aspx?name=DELI_Peace_Through_ Health).

The University of Tromsø in Norway began to offer the world's first graduate course on "Peace, Health, and Medical Work" in 2005 for students in medicine, other health professions, and social sciences. The course builds knowledge about human rights, global health, and disarmament, as well as skills in nonviolent communication, intercultural understanding, advocacy, and media work. In addition, the Health Studies and the Peace and Conflict Studies programs at the University of Waterloo have together developed a full-credit undergraduate course in Peace through Health.

COURSE DESIGN AND IMPLEMENTATION

Course design and content vary for a number of reasons: level, discipline, prior experience in zones of violent conflict or with marginalized people, time available, and whether the course is an elective or a core part of the curriculum. Courses differ in whether they require tuition fees, whether they offer credits, and in terms of their academic rigor and the requirements that students must fulfill.

Getting these courses adopted by health professional schools, especially medical schools, requires explanation of the health consequences of war and violence, enthusiastic support of students, dedicated faculty members, and relevant teaching materials.

Although traditional courses are popular, students seem to have greater appreciation for interactive courses that include group work and applied experiences, in which they are challenged to make decisions and learn practical skills. It usually has proved more effective to begin a course with a small group of students and allow for the subsequent evolution of demand and interest. New technologies may allow students who are geographically and culturally distant to obtain some training involving core ideas but to develop their own training more specific to the context in which they live and study.

If education and training are designed to make professionals more knowledgeable, sensitive, and effective in promoting peace and human rights, courses should be evaluated in terms of both types of effectiveness. Unfortunately, long-term and short-term outcomes are difficult to assess and attribute to specific education. We are therefore left to assess such measures as students' career choices, social activism, and human rights knowledge or attitudes.

THE FUTURE

In order to develop, the field of Peace through Health must build a community of researchers, academics, practitioners, and students and establish common points of reference among them (Böck Buhmann 2005). Both the University of Waterloo and McMaster University are compiling Peace through Health resources, including course materials, case studies, evaluation tools, implementation strategies, and lists of reference materials on fieldwork, research, and education.

Through the Medical Peace Work project http://www.medicalpeacework .org , several European medical peace organizations and educational institutions are strengthening the peace-health field by the development and collection of teaching materials. They are producing an online multimedia course, teaching films, a handbook, and a web-based resource center that will include databases on courses, curricula, syllabi, presentations, film archives, education research, and resource personnel.

In countries such as Bosnia, El Salvador, Costa Rica, and Ecuador, there are movements within family medicine departments, medical schools, other university faculties, and communities to develop Peace through Health training, not just to study the impact of violence, but also to reduce its impact and to strengthen mechanisms for social reconstruction.

And in Sri Lanka, the Faculty of Health Care Sciences at Eastern University in Batticaloa has integrated a module in Peace Medicine into the mandatory training of nurses and physicians. Eastern University, together with the University of Colombo and other medical and public health schools enrolled in the Asia-Pacific Academic Consortium in Public Health (APACPH) collaborate on the development of a peace-health model curriculum for the region. In addition, scholars of this consortium have committed themselves to promoting this new discipline in medical and public health schools, to increasing awareness of it among faculty members, and to giving it due recognition in their training programs.

Education for health professionals worldwide in Peace and Human Rights is continuing to expand. We expect that mainstream medical curricula will increasingly incorporate these subjects. Use of new technology, new methods of teaching, and utilization of cross-disciplinary expertise will be important.

ACKNOWLEDGMENTS

We are grateful to Rob Chase, Andrew Pinto, Dabney Evans, and Joanna Santa Barbara for their review of this chapter, and we thank Kremlin Wickramasinghe, Henk Groenewegen, Sonal Singh, Ed Mills, Aurora Bilbao, and Vince Iacopino for their descriptions of courses in which they have participated.

Adapted from Chapter 27, by Arya, Melf, and Buhmann. In Levy and Sidel, eds. *War and Public Health* 2nd ed. New York: Oxford University Press, 2008.

REFERENCES

Alpert, E. J., R. D. Sege, Y. S. Bradshaw. 1997. Interpersonal violence and the education of physicians. *Academic Medicine* 72 (1 Suppl): S41–50.

Arya, N. 2004a. Peace through Health I: Development and use of a working model. *Medicine, Conflict and Survival* 20: 242–57.

———. 2004b. Peace through Health II: A framework for medical student education. *Medicine, Conflict and Survival* 3: 258–62.

Bandaranayake, D. R. 1993. International health teaching: A survey of 100 medical schools in developed countries. *Medical Education* 27: 360–2.

Bateman, C., T. Baker, E. Hoornenborg, and U. Ericsson. 2001. Bringing global issues to medical teaching. *The Lancet* 358: 1539–42.

Böck Buhmann, C. 2005. The role of health professionals in preventing and mediating conflict. *Medicine, Conflict and Survival* 21: 299–311.

Hoftvedt, B. O., and H. Reyes, eds. 2004. Doctors working in prison: Human rights and ethical dilemmas. World Medical Association. Available online at the www.lupin-nma.net website.

Krug. E. G., L. L. Dahlberg, and J. A. Mercy, et al. 2002. *World report on violence and health*. Geneva: World Health Organization.

Leaning, J. 1997. Human rights and medical education. Why every medical student should learn the Universal Declaration of Human Rights. *British Medical Journal* 315: 1390–1.

Lifton, R. J., and E. Markusen. 1990. *The genocidal mentality: Nazi Holocaust and nuclear threat*. New York: Basic Books.

Mann, J. M. 1997. Medicine and public health, ethics and human rights. *Hastings Center Report* 27: 6–13.

Mann, J. M., L. Gostin, S. Gruskin, et al. 1994. Health and human rights. *Health and Human Rights* 1: 6–23.

McMahon, T., and N. Arya. 2004. Peace through Health. *Student British Medical Journal* 12:438.

Medact. 2002. Global health studies: Proposals for medical undergraduate teaching pack. Available online at www.medact.org/pub_curriculum.php

Melf, K. 2004. Exploring medical peace education and a call for peace medicine. Master's thesis, Centre for Peace Studies, University of Tromsø, Norway.

Miles, S. H. 2004. Abu Ghraib: Its legacy for military medicine. *The Lancet* 364: 725–9.

Rowson, M. 2002. The why, where, and how of global health teaching. *Student British Medical Journal* 10: 215–58.

UNGA. 1978. United Nations Special Session on Disarmament June 30. Available online at the disarmament2.un.org website.

World Health Organization. 1997. Report on the first WHO consultative meeting on Health as a Bridge for Peace. Les Pensières, Annecy, 30–31. Available online at the www.who.int website.

World Medical Association. 1999. Adopted by the 51st World Medical Assembly, Tel Aviv, Israel, October.

27

Looking Ahead

Neil Arya and *Joanna Santa Barbara*

WE HAVE COME THIS FAR . . .

Our aim in this book has been to help you understand how to improve health and peace in situations where they are lacking. We have looked at the pitfalls of intervening with good intentions alone. We hope that this exploration leads to training of future health professionals in peace and conflict transformation principles. We also hope it helps those of you who are working internationally and domestically to clarify your own goals and values and to be aware of your applicable knowledge and skills, assets and deficits. We have tried to provide you with tools to apply these principles and your own unique knowledge, skills, and values to promote peace in your work and daily lives.

The text has expanded beyond narrow concepts of violence to include structures and cultures that perpetrate violence on people and ecosystems. It has provided inspiring examples of individuals acting on peace principles in their lives, working against gun violence and racism, rebuilding societies, and promoting human rights and respect for the natural environment—often at great danger to themselves. Some advocates work locally for public health and deal with marginalized populations, whereas others meet with world leaders and win Nobel Prizes. We believe that "ordinary" people can do extraordinary things. From actions as simple as counting the dead, predicting the effects of war, or documenting torture, their work sometimes attracts the attention of the global press and political leaders. Risking imprisonment while treating people impartially and highlighting violations of human rights in Nepal, health professionals helped to bring down an autocratic government. Others have attained less measurable achievements, working against all odds to promote psychosocial healing in the Middle East, Afghanistan, and Sri Lanka. Peace through Health work has been enhanced by partnerships beyond the health sector—with artists, teachers, or international lawyers—to promote mental health, social healing, and peace. We studied the peacebuilding potential of community-based rehabilitation and of humanitarian organizations and noted how very much students and new technologies have to offer.

CAN WE GO FARTHER?

Those who have learned and worked with the principles of Peace through Health (PtH) may find that these principles illuminate understanding of issues beyond the health arena and point to possibilities of action as citizens, and possibilities of dialogue with decision makers. We need to promote the PtH perspective on violence as a public health problem, to have a voice in public policy (Anderson and Olson 2003; Santa Barbara 2006), and to hold governments to a higher standard in the protection of their citizens' health and of conditions conducive to health (Arya 2008).

CHALLENGES AHEAD

Some writers warn that Western civilization, which many of us imagine to be infinite in duration, is at risk (Diamond 2005). Diamond sees five groups of interacting historical risk factors as important in determining whether a society collapses—all of these risk factors exist for Western nations such as the United States today. The groups of risk factors that Diamond identifies are the damage that people have inflicted on their environment; climate change; enemies; changes in friendly trading partners; and the society's political, economic, and social responses to these shifts. In addition, at least nine states currently possess nuclear weapons of horrendous killing power, and some people believe their use at some point is inevitable. Use of even a fraction of these weapons would escalate human warfare to horrifying levels of mass violence, beyond any conceivable response by health workers.

The primary strategy of the dominant political power at this time, the United States, to address any of these problems is coercive ("hard" or killing) power. The use of persuasive ("soft") power appears only as a prelude to and excuse for the application of coercive power. The instruments of coercive power absorb a large proportion of a nation's scientific and technological intelligence and of the national treasure. Consultation and cooperation with others are not valued. The body of international law governing the behavior of states is seen as arbitrary, and only the interests of the possessor of this power are seen as paramount. The dominant response by the holders of coercive power to the manifest failures of their policies is a frantic application of more of the same. Ordinary people, when asked their opinions, are more reluctant to start war in the first place and are ready to end it long before the holders of power can let go. Maintenance and use of this war system is obviously inimical to health.

In the economic sphere, violence to the Earth is driven relentlessly on by the paradigm of limitless growth. Its obvious inconsistency with the principle of ecological sustainability is ignored, as are the health implications of ecological collapse.

WHAT DO WE HAVE TO OFFER?

"Since wars begin in the minds of men," runs the historic UNESCO Preamble, "it is in the minds of men that the defenses of peace must be constructed." Our examination of actions in PtH has raised many ideas (in the minds of both men and women) of broad applicability—PtH concepts for constructing a peace system in which health can flourish. Those of us in PtH who work in zones of violent conflict (from Afghanistan and Iraq to El Salvador, Haiti, and US inner cities) may have more exposure to real people in the real world than most hard-power specialists. We may therefore be able to provide a more realistic model for work.

In chapter 1 we examined "macro-determinants" of ill health. The obverse of these, the conditions necessary for health, also define peace, or a state of nonviolence, direct, structural, and ecological. We have a clear idea to present on conditions for the health of human populations and of the ecosphere itself.

War	Absence of direct violence
Poverty, inequity	Economic sufficiency, equity
Ecological degradation	Ecological sustainability
Community and cultural disintegration	Community and cultural integrity
Poor governance	Participatory governance, democracy
Human rights abuses	Human rights observance

Some would say the right-hand column describes a state of "human security," but this term is best reserved for favorable contrast with the problematic concept of "state security." The older concept of *basic needs* serves us best; this list corresponds nicely with Galtung's well-known list of security, well-being, identity, and freedom needs.

KNOWLEDGE, SKILLS, AND VALUES

In pursuing these conditions of health and peace, we have examined relevant knowledge, skills, and values. A founding thinker in PtH, Graeme MacQueen (2005), has portrayed knowledge as having particular characteristics.

Knowledge Supporting the Dominant Political and Economic Paradigms

Such knowledge is
1. Short-term: rapid problem solving.
2. Resource hungry: mastery of environment to allow consumption of resources, both renewable and nonrenewable.
3. Expansive: discovering how to spread into available habitat, outstripping competitors and predators, increasing population and/or wealth.
4. In group-based: focus is on limited human in group (existing family, class, tribe, or nation) as moral and cognitive subject, as the only valid "we," and as the backdrop of all decisions.
5. Tool-based: using technology to solve problems.

Knowledge Sustaining Health and Peace in the Broadest Sense

Such knowledge is
1. Long-term: predicting/imagining the future and making present judgments on that basis.
2. Resource-conserving: adaptation through cautious use of resources.
3. Steady-state: equilibrium in relation to habitat and other species.
4. Humanity-based: focus is on the human species (past, present, and future) as moral and cognitive subject, as the "we" that is the context for decisions.
5. Systems-based: focus is on understanding systems, including the logic of collective action, with technology being merely one element in a system.

We have a clear idea of the characteristics of knowledge relevant to increasing and maintaining health and peace in the face of the above challenges.

Skills

Empathic, respectful dialogue is the paramount skill, whether with a single patient, a partner organization, or a militant group discussing a cease-fire. It is the core skill of persuasive power, or "soft power," in political relationships, and it underlies conflict transformation at all levels.

Values

Explicitly or implicitly in many chapters, we have referred to the goal values of peace, health, and human rights observance and participation; to the implementing values of respect, nonviolence, prevention of harm or violence when possible (among others); and to the motivating value of compassion.

APPLYING THESE KNOWLEDGE MODES, SKILLS, AND VALUES TO HEALTH

Healing is being replaced with treating; caring is being displaced by the technical management of disease; the art of listening to the patient is being supplanted by technological procedures. The human body is seen as the repository of unrelated, malfunctioning organs, often separated from the doctor's healing touch by cold, impersonal machines. (McCoy 2002)

Such lessons might be applied first to the health sector (Arya 2006). As many chapters in this book attest, medical care remains a weaker determinant of the health of the population than wealth distribution, education levels, public goods such as potable water, sewage management, housing, environmental integrity (clean air, safe food, and freedom from environmental toxins), personal security, personal risk and lifestyle behaviors, political stability, justice, supportive family relationships and social networks, and personal spirituality. Health-care workers are realizing the limitations of technology in health and exploring the use of holistic methods to improve health. Expensive antibiotics cannot replace interventions such as cleansing wounds with soap and water, good nutrition, restful sleep, stress reduction, meditation, and prayer. Health-care workers are also learning the value of cooperation, relying on the expertise of others, and truly collaborating in health-care teams.

APPLYING THESE KNOWLEDGE MODES, SKILLS, AND VALUES TO PEACE

The many examples of PtH work in this book exemplify the application of long-term, systems-based, humanity-oriented thinking to human problems. The focus on ecological sustainability has not been prominent in PtH work, but it is beginning to be incorporated.

A sustainable model for the future empowers local people and communities to participate in decisions about their own health and security. Although our relationships to family, community, and nation can remain strong, our allegiance must be to humanity and to Mother Earth—to the world we bequeath to our children and descendants.

The dominant strategies of the last 10,000 years will not enable us to survive the next 10,000. We must move beyond tribalism and sectarianism to an interdependent future where we show respect for dignity and human rights. We must cooperate with Nature, live within her limits, and learn from her and each other. Hard power must have a strictly limited role in society if we are to survive. Understanding of interrelationships and a holistic approach will be necessary in medicine, international relations, and our daily lives. Figure 27.1 demonstrates one conception of a model that might effectively be applied in the next era of human development. Let us hope that we in the PtH community are able to help each other successfully through this transition. We hope this book has stimulated you to see exciting possibilities for approaching health work with knowledge of peace processes, broadly conceived, and for approaching peacework in alliance with health professionals.

REFERENCES

Anderson, M., and L. Olson. 2003. *Confronting war: Critical lessons for peace practitioners.* Available online at the www.cdainc.com website.

Arya, N. 2006. The end of biomilitary realism? Rethinking biomedicine and international security. *Medicine, Conflict and Survival* 22 (3): 220–9.

———. 2008. Do no harm: Towards a hippocratic standard for international civilisation. Re-Envisioning sovereignty: The end of Westphalia? ed. Trudy Jacobsen, Charles Sampford, and Ramesh Thakur. 171–92. Hampshire, UK: Ashgate.

Figure 27.1 On the Brink: Development of Humankind

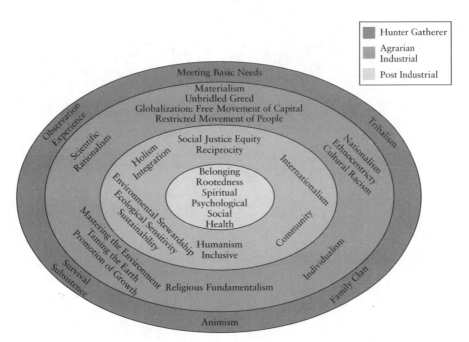

Diamond, Jared. 2005. *Collapse: How societies choose to fail or succeed.* New York: Viking Press.

McCoy, Ronald S. 2002. Restoring the soul of medicine. Address presented at the annual general meeting of the Malaysian Medical Association, June 13.

MacQueen, Graeme. 2005. Peace through Health: An epistemic approach. Paper given at PtH Conference, McMaster University, May. Available online at the www.humanities.mcmaster.ca website.

Santa Barbara, Joanna. 2006. Medicine, peace, and public policy. *Croat Med J.* 47(2): 352–55.

Index

About the Contributors

Neil Arya is a family doctor, assistant clinical professor of family medicine at McMaster University, adjunct professor of family medicine at the University of Western Ontario, and adjunct in both health studies and environmental studies at the University of Waterloo. He has taught Peace through Health in peace studies at McMaster and the University of Waterloo and courses in global health and environmental health at the University of Waterloo. Neil has also served as president of Physicians for Global Survival and vice president of IPPNW; has been involved in projects in Latin America, the Middle East, and South Asia; and has published in various medical, public health, peace, and environmental journals and books. See also www.fes.uwaterloo.ca/ers/faculty/narya/

Caecilie Buhmann received her medical degree from the University of Copenhagen in 2006 and is currently completing her residency. She has a BSc in International Health (University College London, 2005), postgraduate diploma in public health (London School of Hygiene and Tropical Medicine, 2007) and diploma in humanitarian assistance (Fordham University, New York, 2004). She is on the IPPNW board of directors as an international student representative and now as at large member. Caecilie co-founded the Nuclear Weapons Inheritance Project in 2001 and served as a coordinator of the project from 2001 to 2004.

Anne Bunde-Birouste is senior lecturer at the School of Public Health and Community Medicine at the University of New South Wales in Sydney, Australia, and convenor of the health promotion program within the school. Her recent research is in the area of health and peacebuilding, which included a major AusAID-funded program in five countries of the Asia-Pacific region. Her current research involves innovative community development initiatives with refugee youth in the Sydney area.

She is also vice president for advocacy for the International Union for Health Promotion and Education.

Will Boyce is director of the Social Program Evaluation Group at Queens University. He has a joint appointment to the Faculty of Education and the Center for Health Services and Policy Research. Dr. Boyce's focus is in conducting applied research and evaluation of programs in education, health, and rehabilitation for youth and disadvantaged groups. He has major studies under way in youth at risk (smoking, sexuality, mental health, SES, violence), school health policy and curriculum, technology transfer in developing countries (Latin America), HIV/AIDS education in South Africa, and community mental health and social capital in Palestine, India, and sub-Saharan Africa.

Kenneth Bush is a founding professor of the Conflict Studies Program at St. Paul University, Ottawa, Canada. He has developed and taught courses on ethnicized conflict, peacebuilding, post–cold war security, international relations theory, conflict management, forced displacement, foreign policy, and indigenous governance. Dr. Bush has worked with many government and intergovernment organizations and a host of NGOs on the challenges of peacebuilding. Current activities include developing and mainstreaming practical tools and processes that assess the peace and conflict impacts of development projects in conflict zones, and research on the impact of militarized violence on children.

Helen Caldicott is a pediatrician who co-founded Physicians for Social Responsibility, an organization committed to educating medical colleagues about the dangers of nuclear power, nuclear weapons, and nuclear war. She helped start similar medical organizations in many other countries. The international umbrella group IPPNW won the Nobel Peace Prize in 1985. She has authored many books, the most recent being *War in Heaven*. She also has been the subject of several films, including *If You Love This Planet*, which won the Academy Award for best documentary in 1982, and *Helen's War: Portrait of a Dissident*. Dr. Caldicott currently divides her time between Australia and the United States, where she lectures widely. She is founder and president of the Nuclear Policy Research Institute and continues to educate the public about the medical hazards of the nuclear age and the changes necessary in human behavior to stop environmental destruction.

Rob Chase is a community medicine specialist who trained at McMaster University and works in Canada as an occupational health physician in Winnipeg and Toronto. In 1991 he joined the International Study Team's child mortality study in Iraq and then helped form the Health and War program at McMaster University. He has field experience in Sri Lanka helping to start the Butterfly Peace Garden, and he has worked in Afghanistan, Tibet, and Uganda.

Katherine Kaufer Christoffel is professor of pediatrics and preventive medicine at the Feinberg School of Medicine at Northwestern University in Chicago, Illinois. She is an active researcher, clinician, and child advocate; she has published many papers and received many honors for her work. She was the founder of the HELP Network and led its board. She has also served on the board of the International Action Network on Small Arms.

Khagendra Dahal is a physician from Nepal. For the last six years he has been working in IPPNW and spent three years as its international student representative. He has published in international journals, including *The Lancet, BMJ,* and *PLoS Medicine* among others. He has also published in the local media on peace, health, and other social issues. As an intern in 2006, he also participated in the people's movement to restore peace and democracy in Nepal.

Hamit Dardagan developed the Iraq Body Count Project (IBC) jointly with John Sloboda. He is principal researcher for IBC, with responsibility for ongoing development of the method of analysis of media reports, and for the conceptual development of the website. He has written items for *Counterpunch* and has undertaken research for a number of organizations, including Greenpeace. He has been chair of Kalayaan, a human rights campaign for overseas domestic workers in the United Kingdom. Dardagan became ORG's consultant on civilian casualties in war in March 2007.

Ann Duggan is a family physician with a postgraduate diploma in Tropical Medicine and Hygiene, and a Master's in Public Health and honorary Doctorate of Sciences. She has completed sixteen missions with Médecins Sans Frontières. These included assessing and establishing priorities in acute conflict situations in Sierra Leone, Liberia, Sudan (north and south), Rwanda, Zaire (DRC),Congo-Brazzaville, Albania, Macedonia, Azerbaijan, Sri Lanka, Indonesia, and El Salvador.

Dabney Evans is executive director of the Emory University Institute of Human Rights. She is a lecturer at the Rollins School of Public Health at Emory University, teaches courses in human rights, and has trained more than 1000 public health practitioners from over twenty countries. She has engaged in research on trauma, mental health, and perceptions of human rights among adolescent Tibetan refugees. She also serves on the Board of Medical Education in Cooperation with Cuba (MEDICC), a nongovernmental organization whose aim is to improve health-care quality and accessibility in the United States, in Cuba, and throughout the world. Her current research focuses on the nondiscriminatory provision of the right to health in several countries.

Lowell Ewert is a human rights lawyer with a JD from Washburn and an LLM from American University. He directs the Peace and Conflict Studies Program administered by Conrad Grebel University College at the University of Waterloo. Ewert formerly worked for eleven years in the field of international development and has lived in Lebanon, Jordan, Guatemala, Nicaragua, and Kazakhstan. The focus of his research has been on the linkage of human rights to development.

Paul Farmer is a medical anthropologist and founding director of Partners In Health, an international organization that provides direct health-care services and undertakes research and advocacy activities on behalf of those who are sick and living in poverty. He focuses on diseases that disproportionately afflict the poor and has pioneered novel, community-based treatment strategies for AIDS and tuberculosis. He and his colleagues have successfully challenged the policymakers and critics who claim that quality health care is impossible to deliver in resource-poor settings. He has written extensively about health and human rights and has discussed the role of social inequalities in determining the distribution and outcomes of infectious diseases in such works as *Pathologies of Power, Infections and Inequalities, The Uses of Haiti,* and *AIDS and Accusation* and has received numerous awards for his work.

Norbert Goldfield is executive director of Healing Across the Divides, an American not-for-profit. He is on the board of Health Care for All, an organization working for health insurance for all Americans. He is a practicing physician and is medical director of a research group that develops tools to measure quality and pay for health care. He is editor of *The Journal of Ambulatory Care Management*. His most recent book is *National Health Reform, American Style*.

Paula Gutlove is deputy director of the Institute for Resource and Security Studies, where she founded the Health Bridges for Peace (HBP) project. HBP links health care with the prevention and management of intercommunal conflict, using a common interest in public health as an opportunity to bring people together for training, dialogue, collaborative action, and community reconstruction. HBP programs have been conducted in the Balkans, Caucasus, Middle East, and elsewhere. Dr. Gutlove has served as a consultant to international organizations including WHO, OSCE, and UNHCR. She is a program associate of the MIT–Harvard Public Disputes program and a lecturer at Simmons College.

Maria Kett completed her doctorate in social anthropology at the School of Oriental and African Studies, University of London, in 2002. Her thesis focused on health and well-being in suburban China.

Maria is a qualified nurse and has worked in several central London accident and emergency departments. She is also an honorary lecturer on the BSc International Health at IHMEC within UCL and is the task group leader on Conflict and Emergencies for the International Disability and Development Consortium. Areas of research interest include the psychosocial impact of conflict, post-socialist and transitional states, and refugees and internal displacement.

Jim Yong Kim is the François Xavier Bagnoud Professor of Health and Human Rights at the Harvard School of Public Health, professor of medicine and social medicine at Harvard Medical School, chief of the Division of Social Medicine and Health Inequalities at Brigham and Women's Hospital, director of the François Xavier Bagnoud Center for Health and Human Rights, and chair of the Department of Social Medicine at Harvard Medical School. Dr. Kim has twenty years of experience in improving health in developing countries. He is a founding trustee and the former executive director of Partners In Health, a not-for-profit organization that supports a range of health programs in poor communities in Haiti, Peru, Russia, Rwanda, Lesotho, and the United States. He was a contributing editor to the 2003 and 2004 *World Health Report* and edited the volume *Dying for Growth: Global Inequity and the Health of the Poor.* He has won numerous awards for his work.

John Last is professor emeritus of epidemiology at the University of Ottawa. He is the author or editor of 17 books, including *Public Health and Human Ecology* (1987, 1996) and a *Dictionary of Public Health.* He edited four editions of *Public Health and Preventive Medicine* (1980, 1986, 1991, 1998) and four editions of the *Dictionary of Epidemiology* (1983, 1988, 1995, 2001). He co-edited the *Oxford Illustrated Companion to Medicine,* 3rd edition (2001), and the *Encyclopedia of Public Health* (2002) and has written chapters in 49 books, articles in several encyclopedias, 80 original articles in peer-reviewed journals, and over 200 other articles and editorials on a range of issues in public health and human ecology. Dr. Last has been awarded many honors during his long career in public health. His principal research interests are studies of the interactions of ecosystem health with human health and studies of ethical problems arising in public health sciences and practice.

Barry S. Levy, a physician, is an adjunct professor of public health at Tufts University School of Medicine and an independent consultant in occupational and environmental health. He has served as a medical epidemiologist with CDC, as a professor at the University of Massachusetts Medical School, and as a director of international health programs and projects. He has written more than 150 published articles and book chapters and has edited 13 books, including, with Victor Sidel MD, the books *War and Public Health, Terrorism and Public Health,* and *Social Injustice and Public Health.* He has served as president of the American Public Health Association and has received the Sedgwick Memorial Medal, its highest award.

Tarek Loubani is a Palestinian refugee living in Montreal, Canada, where he is doing a residency in family medicine. As a student activist he was well-known for employing the latest in technology and served as technical advisor for Open Medicine and Z Net, among others. He may be contacted at tarek@tarek.org.

Evan Lyon is a long-time clinical volunteer with Partners In Health, with over a decade of experience in rural Haiti. He graduated from Harvard Medical School in 2003 and completed a residency in internal medicine at Boston's Brigham and Women's Hospital (BWH) in 2007. He is currently on the faculty of the Division of Social Medicine and Health Inequalities at BWH. Dr. Lyon's work in Haiti has focused on community-based care for victims of HIV and tuberculosis. In addition to work with Partners In Health, Dr. Lyon is an active member of the People's Health Movement.

Graeme MacQueen taught Buddhist studies in the Religious Studies Department of McMaster University for thirty years, before retiring in 2003. In 1989 he became founding director of the Center for Peace Studies at McMaster, after which he helped develop an undergraduate program in peace studies and co-directed a peacebuilding program with projects in Sri Lanka, Gaza, Serbia, and Afghanistan. He was one of the originators of the Peace through Health concept as it developed at McMaster University.

Ian Maddocks is a palliative care physician who held a number of positions in IPPNW between 1985 and 2004, including vice president, speaker of the council, and chair of the board of directors. He is currently writing the story of a village in Papua New Guinea where he and his family once lived for six years.

Ambrogio Manenti is a medical doctor specializing in health education with a master's in public health care management in developing countries. During the last twenty-five years, he has been working in emergency and development activities, particularly in countries in conflict or postconflict situations such as El Salvador, Nicaragua, Sri Lanka, Somalia, Croatia, Bosnia-Herzegovina, FYR Macedonia, and the occupied Palestinian territory. Since 2003 he has worked in Jerusalem as head of the WHO office for the West Bank and Gaza.

Klaus Melf was trained as a medical doctor in Germany and holds a MPhil in peace and conflict transformation from Norway. He is currently peace-health project manager at the Center for International Health, University of Tromsø. He coordinates the EU-funded pilot project Medical Peace Work, which produces and collects web-based teaching material for health professionals in the field of violence prevention and sustainable peacebuilding.

Viet Nguyen-Gillham has a background in social work and psychotherapy. She has a PhD from Boston University in sociology and social work and has worked internationally in conflict areas (Thailand, Bosnia, Guinea/Sierra Leone, East Timor, Palestine) in programs related to refugees, torture victims, and social development. She is currently working as an independent consultant and researcher in mental health and community development at the Institute of Community and Public Health, Birzeit University.

Wendy Orr was the first and only South African doctor in government employment to reveal police torture and abuse of political detainees, when she successfully obtained a court order to protect detainees from police assault in 1985. In 1995 she was appointed by then President Mandela to the Truth and Reconciliation Commission of South Africa. She organized the TRC hearing into the role of health professionals in human rights abuses and assisted with the investigation into the military doctors who participated in South Africa's chemical and biological warfare program. She currently works as a consultant to the corporate and higher-education sector on transformation, equity, and black economic empowerment strategies.

Andrew Pinto graduated from medical school at the University of Toronto and is currently completing his residency training in community medicine. He has been involved with global health work for a number of years, and his specific interests include small arms/light weapons, Peace through Health, ethics, homelessness, and food security. He is a member of Physicians for Global Survival and hopes to continue to work in solidarity with communities in the future.

Alex Rosen finished his medical studies in 2006 at the Heinrich Heine University in Düsseldorf. He is a German National Academic Foundation scholarship recipient and has also worked for many years with an organization for political youth education. Rosen has lived in Germany, the United States, Israel, Nepal, and Cuba. After founding an IPPNW student group at his university, he became the European student representative of IPPNW, started the IPPNW student website and served IPPNW for two years as international student representative and as a member of the board of directors and executive committee. He currently sits on the IPPNW board of directors as an at-large member.

Simon Rushton is a lecturer in the Department of International Politics at the Aberystwyth University where he is part of the Center for Health and International Relations. He has recently published on the role of the health sector in postconflict peacebuilding, health and international security, the global governance of health, and the role of the UN Secretariat.

Hana Saab has a background in health sciences (BScN) and is currently in the doctoral program in education at Queen's University. Her research is in the area of adolescent health, positive youth development, community development, program evaluation, and the Health Promoting School. She is also a research associate with the Social Program Evaluation Group at the same university and is involved in projects within Canada and internationally. Her interest in global health stems from having lived and worked in the Middle East and Africa. She is project manager for the IDRC-funded project Palestinian Adolescents Coping with Trauma, which is in its second cycle.

Joanna Santa Barbara trained and practiced as a child psychiatrist in Australia and Canada. For 25 years she has been involved with the development of the Center for Peace Studies at McMaster University in Hamilton (Canada). Work from this center on health in war zones evolved into the Peace through Health framework, to which she has contributed theory and practice. She is about to move to an experiment in sustainable living in New Zealand. She has received several awards for peacework and teaching.

Victor W. Sidel, who trained in internal medicine and public health, is Distinguished University Professor of Social Medicine at Montefiore Medical Center and Albert Einstein College of Medicine in the Bronx and adjunct professor of public health at Weill Medical College of Cornell University in New York City. He has been president of the American Public Health Association, a member of the board of directors of the Physicians for a National Health Program, a co-founder and president of Physicians for Social Responsibility, and a co-founder and co-president of IPPNW, which received the 1985 Nobel Prize for Peace. He is co-editor, with Dr. Barry Levy, of *War and Public Health,* of *Terrorism and Public Health,* and of *Social Injustice and Public Health,* all published by Oxford University Press. An all-new second edition (2008) of *War and Public Health,* published by OUP in collaboration with the American Public Health Association, is now available.

Sonal Singh is a board-certified general internist and an assistant professor in internal medicine at Wake Forest University School of Medicine in Winston-Salem, North Carolina. He is also co-founder and associate director of the Center for International Health and Human Rights in Toronto and co-editor-in-chief of the journal *Conflict & Health.* He grew up in Nepal and received his medical degree from the Prince of Wales Medical College in Patna, India, in 1999. He is currently finishing a MPH program at Johns Hopkins University, with a focus on health and human rights. He has published and peer-reviewed extensively in the fields of international health and human rights, HIV, the relationship between conflict and health, and refugee health.

John Sloboda is professor of psychology at Keele University, executive director of the Oxford Research Group, and a co-founder of the Iraq Body Count website. He is author, with Chris Abbott and Paul Rogers, of *Beyond Terror: The Truth About the Real Threats to Our World* (Rider 2007).

Karen Trollope-Kumar is a family physician in the Department of Family Practice at McMaster University and also teaches in the Department of Anthropology. Her interest in anthropology developed during the years that she lived in the Himalayan foothills of northern India, where she worked with her husband on primary health-care projects. After her return to Canada, she continued to pursue studies in anthropology and earned a PhD from McMaster University in 2001. She has a particular interest in health in its cross-cultural context.

Marshall Wallace is director of the Do No Harm Project of CDA Collaborative Learning Projects, based in Cambridge, Massachusetts. Over the past ten years he has worked with local groups in over 20 countries to adapt and use the Do No Harm framework. He also directs the Steps Toward Conflict Prevention Project, which gathers the stories of communities in conflict zones who have developed strategies to exempt themselves from the conflict around them.

Anthony Zwi is professor of public health and community medicine in the School of Public Health and Community Medicine at the University of New South Wales. He has long-standing interests in research on conflict, health, and peacebuilding and seeks to ensure that research feeds into policy and practice. He is especially eager to work with community-based organizations, NGOs, service providers, and policymakers to ensure that the voices of those most marginalized are heard. He believes that universities should be contributing to developing concepts and tools that will be of value in the real world. He also believes that engagement, documentation, and analysis are key first steps in raising issues for debate and system improvement.

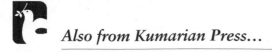

Also from Kumarian Press...

Conflict Resolution and Peacebuilding:

Zones of Peace
Edited by Landon Hancock and Christopher Mitchell

Nation-Building Unraveled? Aid, Peace and Justice in Afghanistan
Edited by Antonio Donini, Norah Niland and Karin Wermester

Transacting Transition: The Micropolitics of Democracy Assistance in the Former Yugoslavia
Edited by Keith Brown

New and Forthcoming:

The World Bank and the Gods of Lending
Steve Berkman

Mobilizing for Human Rights in Latin America
Edward Cleary

**Surrogates of the State:
NGOs, Development and Ujamaa in Tanzania**
Michael Jennings

How NGOs React: Globalization and Education Reform in the Caucasus, Central Asia and Mongolia
Edited by Iveta Silova and Gita Steiner-Khamsi

Visit Kumarian Press at **www.kpbooks.com** or call **toll-free 800.232.0223** for a complete catalog.

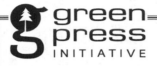

Kumarian Press, located in Sterling, Virginia, is a forward-looking, scholarly press that promotes active international engagement and an awareness of global connectedness.